Dr. Melissa Palmer's Guide To

✱

Hepatitis & Liver Disease

Melissa Palmer, MD

AVERY
a member of Penguin Putnam Inc.

The information, advice, and procedures contained in this book are based upon the research and the personal and professional experiences of the author. They are not intended as a substitute for consulting with your physician or other healthcare provider. The publisher and author are not responsible for any adverse effects or consequences resulting from the use of any of the suggestions, preparations, or procedures discussed in this book. All matters pertaining to your physical health should be supervised by a healthcare professional. It is a sign of wisdom, not cowardice, to seek a second or third opinion.

Cover designer: Phaedra Mastrocola
Editor: Carol A. Rosenberg
Typesetters: Richard Morrock and
            Gary Rosenberg
Printer: Paragon Press, Honesdale, PA

Avery
a member of
Penguin Putnam Inc.
375 Hudson Street
New York, NY 10014
www.penguinputnam.com

Library of Congress Cataloging-in-Publication Data

Palmer, Melissa.
    Dr. Melissa Palmer's guide to hepatitis & liver disease : what you need to know /
Melissa Palmer.
        p. cm.
    Includes bibliographical references and index.
    ISBN 0-89529-922-4
        1. Hepatitis—Popular works. 2. Liver—Diseases—Popular works. I. Title. II. Title:
Doctor Melissa Palmer's guide to hepatitis & liver disease. III. Title: Guide to hepatitis &
liver disease. IV. Title: Guide to hepatitis and liver disease.

RC848.H42 P34 2000
616.3'62 21—dc21

                                                                99-044886

Printed in the United States of America

10   9   8   7   6   5   4   3

Contents

PART III—Understanding and Treating Other Liver Diseases

PART IV—Treatment Options and Lifestyle Changes

This book is dedicated to all of the patients in my practice, without whom this book would not have been possible.

This book is also dedicated to all individuals with liver disease worldwide.

Acknowledgments

To my husband, Alan Pressman, my heartfelt gratitude for the countless hours of unselfish time you spent helping me by revising and editing this book. To the extent that this book is clear and succinct, it is primarily you who deserves the credit. This book would not have been possible without your editorial, legal, and moral support.

To Rags, Augie and Snooper, my supportive companions into the wee hours of the night, you were invaluable throughout the entire process of writing this book. You guys are the cutest creatures on the planet.

To my mother Harriet Palmer, thank you for being a sounding board, for your continuous encouragement and support, and for always being there when I needed you.

To Carol Rosenberg at Avery Publishing, my sincere thanks for your invaluable assistance in editing and fine-tuning this book. Your editorial skills have greatly enhanced its word flow and its comprehensibility.

To Lisa James and the rest of the staff at Avery Publishing, much thanks for your many helpful suggestions, and especially, for your patience.

And, last but not least, to my publisher Rudy Shur, my special thanks. The mindset of this book and the organization of its contents are a reflection of your genius and of your skill as an editor. Thank you because, through this book, we have been able to advance our mutual objective of improving the health, and thereby the lives, of individuals with liver disease.

Preface

Congratulations! By choosing to read this book, you have taken a significant step toward increasing your knowledge of hepatitis and liver disease. The diagnosis of these conditions can have a tremendous impact on the daily lives of many individuals and their loved ones. How do I know this? Because I personally take care of thousands of people with hepatitis and liver disease each year. Who am I? I am a *hepatologist* (liver specialist), and I have perhaps the largest private solo practice devoted to hepatitis and liver disease in the United States.

Many times each day, patients and their family members express to me their fears and concerns about liver disease. Part of my job is to dispel their misconceptions and to correct whatever myths they may have heard. I also supply them with the latest information on hepatitis and liver disease and their treatments. In addition, I provide sound advice on both mainstream and alternative therapies and give my patients the opportunity to avail themselves to promising experimental medications—often before these medications are routinely available in the United States. And, of course, I design and monitor their overall treatments.

Over the past decade, I have spent much of my time educating the lay and medical communities about hepatitis and liver disease through lectures and publications. I have been active in many voluntary societies devoted to the study, prevention, and treatment of liver disease. These nonprofit organizations include the American Liver Foundation (ALF), where I sit on the medical advisory board of the New York chapter as well as on the nutrition education subcommittee of the national chapter. I run liverdisease.com, an Internet website devoted to liver disease. I have appeared on numerous television and radio programs, both locally and nationally, to discuss various aspects of hepatitis and liver disease, as well as the latest available treatments. I have appeared in videos aimed at educating the public about hepatitis and its treatment. I have also actively participated in research studies of the most promising experimental drugs for the treatment of hepatitis. I have been interviewed on various issues pertaining to liver disease for many mainstream publications such as *TIME, Prevention,* and *The Los Angeles Times.* I also serve as a liver disease consultant to four prominent pharmaceutical companies.

I've often been told that I live my life in overdrive. While in the midst of my training in hepatology and gastroenterology, I decided to become a competitive bodybuilder. After a few years of training, I won the title of Ms. Northern States. By then it was time to start my medical practice, so I gave up my short-lived career as a competitive bodybuilder. But I got a whole lot more out of the experience than just a few trophies. I learned a great deal about nutrition and exercise—two power-ful tools that many doctors overlook in their treatment of illness. By combining what I learned as a bodybuilder with what I learned in medical school, I have been high-ly successful in keeping my patients healthy. In fact, I've learned so much about the effects of diet and exercise on liver disease that I am now considered one of the nation's experts on the subject.

I have always believed that it is very important to provide the public with as much information regarding the diagnosis and the treatment of hepatitis and liver disease as possible. My patients constantly ask me, "Where can I get more infor-mation on liver disease?" There is a huge and rapidly increasing population of peo-ple who have liver disease, and most of them are thirsting for more knowledge. There are so many questions that need to be answered honestly and accurately, and there is so much *mis*information that needs to be clarified. Until now, there has been no comprehensive general interest book on liver disease available to the public— no detailed book that could help people navigate the complex and often confusing issues associated with its treatment. That's why I decided to write *Dr. Melissa Palmer's Guide to Hepatitis and Liver Disease.*

I have divided this book into four parts. Part One begins with basic information about the liver's structure and function. Then it takes you step-by-step through the course that a person will follow once he or she has been diagnosed with a liver dis-order. This part will discuss what to expect during the initial visit to the doctor, what types of liver-related blood work and scans will be required, and what their signif-icance is. Part One will advise you of the best ways to find a liver specialist and what qualities to look for in such a specialist. In addition, it will describe how safe and simple a liver biopsy is and will include what everyone needs to know about this procedure. Part One concludes with a discussion of what cirrhosis is and what its potential complications are.

Part Two contains an overall look at hepatitis—a term that is widely misused and misunderstood. This part also discusses the different types of viral hepatitis and their treatments. In particular, it provides detailed information about hepatitis B and C. Part Two also explains the difference between experimental drugs and drugs that have been approved by the Food and Drug Administration (FDA). In addition, this part discusses the potential side effects of drugs, such as interferon, Rebetron, and lamivudine, which are commonly used to treat chronic viral hepatitis. And it explains how the patient can get the most out of these treatments while minimizing potential side effects. Part Two also looks at some exciting new advances in the treatment of chronic hepatitis B and C.

Part Three devotes an entire chapter to the each of the most common liver disorders affecting adults in the United States, including autoimmune hepatitis, primary biliary cirrhosis, fatty liver, nonalcoholic steatohepatitis, alcoholic liver disease, and hemochromatosis. In addition, this part introduces various treatments currently available for these liver diseases. The last chapter in Part Three discusses the differences between benign and malignant liver tumors, and how they are treated.

Part Four addresses specific treatments for some of the more common symptoms, such as fatigue, pain, and itching, that may occur as a consequence of any liver disorder. It also discusses the treatments for some of the complications of chronic liver disease—complications such as internal bleeding and fluid retention. This part also discusses herbs and other alternatives to conventional therapy, and emphasizes what a person needs to know before choosing this route of treatment. Also detailed in this part are the events that lead up to, what takes place during, and what happens after a liver transplantation. Part Four also discusses how proper nutrition and an exercise program can help improve a person's general health and the health of his or her liver. The last chapter in Part Four addresses a core group of questions—on topics such as pregnancy, sexual function, and safety of medications—that individuals with liver disease typically have regarding the illnesses' effect on their personal lives. This final chapter also discusses the extent to which family members and loved ones are at risk of contracting or inheriting specific liver diseases, and how they can best minimize those risks through early detection and prevention strategies—particularly vaccination. The special importance of obtaining the hepatitis A and B vaccinations for everyone with chronic liver disease is stressed in the final chapter as well.

Initially, you may feel the impulse to proceed directly to the chapter that focuses on the specific disease that affects you or a loved one. However, I believe that everyone can benefit from reading the entire contents of this book—especially in light of the overlapping nature of many liver diseases. Although a detailed glossary follows Part Four, you may find it easier to understand the medical terminology in this book by reading it within the context of the chapter in which it is contained.

In writing this book, I've drawn from information that I've obtained during more than fifteen years of extensive research on every aspect of liver disease, and from my firsthand experiences treating thousands of patients with liver disease. The mission of *Dr. Melissa Palmer's Guide to Hepatitis and Liver Disease* is to break through the wall of helplessness that at times surrounds liver disease and to provide people with the genuine hope that they can get better.

Melissa Palmer, M.D.

A Word About Gender

A person with liver disease or hepatitis can be either male or female. The same holds true for a doctor. To avoid using the awkward "he/she" when not referring to a group, and still give equal time to both sexes, the masculine pronouns are used in Parts One and Three and the feminine pronouns are used in Parts Two and Four. This has been done in the interest of simplicity and clarity.

Introduction

I f you're like most people, you've never really thought much about your liver. After all, you can't feel it the way you can feel your heart beating. Your liver doesn't groan with hunger like your stomach, nor does it gurgle during digestion like your intestines. But now your doctor has told you there's something wrong with your liver, and you've suddenly become very much aware of its presence. Perhaps you're recovering from a lifetime of alcoholism and you have alcoholic liver disease, or maybe you've never had an alcoholic drink in your life. Maybe you've been diagnosed with liver cancer, or perhaps you're suffering from a genetic liver disorder. Or maybe—like approximately 4 million other Americans—you've been told that you have just become part of the hepatitis C epidemic sweeping the nation, or that you are one of the almost 400 million chronic carriers, worldwide, of the hepatitis B virus.

You have a lot of questions. Is this disease serious? Am I putting my loved ones in danger? What treatments are available? What are the alternatives to conventional medicine? What medications should I avoid? Will I be able to have children? Is there a diet and exercise program that I can follow to help me get better? This book will help you answer all these questions and more. You'll learn how the liver works to neutralize poisons, to help digest the foods you eat, to combat infection, to control bleeding, and to regulate energy levels. You'll read about the differences between the various kinds of liver diseases and how each affects your body. You'll come to understand why it's critical to fight liver disease as soon as it's diagnosed, even though you may feel fine. You'll also learn what new treatments are available. If you're exploring alternative medicine, you'll learn which herbs, vitamins, minerals, and natural remedies may aggravate your liver disease and which ones may help.

And, if you are a loved one or a friend of someone who has liver disease, you will gain valuable information about how you can actively participate in his or her road to recovery. Plus, you will learn if there are any special measures or precau-

tions you personally need to take in order to reduce your chances of also developing liver disease.

The conventional medical wisdom used to be that doctors couldn't do very
much for their patients with liver disease. But thanks to some remarkable advances
in the field, liver disease is now becoming a readily and successfully treatable condition. The most significant advances, which will be detailed in this book, include
the following:

- **The identification and treatment of the hepatitis C virus.** Soon after the hepatitis C virus was identified in 1989, researchers discovered that one of the body's
  own infection-fighters, an *immunoprotein* called *interferon,* could prove to be an
  effective treatment for some individuals with viral hepatitis. We have also learned
  a lot by reviewing the work of researchers who study acquired immune deficiency
  syndrome (AIDS). Most important, they have shown us the value of combining
  more than one drug in a multi-pronged attack against viruses.

- **Liver transplantation.** The advances that have been made in liver transplantation have been phenomenal. Among them are better drugs for fighting organ
  rejection and improved treatments for potential complications that may occur
  after a transplant. Liver transplantation is no longer viewed as a last resort for
  individuals who experience liver failure. Both physicians and the lay public have
  become increasingly aware of the viability of liver transplantation as a treatment
  option for people who have chronic liver disease. This, in turn, has led to a more
  timely, earlier referral for this life-saving operation. Most liver-transplant recipients lead totally normal, active, productive lives afterwards. In fact, there are
  still people alive today who had undergone some of the first liver transplants
  almost thirty years ago!

- **Gene research.** Researchers have isolated the genes that trigger a number of
  hereditary liver disorders. For example, in 1996 two gene mutations associated
  with the candidate gene for *hemochromatosis*—a hereditary disease of iron overload that occurs in approximately 1.5 million Americans—was identified. This
  will, undoubtedly, lead to readily available screening tests for this disorder, which
  will dramatically increase the number of people and their family members who
  find out about their condition during the earliest, most treatable stages.

- **Vaccines.** The development and availability of highly effective vaccines against
  hepatitis A and B have represented a major advance in preventive medicine and
  public health. Although the first vaccine for hepatitis B was developed in 1982,
  it wasn't until the 1990s that public health officials started pushing the idea that
  all infants and teenagers should be vaccinated. As each new generation becomes
  inoculated, we are that much closer to making hepatitis B a scourge of the past.

  The first vaccine against hepatitis A became available in 1995. Even though
  hepatitis A is generally considered not as serious as hepatitis B, it does make a
  lot of people sick every year. Approximately one hundred individuals die each

year due to this virus. It is especially important for people who already suffer from a liver disease to get the hepatitis A and B vaccinations in order to avoid the potential burden of an additional liver disorder.

This book will introduce you to and help you understand the latest liver-related treatments and advances. It will enable you or your loved one, in conjunction with a specialist, to make educated decisions about the treatment of liver disease. In Part One, you'll learn what you need to know in order to increase your understanding of, and decrease your fears about, liver disease. In Part Two, you'll read about viral hepatitis and its treatment. In Part Three, you'll learn about some common liver disorders occurring in the United States today. Several of the chapters in this part unfold with stories about ordinary people whose lives were changed upon learning of their condition, but who are now benefiting from the latest treatments. (These case studies are composites based on actual people whose names and occupations were changed to protect confidentiality.) Part Four discusses what steps liver disease patients can take to help manage their recovery, and what effect this illness has on their personal lives. In this part, you'll also read about transplantation and alternatives to conventional medical therapy.

Remember, you only have one liver. Liver disease can be treated. You can take part in that recovery. This book, while not a substitute for a doctor's care, can be a guide on the road back to health. (Please note: a person with liver disease is advised to use this book in conjunction with the direct guidance of a liver specialist.)

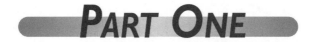

PART ONE

The Basics

A Little Background
on the Liver

Tom, a forty-nine-year-old salesman, was feeling somewhat fatigued. He figured that this was to be expected. He was, after all, working ten-hour shifts, in addition to coaching his son's Little League team. Moreover, he was going to be fifty years old in two months. Perhaps this explained his feeling tired all the time. But, at the insistence of his wife, Tom made an appointment with his family physician for a check-up.

At the doctor's office, Tom told his doctor that he was feeling less energetic than he used to. After asking some questions about Tom's history and conducting a physical exam, the doctor said, "You look fine. But we could use some additional information. I'm going to have my nurse draw some blood from you. Call me in a week to discuss the results of your blood tests."

Tom felt relieved. But when he called for the results of his tests a week later, he heard some hesitation in the doctor's voice. "Tom, you need to come back to the office for further testing. Your blood tests detected a possible problem with your liver."

"My liver?!" Tom responded with some disbelief. "What does this mean? There must be some mistake. What could be wrong with my liver?"

Tom's reaction to finding out there may be a problem with his liver is common among people with liver disease. But what exactly is liver disease? Most people know that drinking too much alcohol is bad for the liver and that it can lead to alcoholic liver disease. But few people know that there are viruses, genetic factors, medications, herbs, and vitamins—among other variables—that can adversely affect the liver. Even having too much body fat can cause liver damage. Also, few people know that without a healthy liver, you would not have the energy to work or do simple daily chores; or that if you cut yourself shaving, you would not be able to stop bleeding; or that if you were exposed to toxic chemicals, your body could not filter out these dangerous, potentially life-threatening substances; or that if approximately 85 percent of the liver stops functioning, practically every other organ in the body would eventually deteriorate.

In order to understand liver disease, you must first learn about the structure and functions of the liver—nature's most miraculous life-giving machine. To help you do this, this chapter discusses the anatomy of the liver and the liver's many functions. It finishes up by explaining exactly what liver disease is.

THE LOCATION AND STRUCTURE OF THE LIVER

The liver is a wedge-shaped gland located on the upper right side of the body, lying beneath the rib cage, which functions as its personal protective barrier. (See Figure 1.1.) Making up about 2 to 3 percent of the body's total weight, the liver is the largest organ in the body. It is crisscrossed by a densely packed web of blood vessels and special passageways called bile ducts. This organ's blood supply is a complicated superhighway with two main "thoroughfares" allowing blood to enter the liver—one called the *portal vein* and the other called the *hepatic artery*. Blood exits the liver through the *hepatic vein*. The cells that make up the liver are known as *hepatocytes*. Nestled beneath the liver lies a pear-shaped organ called the *gallbladder*. Its main function is to store and concentrate bile. The liver and the gallbladder are connected by *bile ducts*. The bile ducts, as their name suggests, carry *bile*—a bitter, greenish mixture of acids, salts, and other substances—into the intestines. The liver is strategically located in the body so that it can communicate efficiently with all of the other organs, in addition to performing numerous vital functions essential to daily living.

THE LIVER'S MANY FUNCTIONS

The brain *thinks*. The heart *beats*. The stomach *digests*. But there's no single active verb to describe what the liver does. This is because the liver has so many different jobs to perform. In fact, if you were to write a classified ad that covered all the liver's responsibilities, it might read something like this:

WANTED—One highly reliable, extremely flexible organ that can act as watchdog, grocer, housekeeper, bodybuilder, energy plant supervisor, and sanitation engineer. Will be required to process and sort gallons of digested food from the stomach and intestines each day. Must discriminate among fats, proteins, and carbohydrates and send them wherever they are needed in the body. Must be able to detoxify thousands of substances—ranging from alcohol to bug spray to turpentine fumes—that may be ingested with food and drink, absorbed through the skin, or

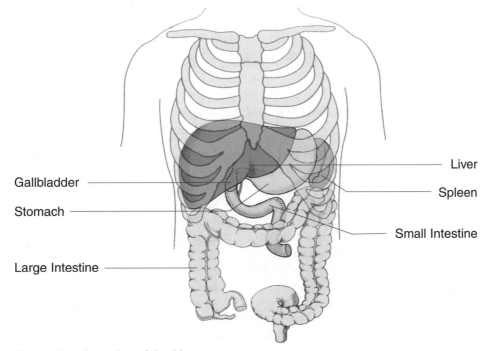

Figure 1.1. Location of the Liver

breathed in the air. Should be able to dismantle old worn-out blood cells and recycle whatever parts are salvageable and prepare the rest for elimination. Must transform cholesterol into steroid hormones, such as androgens and estrogens, and share responsibility with the kidneys to control thyroid hormones, which influence metabolism. Must regulate sugar levels for proper energy management and create clotting factors that stop bleeding from cuts or other wounds. Additional duties will include—but are not limited to—building reserves of vitamins A, D, E, K, and B_{12} as well as of iron and copper. Must be able to accomplish all of the above without weighing more than three to four pounds.

That's a pretty tall order. But the liver accomplishes it all silently, working in the background, never advertising its presence. Sometimes, when a part of the liver is damaged or removed, it is even called upon to perform the incredible task of "regenerating" itself! (See the inset "The Myth of the Regenerating Liver" on page 10.)

The following material discusses the liver's many functions. It also covers some of the problems that can arise when liver disease exists. In general, it is important to always keep in mind two basic functions of the liver. First, virtually everything that enters the digestive tract—foods, drinks, and medicines, for example—and everything that is breathed in the air or absorbed through the skin must pass through the liver in an attempt to be purified and detoxified. Second, the liver ensures that the other organs in the body are supplied with sufficient amounts of the various fuels, such as carbohydrates, proteins, and vitamins, that are necessary to get a person successfully through each day.

The Importance of Bile, Bilirubin, and Bile Acids

Bile does double-duty both as an aid in the digestion of fats and as a neutralizer of poisons. The importance of bile was recognized as far back as 400 B.C., in the days of Hippocrates, who suggested that an imbalance of the four body humors, or fluids —blood, phlegm, black bile, and yellow bile—signified disease. Bile is formed in hepatocytes (liver cells) and consists mainly of bile acids and pigments; cholesterol; electrolytes, such as sodium, potassium, and calcium; and proteins. Bile is released from the liver cells into the *duodenum*—the first part of the small intestine—to aid in digestion. The liver's bile ducts collect the bile and transport it to the gallbladder. There, the bile is concentrated and stored until the cells along the inside lining of the small intestine send a hormonal signal that some fatty food, say a double-fudge brownie, has entered the digestive system. A muscle surrounding the gallbladder contracts and a little bile is squirted into the intestines through the bile ducts. In much the way detergent helps to lift grease off a dirty plate, bile surrounds the fats and helps to break them apart so that the body can digest them. Pretty soon that brownie starts to dissolve into clumps that are small enough to pass through the rest of the intestines and out of the body. Therefore, when liver disease exists, there may be trouble digesting fatty foods. Similar to its action on fat, bile envelops some poisons in a protective barrier until they can be safely carted out of the body in the feces.

The yellow color that is commonly associated with bile is mainly due to one of its components known as *bilirubin*. Bilirubin is actually a waste product of worn-out, old red blood cells. When the bilirubin level rises in the blood from hepatitis

---

The Myth of the Regenerating Liver

The liver is commonly known by its remarkable ability to regenerate itself. But this statement is somewhat misleading. The liver does not really regenerate itself the way in which a starfish re-grows a missing arm. If an individual has up to 80 percent of a healthy liver removed, the remaining portion of the liver will expand to fill the empty space until its original weight is achieved. In this scenario, the liver will be fully functioning. However, if the remaining portion of a liver is permanently scarred (cirrhosis), this expansion process cannot occur and "regeneration" is therefore impossible.

or liver disease, an individual becomes *jaundiced.* This is noted as a yellow tint to the skin and eyes. Jaundice is discussed more in Chapters 2 and 3.

Bile acids are a major component of bile and are closely involved in both the production and the elimination of *cholesterol.* However, what many people do not realize is that cholesterol also is a significant component of all living tissues and is involved in the processing of vitamins and hormones. Most people associate cholesterol with something that you do not want to have too much of. This is partly correct, as virtually everyone knows that too much cholesterol clogs the arteries. If a person's diet contains an excess of cholesterol-containing foods, it is the job of the bile acids to scavenge this surplus of cholesterol particles and eliminate them from his body. Some types of liver disease are marked by abnormally high cholesterol levels. This will be discussed in detail in Chapter 15.

The Liver's Role in Processing Vitamins and Minerals

The liver is a warehouse for the storage of many vitamins and minerals, including vitamins A, B_{12}, D, E, and K; copper; and iron. For example, a normal liver contains approximately a two years' requirement of vitamin A. Centuries ago, Asian physicians were known to remove the livers from wild animals and place them on the eyes of people complaining of visual problems. While this may sound barbaric, it is now known that vitamin A may help alleviate night blindness—a condition resulting from vitamin-A deficiency. Since the liver stores these vitamins and minerals, beware of overloading its storage capabilities. For instance, people who supplement their diets with too much vitamin A or iron can actually damage their livers. This can occur even in people who have normally functioning livers. So, you can imagine what too much of a good thing could do to someone who already has liver disease. Don't add insult to injury! The toxic effects of too much iron are also demonstrated in the liver disease *hemochromatosis*—a disorder of iron overload. See Chapter 18 for more on this disorder.

You may already know that the body uses fats as a kind of storehouse for excess calories. But did you know that fats are also necessary for the absorption of vitamins A, D, E, and K? These vitamins can exist only in a fatty solution. So if the bile ducts are blocked, as sometimes happens in liver disease, the body cannot digest the fats it needs to absorb these vitamins. This is particularly serious in the case of vitamin K, which the body needs to make the blood clot. It's one reason why some people with liver disease have a pronounced tendency to bleed. Unfortunately, the liver is such a complicated organ that simply taking more vitamin K doesn't correct this problem. For more information on vitamins and minerals and your liver, see Chapter 23.

The Liver's Role in Attacking Poisons

It's one thing to break down fats and help absorb vitamins. It's quite another, however, to neutralize poisons. You might be surprised at just how vigilant the liver can be in this regard. Everything from aspirin to herbs to chemical solvents to recreational drugs is considered potentially dangerous. Therefore, in addition to the actions of bile, some cells in the liver are individually equipped to dismantle potentially toxic molecules piece by piece, or to alter them in such a way that they can be more easily eliminated from the body. That is why many people compare the liver to a giant filter that helps keep your insides clean. If that filter should ever get broken or damaged by a liver disorder, the rest of your body would slowly turn into the biological equivalent of a toxic dump.

The Liver's Role in Building Muscles

You don't have to be Arnold Schwarzenegger to appreciate the liver's role as a bodybuilder. All the muscles in the body are made up of compounds called *proteins,* which are in turn composed of *amino acids* linked together like paperclips in a chain. It's up to the liver to produce enough of the right type of amino acids for the body to build good, healthy muscles. Without these building blocks, your body would have trouble maintaining your muscles, such as those in your arms, legs, neck, and even your heart. In fact, if your liver is too damaged to metabolize proteins correctly, your muscles may literally waste away. This makes you prone to bone fractures, as bones easily become brittle when their protective muscle lining is diminished. For more information on how you can slow, or possibly even prevent this process, see Chapter 23.

The Liver's Role in Regulating Energy

A car runs on gasoline. A computer depends on electricity. The body uses its own special kind of fuel, a carbohydrate molecule called *glucose.* The liver's job is to keep the right amount of glucose in the blood and to keep it flowing to the organs that need it at all times. One of the ways it does this is by storing excess glucose in the form of another carbohydrate called *glycogen.* Whenever the body runs low on glucose, it can tap the glycogen in the liver for a little extra energy boost. If your liver is inflamed or damaged, your body will have trouble regulating the glucose levels in your blood. This is one of the reasons that many people with liver disease tire so easily.

The Liver's Role in Maintaining Hormonal Balance

The liver also has an intricate relationship with hormones, including steroid and thyroid hormones. Did you know that the hormones that give us feminine and masculine traits—that is, estrogens and androgens—are actually made from cholesterol? Since it's the liver's job to regulate the production and breakdown of these substances, liver disease can lead to hormonal imbalances. One effect of such an imbalance is the appearance of feminine characteristics in men, such as *gynecomastia* (breast enlargement). See Chapter 2 for more information on physical abnormalities and liver disease.

The Liver's Role in Processing Drugs

Most drugs that are taken orally must be processed by the liver in order to be absorbed and used efficiently by the body. Those drugs that are best absorbed by the body have the characteristic of being fat-soluble. Drugs that are not fat-soluble are known as water-soluble drugs. Water-soluble drugs are poorly absorbed when swallowed, have difficulty getting into the bloodstream, and are promptly eliminated from the body. Thus, most drugs are fat-soluble. When a fat-soluble pill or tablet is swallowed, it is readily absorbed by the fat (lipid) cells lining the walls of the stomach and intestines, and is able to easily gain access into the bloodstream. A drug must enter the bloodstream in order for it to have its desired effect. After a drug has produced its effect, it must be eliminated from the body. Fat-soluble drugs circulate through the bloodstream, either attached to proteins or trapped by fat cells. They are not easily eliminated. In order to eliminate these drugs from the body, they must be converted into water-soluble products. This job is efficiently accomplished by the liver.

The liver is the only organ in the body whose blood vessels contain wide-open holes, called *fenestrations.* This unique characteristic allows the entrance of most drugs and other substances through these blood vessel holes and into the liver cells. Once inside the liver cells, fat-soluble drugs are converted into water-soluble drugs with the help of a complex group of specialized enzymes known as the *cytochrome P450 system.* Once this has been done, the drug, now rendered water-soluble, is excreted back into the bloodstream and is capable of being efficiently eliminated by the body.

When the liver has been damaged, the metabolism (breakdown) of certain drugs and medications may be altered. Dangerous levels of these drugs may accumulate in the body, potentially causing serious adverse consequences. Therefore, it is essential that a person who has liver disease inform his doctor of the drugs and medicines he is taking, including any over-the-counter drugs or remedies and herbal preparations.

WHAT IS LIVER DISEASE?

So far you've learned that the liver is an extraordinarily complex organ that controls virtually every aspect of your body's daily functions, and that it accomplishes this feat efficiently and quietly. So what exactly is liver disease? Unfortunately, due to the complexities of the liver, this question cannot be answered in just a few simple sentences. Instead, it will take an entire book to explain the intricacies of liver disease. Fortunately, you're reading the right book!

Although the liver is such a robust organ, it can become overworked and overstressed by a variety of factors, including viruses, autoimmune disorders, obesity, alcohol, inherited diseases, benign and malignant tumors, medications, some herbal remedies, and certain vitamins when taken in excess. Liver disease occurs when one of these variables overwhelms the liver's functional capacity, resulting in injury, damage, and/or destruction of liver cells. While these factors—each of which will be discussed in later chapters—can all cause liver disease, there are many different degrees and manifestations of liver disease. The liver is such a complex organ that its injury and damage cannot be neatly divided into specific stages.

Liver disease can mean that a person has *fibrosis, cirrhosis,* or *hepatitis.* These conditions are not diseases per se, but rather the result of injury and/or damage caused by one of the variables mentioned above. *Fibrosis* is the initial stage of the formation of scar tissue in the liver. *Cirrhosis* is irreversible scarring of the liver. Cirrhosis and its complications will be discussed in Chapter 6. *Hepatitis* simply means *inflammation of the liver* and may be caused by a variety of factors, such as infections or toxins. An overall look at hepatitis will be discussed in Chapter 7. What can make matters even more confusing is that more than one of these conditions can exist at the same time!

Disease can be *acute* (occurring for less than six months) or *chronic* (occurring for more than six months). A person's liver disease may totally resolve and never return, or he may have one or more relapses of the initial disease. Someone can live a full lifetime with liver disease in good health. Or he can be constantly ill, his liver disease manifesting its many symptoms, physical signs, and complications. Liver disease may be silent, or a person may have some or all of its many symptoms and physical signs. For example, a person with cirrhosis may not exhibit any signs of liver disease, or he may be drastically ill with symptoms such as *ascites* (an abnormal accumulation of fluids in the abdomen); *encephalopathy* (mental confusion); and/or jaundice.

A person may become severely ill with excessive fatigue, stomach discomfort, and jaundice within a few weeks of becoming infected with a virus that affects the liver, such as hepatitis virus A, B, or C. Or the person may not exhibit any symptoms of infection for up to thirty years! And even when symptoms do occur, they may be as subtle as feeling a little more tired than usual—like Tom, in the beginning of this chapter.

As you can see, due to the complex nature of the liver's structure and functions, liver disease is far from easy to define succinctly. It can manifest itself in so many different ways, some of which are not apparent. In fact, the liver is such a resilient organ, it normally produces no clear, outward signs of distress until it's almost on the verge of collapse.

CONCLUSION

Now that you've read this chapter, you are more aware of the liver's anatomy and the innumerable crucial functions that this organ performs in order to keep you alive and healthy. You should also have a better understanding of what liver disease is. In Chapter 2, the first symptoms, signs, and other clues that something is wrong with the liver will be discussed. In addition, some of the physical manifestations that indicate that a person has liver disease will be described in detail.

2

Signs, Symptoms, and Other Clues of a Liver Problem

In Chapter 1, we met Tom, whose feeling of fatigue was the first clue that something was wrong with his health. This prompted him to make an appointment with his family doctor. Through the process of taking a history, performing a physical exam, and drawing some routine blood work, Tom's doctor was able to determine that his problem was liver related. Tom's wife was wise to urge him to see his doctor so quickly. Since liver disease can sometimes exist for a long time without exhibiting any obvious symptoms, Tom may have continued to remain unaware of his condition.

Of all the organs in the body, the liver is truly the strong, silent type. Whether it's fighting a viral infection or struggling under the burden of excess scar tissue, the liver rarely complains. It just keeps performing its many functions the best it can. That is why liver disease can progress for years before it's noticed. In fact, in most cases of liver disease, the first clues that something is wrong are virtually imperceptible. It is often when the liver is on the verge of collapse and can no longer perform its duties that its deterioration becomes apparent.

So how do most people find out they have liver disease? Well, sometimes—as in Tom's case—there is a subtle clue that something is wrong, such as feeling fatigued. But even these warnings may be so vague and evolve so gradually that they go unnoticed by the person with the disease and the people he comes in contact with on a daily basis. In fact, sometimes an infrequent acquaintance will be the first to detect a change in a person's appearance or personality. In other cases, a doctor may recognize the physical manifestations of liver disease while performing a routine physical examination. Or, through eliciting specific information from the patient, the doctor will make a connection between his responses and liver disease.

This chapter discusses some of the symptoms associated with liver disease—symptoms that may result in a visit to the doctor's office. It explains what to expect at the doctors' office during the initial visit; what the doctor is looking for during the exam; and the significance of what he may find.

SYMPTOMS OF LIVER DISEASE

Symptoms of liver disease are very nonspecific. There is no distinct symptom that accurately indicates that something is wrong with the liver, or what kind of liver disease someone has, or how serious the problem might be. In fact, many people with liver disease have absolutely no symptoms whatsoever. That's right! Sometimes even in the advanced stages. This is known as being *asymptomatic,* or as having a silent disease. So feeling fine doesn't always mean that nothing is wrong.

Often the first clues that something is wrong with the liver may include fatigue, pain, fever, flu-like symptoms, jaundice, altered mental status, itching, abdominal distention, and weight gain. Any one of these symptoms may prompt someone to make a doctor's appointment. In general, a person may encounter some or all of these symptoms at any time during his disease—either intermittently or consistently. To learn about the treatments for these symptoms, see Chapter 20.

Fatigue

Fatigue is a symptom characterized by a diminished ability to exert oneself, usually associated with a feeling of being tired, bored, weak, and/or irritable. Fatigue is probably the most common and debilitating symptom of liver disease. It is universal to all types and stages of liver diseases. In some people, fatigue begins several years after the liver disease diagnosis has been made. In others, it is the primary reason for seeking medical attention in the first place. Oftentimes, multiple visits are made to a variety of different types of doctors in search of the cause of the fatigue before it is connected with liver disease. Some people even seek psychiatric evaluation since depression often accompanies fatigue.

Fatigue may occur at any time of day, but it is most common in the morning. Often, little more than an hour after awakening, a person may already feel the exhaustion of having worked an entire day. Others describe weakness and lack of energy throughout the whole day. Their usual "pep" is gone. Even little tasks become more trying, and around 4:00 PM, they simply must lie down to take a nap.

Fatigue can be caused by the liver disease itself or from disorders—such as thyroid disease or vitamin deficiencies—often associated with liver disease. The doctor must carefully look at all of the factors possibly contributing to his patient's feeling of fatigue, as some factors can be corrected easily.

Pain

Most people with liver disease expect to feel pain over their liver, known as *right upper quadrant pain or tenderness* (RUQT). However, this type of pain is rarely due to chronic liver disease. RUQT occurs most commonly in the acute stages of liver disease, such as in acute viral hepatitis. It may occasionally occur when one experiences a flare-up of a chronic liver disease, although these flare-ups are uncommon. It is most often caused by acute inflammation, irritation, and distention of the liver's surface. Otherwise, the liver is rarely tender.

If pain in the region of the liver is experienced, other causes must be considered. For example, it may indicate gallstones, which happen to be associated with many liver diseases. Or it may indicate liver cancer—also known as *hepatoma* or *hepatocellular carcinoma* (HCC). Scar tissue from prior abdominal surgery known as *adhesions* is also a cause of abdominal pain. Intestinal pain must also be considered, as the right side of the large intestine lies in close vicinity to the liver (see Figure 1.1 on page 9). Many people claim that although they do not actually feel pain in the liver region, they experience a rather vague sense of "fullness" or an "awareness" of the liver. The cause for this is unclear. If a person experiences abdominal pain associated with swelling of the abdomen, *ascites*—the accumulation of fluid in the abdomen—must be considered. Ascites is associated with advanced liver disease and is discussed in Chapter 6. Other causes of abdominal pain include those related to the stomach, such as peptic ulcer disease and gastritis, which are not necessarily indicative of liver disease and are readily treatable when discovered.

Fever

Fever is seen in some people with acute viral hepatitis—especially hepatitis A—and in some people with alcoholic hepatitis, which will be discussed in Chapters 8 and 17 respectively. Fever is also experienced by some people with medication-induced hepatitis, which will be discussed in Chapter 24. However, this symptom is uncommon in people with chronic liver disease.

If fever occurs in a person who has ascites, an infection of this fluid may be present. This is a serious condition known as *spontaneous bacterial peritonitis* (SBP) and will be discussed in Chapter 6. *Cholangitis* is an infection in the bile ducts and can occur, for example, in a person with gallstones, or with a liver disease known as *primary sclerosing cholangitis*, which will be discussed in Chapter 15.

Flu-Like Symptoms

During the acute stages of liver disease, a person may experience symptoms similar to those of the flu. These symptoms, which include fever, muscle and joint aches, decreased appetite, nausea, rashes, headaches, weight loss, and generalized weakness, may last anywhere from several days to several weeks before they are completely resolved. In a person who has chronic liver disease, these symptoms are not as common, but may occur intermittently throughout the course of the disease. If any of these flu-like symptoms are constant in a person with chronic liver disease, a cause other than a liver problem should be investigated by his doctor.

Jaundice

Jaundice—noted by a yellow tint to the skin and eyes—is not actually a symptom, but a sign of liver disease, which is usually detected during a physical exam. It becomes apparent when the bilirubin rises to a level greater than 2.5 milligrams per deciliter (2.5 mg/dl). (A normal bilirubin level is lower than 1.5 mg/dl.) When a person's bilirubin level is elevated, stools may become a light clay color and urine may become a dark tea color.

Many people think that if they have never been jaundiced, then they have never had and do not currently have liver disease. This is far from the truth. In fact, many people who have liver disease may never experience jaundice. But in others, it may be the first clue that something is wrong. In these cases, jaundice may occur as a manifestation of acute hepatitis or may be an ominous sign of deteriorating liver disease. It is important to keep in mind that jaundice can be due to a myriad of causes, some of which are not even related to the liver. These causes are discussed in more detail in Chapter 3.

Altered Mental Status

For some people, the first clue that something is wrong may be *encephalopathy*— altered mental status. A person experiencing a mild, chronic form of encephalopathy may constantly forget simple things, such as where he placed his glasses or whether he already took his medication. Or he may get irritable over insignificant things or experience other behavioral changes. A person experiencing a more severe, acute form of encephalopathy may forget major information, such as what year it is or even his own name and address. Or the person may react in a strangely inappropriate or even violent manner. Encephalopathy is a sign of severe liver deterioration. It is discussed in more detail in Chapter 6.

Itching

Pruritus is the medical term for itching. It is commonly the first clue that something is wrong in people with primary biliary cirrhosis, which will be discussed in Chapter 15. Pruritus can also occur in any liver disease complicated by cholestasis—impairment or failure of bile flow—such as in people with cirrhosis complicated by jaundice. Pruritus is a symptom that can be extraordinarily annoying and extraordinarily difficult to treat. It can range in intensity from being so mild that it does not interfere with daily activities, to being so intense that it inhibits a person from sleeping at night or even holding down a regular job. The itching can occur all over the body or be limited to specific areas, such as the palms of the hand or the upper back. Some people describe this sensation as a tingling or burning sensation beneath the skin, which is not relieved by any amount of scratching. Sometimes itching can become so severe that patients will resort to scratching themselves with sharp objects, thereby causing permanent scars. The cause of this intense itching is not entirely understood, but is probably due to a combination of factors.

Abdominal Distention and Weight Gain

One liver-related symptom that often leads a person to seek evaluation from a doctor may be abdominal distention associated with an unexplained weight gain. As discussed previously, abdominal distention may be due to ascites—the accumulation of fluid in the abdomen. This is a sign of severe deteriorating liver disease and must be clearly distinguished from other causes of abdominal distention.

Many patients with liver disease become bloated due to *malabsorption* or *maldigestion*—impaired or inadequate absorption or digestion of certain foods. Abdominal distention will result as the digestive tract fills with gas. This is a readily reversible condition treatable by specific food avoidance, but to the untrained eye, it may look like ascites.

Fatty liver is another condition leading to abdominal distention and liver abnormalities. In people with fatty liver due to being overweight, a distended abdomen is due solely to excessive *adipose* (fatty) tissue. This condition, which is discussed in Chapter 16, is often easy to reverse with weight loss.

Other Symptoms

Other symptoms that can be the first clues that something is wrong with the liver include altered sleeping habits, joint aches, a persistent rash, and/or depression. These symptoms are not specific for liver disease, and, as always, a full evaluation should be conducted by a doctor in order to specifically determine their causes.

THE INITIAL VISIT TO THE DOCTOR

The initial visit to the doctor is composed of a consultation and a physical exam. Typically, blood is drawn for testing. During the consultation, the doctor will ask the patient a variety of questions. Some of the responses may provide the doctor with clues that something is wrong with the patient's liver. After the consultation, the doctor will perform a physical exam to look for other clues that may indicate a liver-related disorder. Blood tests, which provide additional information, will be discussed in Chapter 3.

The Consultation—Questions, Questions, Questions

So many things can go wrong with the liver that the doctor must ask many questions to accurately assess the cause and severity of the liver problem, as well as what type of treatment may be necessary. The list below details potential questions that the doctor may ask on the initial office visit to help determine the nature of the liver disorder. This list is provided so that the patient will know what to expect at the consultation and will be prepared to answer these questions during the visit. Answering these questions may also help trigger the patient's memory of past incidents or family history of liver disease, so as to give him some insight as to why he has a liver disorder.

- What symptoms brought you here? When did they start? Are they getting worse?

- Have you ever been told that something is wrong with your liver?

- Have any of your family members ever been told they have liver disease?

- Do you have a history of sexual promiscuity?

- Have you ever had sex with someone of the same gender?

- Have you ever used recreational drugs like cocaine or heroin? Have you ever shared an intravenous needle? A cocaine straw?

- Have you ever had any tattoos or are any of your body parts pierced?

- Have you ever received or donated blood or blood products?

- Did you serve in the military?

- What is your occupation?

- Where were you born?

- How much alcohol do you drink?

- What's your usual diet like? Has your appetite changed recently?

- Have you recently eaten shellfish or wild mushrooms?

- Have you gained or lost weight in the past few months?

- Have you recently traveled outside the United States?

- What is your past medical, surgical, and anesthetic history?

- Do you have a bleeding problem or excessive bleeding?

- Do you use paint thinners, pesticides, or other toxic substances as part of your job or around the house?

It's a good idea for the patient to provide the doctor with a list of any over-the-counter medications, herbal remedies, and vitamins or diet pills that he may be taking. Although these substances do not require a prescription and are not thought of as dangerous, they can adversely affect the liver in some cases.

As indicated by the above list, the patient should expect to answer some highly personal questions. It is extremely important for the patient to tell the doctor the whole truth—whether it happened in the past or is occurring in the present. Of course we all have done things we would rather forget. It is convenient to think that certain episodes from the past don't count anymore, but everything counts even if it occurred a long time ago. Remember, all patient records are kept strictly confidential. The patient must sign a written, witnessed request before any information is released to anyone. Therefore, keeping the doctor in the dark about past events can only hurt the chances for getting better.

The Physical Exam—Signs of Liver Disease

After the consultation, a thorough physical examination will be performed in order to look for *signs*—the physical clues or findings—of liver disease. However, the liver is so adept at hiding what's wrong—especially in the earliest stages of the illness—that even a doctor can't always tell from a physical exam that something is wrong with the liver, what specific type of liver disease a patient has, or how damaged the liver is. Consequently, many patients with liver disease, even those with cirrhosis, pass their physical exams with flying colors.

If liver disease is so hard to detect, why does the doctor bother examining the patient? First, it gives the doctor a baseline against which to compare any future changes. Second, although there are no obvious outward signs in the earliest stages of chronic liver disease, there are some subtle changes in appearance that may be present when someone has developed cirrhosis, which an astute doctor will detect. Third, there are a few physical findings that are actually suggestive of specific types of liver disease. These will be discussed below. Lastly, and most important, there are numerous physical clues that are associated with a more serious outcome—cirrhosis and liver failure.

The Baseline Exam

The doctor will commence the exam by assessing the patient's overall appearance. Are there signs of chronic weight loss or do the muscles appear to be withering away? How's the blood pressure, pulse, and breathing? Is there a fever? Does the breath smell of alcohol? Is there any mental confusion? Are there track marks from intravenous drug use? Are there any rashes, lesions, or unusual masses? Is the skin or are the eyes jaundiced? Do the hands and nails have signs of liver disease? (By the way, the brown spots on the back of the hands that many people call *liver spots* actually have nothing to do with the liver.) Are there signs of fluid retention, such as pedal edema (swollen ankles) or ascites? Is the liver hard and nodular (a sign of trouble) or is its texture smooth (a sign of health)? If the liver is either too big or too small, disease may be indicated. An enlarged liver is known as *hepatomegaly.*

Now that the doctor has assessed the general appearance of the patient, let's discuss the physical findings suggestive of cirrhosis. Three points must be stressed. First, a person with cirrhosis may manifest one, none, all, or any combination of these signs. Second, some of these signs may occur in people with liver disease, who have not yet progressed to cirrhosis. And third, many of these signs may also be seen in people without liver disease at all.

Signs That Suggest Cirrhosis

When the liver becomes *cirrhotic*—irreversibly scarred and damaged—it cannot properly execute its many important functions, which were discussed in Chapter 1. This may become apparent during the physical exam. As the liver struggles to manufacture proteins, there may be evidence of general deterioration in a person's health—predominantly noted by the loss of muscle mass known as *muscle wasting*. This is usually most prominent on the upper body and arms.

The spleen may enlarge to compensate for the decreased functional abilities of the damaged liver. This is known as *splenomegaly*. The *spleen* is an organ lying directly opposite the liver under the ribcage on the left side of the body. The spleen plays a role in the storage of platelets. *Platelets* are blood cells that help blood to clot. Thus, an enlarged spleen is often associated with *thrombocytopenia*—a low platelet count. This is discussed in Chapter 3.

Many abnormalities may become evident due to the failure of the liver to metabolize endocrine hormones properly. Liver palms *(palmar erythema)* is the bright red coloring of the palms, particularly at the base of the thumb and pinky. It may be associated with some throbbing or warmth of the hands. Enlarged blood vessels found on the upper chest, back, face, and arms, resembling little red spiders, are known as *spider angiomatas*. They characteristically blanch (turn white) if light pressure is applied to their centers. Body hair patterns may change. Men note that they need to shave less often. Hair becomes sparse on the chest, face, and pubic region. Women may have decreased underarm hair. *Gynecomastia* (breast enlargement) may become noticeable in men, and breasts may also feel tender.

There are other manifestations of cirrhosis that do not have a clear explanation. These include *Terry's nails,* a condition in which the normal pinkish color of the nail bed turns completely white and the half-moon circles at the base of the nails disappear; and *paper money skin,* a condition in which the upper body is covered with numerous thin blood vessels that resemble the silk threads in a United States dollar bill.

Signs That Suggest a Specific Liver Disease

Most manifestations of liver disease are universal to all liver diseases, independent of their cause. However, there are a few findings that may suggest a specific liver disease. *Xanthomas* (an irregular yellow nodule or patch usually found on the ankles, elbows, and knees) and *xanthelasmas* (a yellow nodule or patch on the eyelids) are associated with very high cholesterol levels and are found in people with primary biliary cirrhosis (see Chapter 15). These irregular patches can be very disfiguring and painful. These lesions can also be found in other liver diseases and in other diseases associated with elevated cholesterol levels.

People with cirrhosis due to alcoholic liver disease will likely have many visible physical findings. *Dupuytren's contracture* is a puckering of the palm that prevents a person from totally straightening out his hand. The severity of this deformity may correlate with the quantity of alcohol consumed. *Parotid gland enlargement* may also occur. The parotid gland is a gland on the face located under the ear. When it becomes enlarged, it causes the earlobes to protrude at right angles to the jaw. In addition to gynecomastia, the testicles may shrink, a condition known as *testicular atrophy.* Testicular atrophy may also be a manifestation of hemochromatosis.

An *hepatic bruit*, a harsh, musical sound heard when a stethoscope is placed over the liver, is suggestive of liver cancer (hepatoma).

Signs That Suggest Liver Failure

Liver failure is defined as cessation of normal liver function. It can occur in a previously healthy individual without prior evidence of liver disease. This is known as *acute* or *fulminant liver failure.* Or it may occur as the end result of cirrhosis. Signs of liver failure indicate a poor outcome and are the most ominous findings of a physical exam.

Encephalopathy, which was discussed on page 18, virtually always accompanies liver failure. Sometimes, people with encephalopathy are initially seen by a doctor in a hospital setting after a family member discovers them unconscious in a coma. *Fetor hepaticus* is a foul, sweetish, or feces-like smell on the breath (often referred to as a "dead mouse" or "corpse"). This can be a sign of either acute or chronic liver failure and often precedes encephalopathy. *Asterixis,* which occurs with encephalopathy, is an uncontrollable flapping of the hands that becomes noticeable when a patient stretches out his arms, palms out, as if stopping traffic.

Scleral icterus is the yellow discoloration of the sclera (whites of the eyes) and jaundice, as you've learned, is the yellow discoloration of the skin and eyes. Both of these conditions are manifestations of an elevated bilirubin level. Ascites is the accumulation of excess fluid in the abdomen. When ascites is associated with fever and abdominal pain, spontaneous bacterial peritonitis (SBP) may be present. If there is a massive amount of ascites, one may even have a protrusion of the umbilicus (belly button), known as an *umbilical hernia.* In severe cases, the belly button can actually burst open causing a massive leak of ascitic fluid. Dilated blood vessels can snake out from the belly button—an appearance appropriately termed *caput medusa.* Edema is fluid accumulation in the legs, especially the ankles (pedal edema). Immediate evaluation and treatment of these manifestations of liver failure—which will be addressed in Chapters 6 and 20—is crucial.

CONCLUSION

After reading this chapter, you should know what to expect when you or your loved one goes to the doctor for an evaluation of a liver-related problem. Also, you are now more knowledgeable about the symptoms and signs of liver disease. Depending upon which signs and symptoms a patient mentions or displays at the time of the initial evaluation, the doctor may have a general idea of what is wrong with his liver. On the other hand, the doctor still may not be able to determine whether a liver disorder actually exists. In either case, the next step is to perform some routine blood tests to obtain additional diagnostic information. Chapter 3 will introduce you to the basic blood tests and imaging studies that doctors utilize in their efforts to diagnose individuals who have liver disease.

3

Tests, Tests, Tests— Learning What You Need to Know

After consulting with Tom and conducting a physical exam, Tom's doctor decided that some blood tests were in order to gather additional information. Included in all or most routine panels of blood are tests pertaining to the liver. These tests are commonly referred to as liver function tests (LFTs). Some of Tom's LFTs were abnormal, which led his doctor to the conclusion that there was a problem with Tom's liver. Tom also had a sonogram of his liver, which was normal. He assumed that since his liver sonogram was normal that there was nothing wrong with his liver. Tom subsequently learned that this was not necessarily the case.

The significance, usefulness, and limitations of liver function tests (LFTs) are discussed in this chapter. Unfortunately, LFTs cannot identify a specific liver problem. However, there are some special blood tests, which are not included in routine blood work, that can be ordered if a certain liver disease is suspected. (The table on page 31 details these special blood tests.) In addition, this chapter discusses the various imaging studies, such as sonograms, CT scans, and MRIs, which are used to visualize the liver.

UNDERSTANDING LIVER FUNCTION TESTS (LFTS)

Wouldn't it be nice if your liver came equipped with a dashboard, like the one in your car that tells you that the oil needs changing, that the engine's overheating, or that you need to find a gas station in hurry? Since it doesn't, doctors have come to rely on a number of blood tests—known as liver function tests (LFTs)—to give them some indication of what's going on inside the liver. But don't be fooled by this name. While LFTs are commonly used to reflect how well the liver is working, this name can be misleading, as it is impossible for any blood test to accurately assess all of the liver's varied functions. Thus, like the indicator lights and gauges in a car, the LFTs are not a perfect indication of exactly what's wrong. They can, however, alert the doctor that something is amiss with the liver. Furthermore, they can help determine which additional tests are necessary. And, when used in conjunction with these additional tests, LFTs give the doctor a better idea of what is wrong with the liver and how well the liver is working. By keeping track of the results from the LFTs over the months and years ahead, both the patient and the doctor may—in some cases—have an idea whether the liver condition has stabilized, improved, or worsened; whether a specific treatment is working; or if something different needs to be tried.

LFTs consist of many different blood tests that check for the levels of liver enzymes (transaminases and cholestatic liver enzymes); bilirubin; and the liver proteins. The following is a discussion of these tests.

Liver Enzymes

There are four liver enzymes included on most routine laboratory tests that can indicate the presence of liver disease. They are *aspartate aminotransferase* (AST or SGOT) and *alanine aminotransferase* (ALT or SGPT), which are known together as *transaminases*; and *alkaline phosphatase* (AP) and *gamma-glutamyl transpeptidase* (GGTP), which are known together as *cholestatic* liver enzymes.

AST and ALT (Transaminases)

AST and ALT are jointly known as transaminases. They are associated with inflammation and/or injury to liver cells, a condition known as *hepatocellular liver injury*. Damage to the liver often results in a leak of AST and ALT into the bloodstream.

Because AST is found in many other organs besides the liver, including the kidneys and the heart, having a high level of AST does not always (but often does) indicate that there is a liver problem. For example, even vigorous exercise may elevate AST levels in the body. On the other hand, because ALT is found only in the liver, high levels of ALT almost always indicate that there's a problem with the liver.

Despite what one might expect, high levels of transaminases in the blood don't always reveal just how badly the liver is inflamed or damaged. This is an extremely important point to keep in mind. The normal ranges for AST and ALT are around 0 to 40 IU/L and 0 to 45 IU/L respectively. (IU/L stands for international units per liter and is the most commonly accepted way to measure these particular enzymes.) But someone who has an ALT level of 50 IU/L is not necessarily in better condition than someone with an ALT level of 250 IU/L! This is because these blood tests measure inflammation and damage to the liver at an isolated point in time. For instance, if the liver is inflamed on the day that blood was drawn—let's say if a patient consumes an alcoholic drink a few hours prior to blood being drawn—the levels of the transaminases may be much higher than if the alcohol had not been consumed. Following the same reasoning, if the liver was damaged years before—

by excessive alcohol use—the results of a blood test done today may be normal, but a damaged liver may still be present. Also, even the time of day that a blood sample is drawn may influence the level of transaminase elevation. People appear to have higher transaminase levels in the morning and in the afternoon than in the evening.

Elevations of the transaminases occur due to so many causes that they give the doctor only a vague clue of the diagnosis. Some possible causes are as follows:

- Viral hepatitis

- A fatty liver

- Alcoholic liver disease

- Drug/medication-induced liver disease

- Autoimmune hepatitis

- Herbal toxicity

- Genetic liver diseases

- Liver tumors

- Heart failure

However, additional testing is required in order to determine more precisely what is wrong with the liver.

GGTP and AP (Cholestatic Liver Enzymes)

High levels of the GGTP and AP hint at a possible blockage of the bile ducts or of possible injury or inflammation of the bile ducts. In either case, there is an impairment or failure of bile flow, which is known as *cholestasis*. This type of liver injury is known as *cholestatic liver injury*, and this type of liver disease is known as *cholestatic liver disease*. (Primary biliary cirrhosis, discussed in Chapter 15, is an example of a cholestatic liver disease.) *Intrahepatic cholestasis* refers to bile duct blockage or injury within the liver. Intrahepatic cholestasis may occur in people with primary biliary cirrhosis or liver cancer (see Chapter 19), for example. *Extrahepatic cholestasis* refers to bile duct blockage or injury occurring outside the liver. Extrahepatic cholestasis may occur in people with gallstones.

When a blockage or inflammation of the bile ducts occurs, the GGTP and AP can overflow like a backed up sewer and seep out of the liver and into the bloodstream. These enzymes typically become markedly elevated—approximately ten times the upper limit of normal.

GGTP is found predominantly in the liver. AP is mainly found in the bones and the liver but can also be found in many other organs, such as the intestines, kidneys, and placenta. Therefore, elevated levels of AP will indicate that something is wrong with the liver only if the amount of GGTP is raised as well. Conversely, GGTP can be elevated without AP being elevated, as it is a sensitive marker of alcohol ingestion and certain *hepatotoxic* (liver toxic) drugs. Once again, this demonstrates the complexities that arise when evaluating the LFTs.

Normal levels of AP range from 35 to 115 IU/L and normal levels of GGTP range from 3 to 60 IU/L. Some causes of elevated AP and/or GGTP include the following:

- Primary biliary cirrhosis

- Primary sclerosing cholangitis

- A fatty liver or nonalcoholic steatohepatitis (NASH)

- Alcoholic liver disease

- Liver tumors

- Drug-induced liver disease

- Gallstones

Bilirubin

Bilirubin is the yellow-colored pigment that the liver produces when it recycles worn-out red blood cells. Normal bilirubin levels are less than 1 mg/dl (milligram per deciliter). When levels become elevated, eyes and skin may turn yellow (jaundice), urine may appear a dark-tea color, and stools may look like light colored clay. Elevated bilirubin, while not the most common abnormality in blood tests pertaining to the liver, is quite obvious on a physical exam, and it is the most familiar liver-related abnormality generally known.

A common phrase doctors often hear from their patients is, "I can't have liver disease, I'm not yellow." People are often surprised to discover that most people with liver disease will never become yellow. In fact, many bilirubin elevations are not even related to liver disease at all. Bilirubin metabolism is very complex and consists of many steps. A problem with any one of these steps results in an abnormally high level of bilirubin. As it pertains to the liver, an elevated bilirubin level is usually associated with worsening liver disease or with bile duct blockage (cholestasis). Some possible causes of a high bilirubin level include the following:

- Primary biliary cirrhosis

- Primary sclerosing cholangitis

- Alcoholic hepatitis

- Hemolysis—red blood cell (RBC) destruction

- Drug-induced liver disease

- Choledocholithiasis (gallstones in the bile duct)

- Liver failure or general worsening of liver disease

- Tumors afffecting the liver, bile ducts, or gallbladder

- Viral hepatitis

- Benign familial disorders of bilirubin metabolism, such as Gilbert's disease

Bilirubin elevations are often associated with GGTP and AP level elevations (discussed on page 27). When elevated levels of both bilirubin and GGTP and AP occur, a person is referred to as being *cholestatic*. However, if the bilirubin level remains normal and the GGTP and AP remain elevated, the person is known as having *anicteric cholestasis*. Diseases in which these events typically occur are known as *cholestatic liver diseases*.

Liver Proteins

Albumin, prothrombin (factor II), and immunoglobulins are proteins that are made primarily by the liver. Abnormal levels of these proteins can help determine whether there is a serious liver disorder present.

Albumin

Normal blood levels of albumin are about 4 g/dl (grams per deciliter). When the liver becomes severely damaged, it loses its ability to make albumin. People with chronic liver disease accompanied by cirrhosis often have levels of albumin below 3 g/dl. A low albumin level in general is an indicator of poor health and nutrition, and is not specific to liver disease.

Prothrombin Time

The liver manufactures most of the clotting factors that the body uses to stop bleeding. The time it takes to produce a clot, called the *prothrombin time* (PT), generally runs from nine to eleven seconds. Vitamin K is an important factor in the blood clotting process. If the liver is very seriously damaged or if a vitamin K deficiency is present (as sometimes occurs in cholestatic liver diseases such as primary biliary cirrhosis), the PT will run much longer than normal, thereby increasing the risk of excessive bleeding. In some cases, injections of vitamin K can help the PT return to normal. Improvement of the PT with a vitamin K injection indicates the liver is still functioning. When the PT does not normalize after a vitamin K injection, a condition known as a *coagulopathy* (a tendency to bleed excessively), severe liver damage, and/or liver failure may exist.

Immunoglobulins

Immunoglobulins are proteins associated with the immune system, some of which are made by the liver and some of which are made by *leukocytes*—white blood cells (WBC). A variety of immunoglobulins are increased in many people who have chronic liver disease. Elevations of the *immunoglobulins* A, G, and M (IgA, IgG, and IgM) can be suggestive of specific liver diseases (see Table 3.1 on page 31).

Platelets

Platelets are blood cells that help the blood form clots. The spleen plays a role in the storage of platelets. In people with cirrhosis, the spleen works overtime to compensate for the decreased functional abilities of the damaged liver. This is associated with a low platelet count known as *thrombocytopenia*. The normal platelet count is 150 to 450×10^3/microliter. If a patient has a value lower than 150×10^3/microliter, thrombocytopenia is said to be present.

Some Final Thoughts on Blood Work

Remember, an isolated group of blood test results cannot be used to predict the future of a person with liver disease. The actual numbers themselves may have little significance. Their meaning is only important in conjunction with a multitude of other factors, each of which must be carefully interpreted by a doctor. In other words, don't get too hung up about the individual numbers. Each is just one piece of a very large puzzle. In most cases, the numbers are just a clue that something is wrong—only the first step toward a correct diagnosis.

After the routine blood tests are evaluated, more specific blood work is usually required in order to pinpoint an exact cause of liver abnormalities. Table 3.1 on page 31 lists the blood tests that are used to diagnose specific liver diseases. These blood tests will be discussed in more detail throughout the book. Usually, the laboratory provides the doctor with the results of routine blood work within a day or two; but the results of more specific blood tests may take up to two weeks, depending on the laboratory. The waiting period may not be easy. (Try to be a patient patient.)

UNDERSTANDING IMAGING STUDIES

After the blood tests have been performed, the doctor will want to visualize the liver as a whole. Therefore, the next step is a trip to the radiologist's office to obtain one or more imaging studies of the liver.

There are several methods that can be used to obtain an image of the liver. They include taking a *sonogram,* also known as an ultrasound or sono; a *computerized axial tomography scan*, also known as a CT scan or CAT scan; or a *magnetic resonance image* (MRI). All of these imaging scans are noninvasive (no surgery required), they do not hurt, and they can be done while the patient is awake and lying

Table 3.1. Blood Tests Used to Diagnose Specific Liver Diseases

Liver Disease	Blood Test	Chapter Reference
Hepatitis A	Hepatitis A Antibody IgM and IgG	8
Hepatitis B	• Hepatitis B core Antibody (HbcAb) • Hepatitis B surface Antigen (HbsAg) • Hepatitis B surface Antibody (HBsAb) • Hepatitis B e Antibody (HBeAb) • Hepatitis B e Antigen (HBeAg) • Hepatitis B viral DNA (HBV DNA)	9
Hepatitis C	• Hepatitis C Virus Antibody (HCVAb) • Hepatitis C Virus Ribonucleic Acid (HCV RNA) • Elevated Immunoglobulin G (IgG)	10
Autoimmune Hepatitis	• Antinuclear Antibody (ANA) • Smooth Muscle Antibody (SMA) • Antiliver/Kidney Microsomal Antibody (LKMAb) • Elevated Immunoglobulin G (IgG)	14
Primary Biliary Cirrhosis	• Antimitochondrial Antibody (AMA) • Elevated Immunoglobulin M (IgM) (PBC)	15
Alcoholic Liver Disease	• Blood Alcohol Level • Elevated Immunoglobulin A (IgA) • Mean Corpuscular Volume (MCV) > 95 fl • Vitamin B_{12} and Folate Deficiency • Desialylated Transferrin Level	17
Hemochromatosis	• Iron (Fe) • Ferritin • Percent Transferrin Saturation • Total Iron Binding Capacity (TIBC) • Gene Testing—Histocompatibility Leukocyte Antigens (HLA-H) and DNA Probe Analysis by PCR	18
Liver Cancer (Hepatoma)	Alpha-Fetoprotein (AFP) > 400ng/dl	19

on his back. One or more of these imaging studies are usually performed to make sure the liver is located where it is supposed to be in relation to the other organs; to determine if there are any abnormal masses in the liver; or to find out if gallstones are present in the gallbladder.

Sonograms

While sonograms are most commonly thought of as the imaging study used to see the fetus in a pregnant woman, they are, in fact, the most frequently used imaging study to visualize the liver. A sonogram is a fast and inexpensive way to get a look at this organ. Although they are performed in a radiologist's office, no radiation is actually used—sound waves produce the image.

Sonograms are usually performed on a patient with an empty stomach to allow the gallbladder to remain full of bile, which makes it easier to spot gallstones. In fact, more than 95 percent of all gallstones are discovered during a sonogram. Sonograms are also used to detect masses on the liver, which can be either benign (noncancerous) or malignant (cancerous), but they cannot definitively distinguish between the two. Furthermore, sonograms can estimate the size of a detected mass. However, even if a sonogram appears normal, it doesn't mean that there is no problem with the liver. In fact, many people who have liver disease have had sonograms that look perfectly fine, as Tom's did in the beginning of this chapter. Therefore, don't be surprised if the doctor orders more tests after the sonogram.

CT Scans and MRIs

CT scans and MRIs provide more comprehensive views of the liver in relation to its adjacent organs. They are most often utilized to further evaluate a mass found on sonogram. CT scans utilize gamma radiation by transmitting an x-ray beam through the liver. Any abnormal masses will stop the x-ray beam in its tracks, and an image will be recorded. With an MRI, electromagnetic radiation creates a picture of the liver. MRIs are useful in detecting a fatty liver, iron overload, and *hemangiomas*—a benign blood tumor (see Chapter 19).

Some Final Thoughts on Imaging Studies

Many exciting breakthroughs have been made that have enhanced the diagnostic accuracy of these imaging studies. However, even these advanced techniques don't tell the whole story of what's going on with the liver. It is very important to understand that the liver is a master of camouflage. Even people with severe liver disease and cirrhosis may have normal imaging studies. This is a key point to remember, and it bears repeating. Sonograms, CT scans, and MRIs can look totally normal at any stage of liver disease. That is why doctors have come to rely on the liver biopsy, which will be discussed in Chapter 5, as the gold standard for evaluating liver disease.

CONCLUSION

After reading this chapter, you should now understand that blood tests and imaging studies typically used to visualize the liver don't always help to determine what is wrong with the liver or may not help assess the degree of inflammation or the damage that has occurred. A liver biopsy, which is usually performed by a specialist, is the only test that can accurately determine this information. Chapter 5 is devoted to discussing this procedure in detail. But first, it is crucial to find a specialist who is skilled at performing the liver biopsy and has the knowledge to accurately interpret the results. The next chapter discusses the different types of doctors that a person may choose for his specialized care, and assists him in choosing the right one. It also explains what qualifications to look for in a specialist, and where and how to obtain this information.

4

Choosing the Right Doctor

Tom's doctor advised him to consult a specialist for further evaluation of his liver disorder and referred him to a gastroenterologist who was conveniently located only a couple miles from Tom's house. At the gastroenterologist's office, Tom noticed that the waiting room was chock full of pamphlets and other literature on stomach and intestinal disorders, but there was nothing on liver disease.

Tom was taken into the consultation room by the receptionist. There, the gastroenterologist asked Tom some questions about his health before leading him to another room for the physical exam. At the end of the exam, the gastroenterologist said, "You look healthy, Tom. I've reviewed your blood work and the sonogram report from your doctor. Since your LFTs are only slightly elevated, you don't need further evaluation with a liver biopsy and you do not need to start on any treatment. See me again in six months and we'll repeat the tests. But if you start to feel worse, call me."

"Why do I feel so fatigued?" Tom asked. "What should I do?"

"Get more rest and just take it easy for a while," was the gastroenterologist's reply.

Tom left with mixed emotions. On the one hand, he was relieved that the doctor thought he didn't need a biopsy. On the other hand, Tom recalled reading an article stressing the importance of liver biopsies and early treatment of liver disease. Tom felt a little uneasy. "Does this gastroenterologist really focus his practice on liver disease? Is there a specialist in my town whose practice is concentrated on liver disease? And can I find such a doctor?"

Looking for answers, Tom searched the Internet (which had many websites devoted to liver disease), called several nonprofit organiza-

tions, and even conducted some research at his local library. He also asked people he knew to recommend a liver specialist. Tom's hard work led him to a hepatologist—a liver specialist—in his area. At the initial visit, the hepatologist strongly recommended a liver biopsy to further evaluate Tom's condition, and began to discuss possible treatment options. Tom was surprised at how different the two doctors' opinions were.

For a person with liver disease, finding the right doctor is no simple task. It may require both time and effort. In many instances, someone with chronic liver disease will be under the care of the same doctor for many years or possibly for his entire life. Therefore, choosing the right specialist is a decision of extraordinary importance. But finding "Dr. Right," unfortunately, is not always so easy.

This chapter takes you step-by-step through the process of finding a qualified specialist in liver disease. It discusses the differences in expertise among the various types of doctors who treat liver disease. It explains what qualifications to look for in a specialist, and where and how to obtain information regarding the specialist's qualifications and credentials. It will also cover what a patient should expect from the doctor's office and the office staff, and what to do if a specialist does not participate in the patient's insurance plan. Finally, included are some tips on how to prepare for, and get the most out of, the initial consultation with a specialist.

WHAT KINDS OF DOCTORS TREAT LIVER DISEASE?

There are many different kinds of doctors who evaluate and treat people with liver disorders. First, there is the family physician or internist. These doctors are also referred to as primary care physicians (PCPs). They are often the first ones to discover that something is wrong with the liver. From there, the patient is customarily referred to a specialist—either a gastroenterologist or a hepatologist—for further evaluation and treatment. This specialist may be at an academic institution or in a private practice. The difference between the various types of doctors a patient with liver disease encounters may sometimes be confusing. Hopefully, this section will clarify these differences in order to eliminate any future confusion.

The Medical Doctor (MD)

Medical doctors (MDs) are physicians who have successfully completed four years of medical school training. After graduating from medical school, these doctors must complete a minimum of one additional year of training in a hospital in what is known as an internship. They must then pass a state-licensing exam in order to practice medicine in that state. After obtaining their license, they have the right to practice general medicine in that state. However, many doctors choose to continue their training in a hospital by undergoing a residency—typically an additional two years.

After completing their residency, these doctors must take an exam in order to become board certified in a specialty, such as family medicine or internal medicine. At this time, a doctor may decide to undergo additional specialty training, known as a fellowship, in a specific area of internal medicine, such as gastroenterology and/or hepatology.

The Doctor of Osteopathy (DO)

Doctors of osteopathy (DOs) are commonly referred to as *osteopaths*. These are doctors who graduated from a four-year osteopathic school. They must also complete a one-year internship in a hospital in order to be eligible to obtain a license to practice medicine. Osteopaths can also choose to undergo an additional two-year residency, and may thereafter undergo specialty training in a specific area of medicine.

Osteopaths tend to focus on treating "the body as a whole," particularly on the body's ability to heal itself. Osteopaths typically center their treatment on the musculoskeletal system, the muscles and bones, often using techniques such as bone manipulation and a form of massage.

The Family Physician

A family physician is a doctor—either an MD or a DO—who has been trained to prevent, diagnose, and treat medical conditions in people of all ages. The family physician takes care of the general health of the patient and his entire family. Their training is not limited to internal medicine, but includes some training in psychiatry, obstetrics, gynecology, and surgery. These are the "Marcus Welby" doctors, seemingly able to handle almost any general problem.

There is a separate board certification examination specifically for family practitioners. This is known as the family practice boards. Specializing in family practice medicine requires an additional three years' training beyond medical school. The amount of exposure and degree of expertise in liver disease varies among family practitioners. However, family physicians have not undergone additional specialized training in liver disease.

The Internist

An internist is a doctor—an MD or a DO—who is trained to prevent, diagnose, and treat medical conditions in adolescents and adults, including the elderly. Internists have received some basic training in subspecialty areas of internal medicine, including gastroenterology and hepatology. Internists are trained to treat both straightforward and complex problems of the internal organs. They are also trained in emergency medicine and critical care medicine. There is a separate board certification examination specifically for internists. It is known as the internal medicine boards. Specializing in internal medicine requires an additional three years' training beyond medical school.

The amount of exposure and degree of expertise in liver disease varies among internists. Internists have the option of continuing their training in a subspecialty of internal medicine. This requires applying for, and being accepted into, a fellowship in the subspecialty of their choice. Both gastroenterology and hepatology are among the many subspecialties of internal medicine.

The Gastroenterologist

A *gastroenterologist* is an internist who has completed specialty training in the treatment of digestive disorders. Digestive disorders include disorders of the esophagus, stomach, small and large intestines, pancreas, gallbladder, and liver. In order to become board certified in gastroenterology, the doctor must first become board certified in internal medicine. In order to become eligible to even take the examination for board certification in gastroenterology, a gastrointestinal (GI) fellowship lasting an additional two to three years beyond an internal medicine residency must be completed.

During the course of their two to three years of training in gastroenterology, some gastroenterologists have little exposure to patients with liver disease. On the other hand, some gastroenterologists have had a great deal of exposure to patients with liver disease during the course of their gastroenterology specialty training. Thus, the level of experience and expertise among gastroenterologists in diagnosing and treating liver disease varies greatly. It is important for the patient to determine the gastroenterologist's level of expertise in liver disease prior to establishing a long-term medical relationship with this type of doctor. This will be discussed on page 42.

The Hepatologist

A hepatologist is the most experienced and qualified type of doctor to treat people with liver disease. Since there is currently no separate board certification examination in the field of hepatology, there is no official definition of a hepatologist. However, there are specialized training programs for doctors who are focused solely on liver disease. These are known as hepatology fellowships and typically last from one to two years. Over the course of a hepatology fellowship, a doctor receives comprehensive training in the diagnosis and treatment of liver disease. This specialty training typically includes extensive exposure to all liver diseases, including those that are rare and infrequently seen. This intense training in liver disease is rarely matched in a gastroenterology fellowship.

A physician who successfully completes a hepatology fellowship is considered a hepatologist. Most hepatologists, although not all, are also gastroenterologists. These doctors have successfully completed both a hepatology and a gastroenterology fellowship. Occasionally, gastroenterologists who have not completed a fellowship in hepatology, nonetheless focus their medical practice primarily on the diagnosis and treatment of people with liver disease. While these physicians do not have a separate diploma in the field of liver disease, they may also be considered hepatologists.

For many reasons, it is to the patient's advantage to choose a hepatologist to treat his liver disease. The patient can be virtually assured that the hepatologist will have substantial experience in the diagnosis and treatment of the full range of liver diseases. Furthermore, hepatologists are likely to be the first to learn about the most up-to-date therapies—both FDA-approved and experimental—and to incorporate them into their practices. However, whether someone chooses to see a gastroenterologist or a hepatologist, it is important to find a doctor who is willing to work with him as an equal partner in the healing process.

Academic Physicians Versus Private Practitioners

People searching for a doctor should be aware of the differences between academic physicians and private practitioners. Each type of doctor has pros and cons that must be carefully weighed by the patient as part of the process of choosing a physician.

The Academic Physician

An academic physician is a doctor who has accepted a faculty position on staff at a hospital. Often, though not always, the hospital will be associated with a medical school. These doctors spend a portion of their time teaching medical students and physicians-in-training (interns, residents, and fellows) about their specialty—in this case hepatology. Also, some of these doctors conduct research that can make up a considerable percentage of his workload. Some of this research is performed in a laboratory and some is within the context of a clinical trial involving patients. (See Chapter 11 for a discussion of clinical trials.)

These physicians are usually board certified in their specialty, and some have contributed significantly to the advancement of the medical profession in their specialty. However, this is not always the case. No one should ever assume that the qualifications of a given academic physician (even of the department chairman) are superior to those of a given private practitioner merely based on the academic physician's employment by a hospital.

Academic physicians are generally expected to stay abreast of the newest developments in their field. Such a physician may have initiated or prompted the investigation of a new drug or may have played a significant role in the development of a new medical procedure. Frequently, academic physicians are involved in conducting investigational trials on the most promising experimental drugs. However, the requirements of entering a study at an academic center may be very rigid and typically involve a risk that the patient will be given a placebo (dummy drug).

Doctors at an academic institution usually allot some time to patient care. However, since these physicians must also teach, the patient will sometimes be evaluated and treated primarily by a doctor-in-training rather than the more experienced faculty member he was expecting. Although these doctor trainees must discuss the patient with the academic physician, the patient will be given no assurance of ever meeting with the academic physician, or he will only briefly meet with this academic doctor whose credentials prompted his visit in the first place. This may occur on the initial consultation and/or on subsequent visits. Thus, the patient cannot count on a close personal relationship with this doctor. Therefore, it is important for a patient making an appointment with a physician who is on staff at a hospital to inquire whether he will be seeing the doctor in a clinic setting or in some type of private office.

Finally, since these physicians are typically based within a hospital, their office hours are often limited. Rarely, if ever, will these physicians make themselves available for appointments after 5:00 PM, before 8:00 AM, or on weekends. And since these doctors have so many other duties in the hospital, such as meetings, teaching, and lecturing, typically only two or three days will be devoted to seeing patients and only for a limited number of hours. The result of such limited hours is that the patient will generally only be able to book an appointment several weeks, if not months, in advance. Furthermore, hospital-based physicians are typically away from their practice many weeks out of the year attending meetings and lecturing.

The Private Practitioner

A private practitioner is a physician who typically focuses his career on patient care. Usually, but not always, private practitioners take care of people who are admitted to local hospitals in their communities. That is, these private practitioners have either admitting or consulting privileges at one or more local hospitals. Some private practitioners may also be affiliated with an academic institution, where they also treat patients and occasionally teach.

Private practitioner physicians may be in solo practice, wherein only one doctor is running the practice; in a partnership, wherein two or more physicians share the responsibilities of the practice; or in a group practice, wherein several doctors are affiliated across an array of different medical specialties. As compared with an academic setting at a large hospital, a more personal relationship with the physician is more likely to develop in a private-practice setting. However, if the physician is not a solo practitioner, the patient should inquire whether he will be seen by the same physician on each visit.

Private practitioners typically have much longer and more flexible office hours than physicians who are hospital staff members. Thus, early morning, evening, and weekend hours are often available. Of course, the actual hours of availability vary considerably among private practitioners. Also, as compared with hospital-based physicians, private practitioners are less likely to be away from their offices for extended periods of time. Thus, it is possible to obtain an appointment with a highly qualified hepatologist in private practice much quicker (usually within a week or two) than with an academic hepatologist of similar stature.

A person doesn't necessarily have to be treated at an academic institution in order to enroll in a clinical trial of an experimental drug. Some private practitioners conduct clinical studies as part of their practice, in the same manner as would an academic physician. However, this is not especially common and generally applies only to the most knowledgeable privately practicing hepatologists. This is an important area to inquire about prior to making an appointment with the doctor. Typically, studies run in a private practitioner's office are less rigid in terms of criteria for including or excluding subjects and are less likely to involve the use of a placebo as compared with those conducted at an academic institution. It is important to thoroughly research the credentials of the physician conducting the study, whether the study is conducted in a private practice setting or at an academic institution. This will be discussed in further detail in Chapter 11.

Finally, many people with liver disease incorrectly assume that, if they are treated by an academic physician who is affiliated with a transplant center, this will automatically increase their chances of obtaining a new liver, should one be required. This is a total misconception, as all people are subject to identical rules, regulations, and criteria for liver transplantation—regardless of whether the patient is being treated within an academic or private practice setting.

WHAT TO LOOK FOR IN A SPECIALIST

Now that you a familiar with the different kinds of doctors, the next step is to find out about and evaluate the chosen doctor's qualifications. It is best for the patient to independently verify the doctor's qualifications and credentials prior to making an appointment for the initial consultation. Time with the doctor is valuable and should be focused mainly on determining a plan of action to treat the patient's liver disease, not on questions concerning the doctor's credentials. Also, there is no guarantee that the doctor will be totally forthcoming about his level of experience. It's very important to remember that just because the doctor's business card or door sign says liver disease, it shouldn't be assumed that his practice focuses on liver disease. The printer and the sign maker do not verify the doctor's qualifications and credentials. What are the criteria to use when choosing a specialist, and how do you determine whether the doctor meets these criteria? The following pages will guide you in the right direction.

Determining Board Certification

Determining the doctor's board certification status should be considered an essential first step in the search for a specialist. *Board certified* indicates that the doctor has completed rigorous training in the specialty and has passed an intensive set of boards (exams) in that specialty. Being board certified in a specialty indicates that the American Board of Medical Specialties has certified that the doctor has successfully completed an approved educational training program and possesses adequate knowledge to competently practice and provide a high quality of patient care in that specialty. *Board eligible* indicates that the doctor has completed training in the specialty, but either has not taken or has not passed the boards in that specialty.

All board-certified gastroenterologists must first become board certified in internal medicine. Thus, all board-certified gastroenterologists are also board-certified internists. Remember two important points: First, although a doctor may be board-certified in gastroenterology, this doesn't mean that his medical practice is focused on liver disease. And second, there is currently no board-certification exam solely in hepatology. As such, there is no such thing as a board-certified hepatologist. Therefore, the patient must search for either a board-certified gastroenterologist who did an additional, separate fellowship in liver disease, or a board-certified internist who did a fellowship in liver disease. Finally, a patient may search for a board-certified gastroenterologist who did not complete a hepatology fellowship, but who focuses his practice on liver disease.

Information about a doctor's board-certification status is available through a variety of channels. In most main library branches, there are sets of reference books that provide a list of board-certified doctors in the United States. Be careful, however, as some types of directories list only doctors who have paid to be listed. The most reputable directory is *The Official American Board of Medical Specialties (ABMS) Directory of Board-Certified Medical Specialists.* This is an excellent starting point for choosing a suitable specialist. Be sure to look in the most recent edition. This directory will also provide some useful information concerning the specialist's medical background, including where and when the specialist completed medical school, internship, residency, and fellowship training. It will also state if the doctor completed a hepatology fellowship. If a doctor is not listed in the ABMS directory, then that doctor is not board certified.

Since a doctor must be board certified in internal medicine in order to become board certified in gastroenterology, the patient should try to find a doctor who is certified in both specialties. In fact, gastroenterologist and hepatologist are listed in the section on internists in the ABMS directory. (Don't forget, there is the rare exception of the hepatologist who, having done no specialty training in gastroenterology, will be board certified only in internal medicine.)

All of the information in ABMS directory can also be obtained by personally contacting the American Medical Association (AMA) or the American Board of Medical Specialties to inquire specifically about the credentials of a doctor. (See Appendix for mailing addresses, phone numbers, and Internet website addresses.)

Determining the Doctor's Experience With Liver Disease

It is essential to find a doctor who has a significant amount of experience in taking care of people who have liver disease. In this regard, the patient should pose some basic questions to the doctor. See the sample questions on page 43. Remember, however, that it is difficult to verify the doctor's answers—in this case, there are no associations or books in which to look for verification.

• *Approximately what percentage of your practice is devoted to liver disease, and about how many liver disease patients are you presently treating?*

Some doctors have a very large practice but treat very few individuals with liver disease. Other doctors have a relatively small practice, but it may be one that is devoted primarily to taking care of people with liver disease. And some doctors—despite being well known in the field of hepatology—have not actually treated many people with liver disease. These doctors, who often work at large, well-respected hospitals, have devoted their careers to liver disease *research* rather than patient care.

• Approximately how many liver biopsies have you performed within the past year?

Some doctors have little experience performing this relatively simple procedure, which will be discussed in great detail in Chapter 5. Other doctors perform liver biopsies regularly. Although there is no "right" number, you can consider a doctor sufficiently experienced if he performs between 50 and 100 liver biopsies per year. Also, it's important to determine if the doctor will actually be performing the biopsy, or if a trainee, associate, or radiologist will be performing the procedure instead.

• Are you involved in liver disease research?

It is advisable to ask the doctor whether he has participated in or is currently conducting research devoted to liver disease. For example, a doctor may be involved in experimental trials to evaluate a promising new form of diet or drug therapy for liver disease or may be involved in evaluating a new method of diagnosing liver disease. A doctor involved in such investigations will afford the patient the opportunity not only to learn firsthand about the most up-to-date therapies, but also may enable the patient to begin using a promising form of therapy before it becomes readily available.

• Have you written any articles on liver disease?

A patient should feel free to inquire about the doctor's medical research experience and also about whether the doctor has written any articles that have appeared in any well-respected peer-review medical publications, such as *Hepatology, Gastro-enterology,* or *Seminars in Liver Disease.* This information can be independently checked by accessing MEDLINE on the Internet (see Appendix for website address) or by asking for a copy of the article. Doctors are usually more than happy to comply with such a request. Remember, however, medical articles are written for other physicians and other members of the medical community. These articles will, therefore, contain technical medical terminology.

• Are you aware of alternatives to conventional medical therapies?

While a liver specialist is primarily involved in prescribing mainstream medical treatments, a good doctor should also be well aware of the available alternatives to conventional medical therapy. Extensive evaluation of the alternative treatment in question must be reviewed before the doctor labels it bogus. How familiar is the doctor with the alternative therapy in question? What type of evaluation of this alternative therapy did the doctor conduct to reach his recommendation? How many of the doctor's other patients tried this alternative treatment, and what were the results?

Remember that just because the doctor didn't learn about alternative medicine in medical school doesn't mean he doesn't have to stay up to date on at least the most popular alternatives for treating liver disease. While the doctor may not necessarily support its use, he should be well aware of the potential positive and negative effects that alternative therapies have on the liver and the rest of the body.

While you may be tempted to ask the doctor his age or how long he has been in practice, these questions are of questionable usefulness. Though most people would prefer not to be treated by a doctor who has just completed specialty training, the actual amount of years in practice may not be a reliable indicator of the doctor's experience with liver disease. For example, a doctor who has been in practice for thirty years may treat only ten individuals with liver disease each week. While another doctor, who may have been in practice for ten years, treats thirty people with liver disease each week. Who is more qualified? The answer is they both may be sufficiently qualified. The bottom line is that the age of the physician and the actual number of years he has been in practice are not reliable criteria by which to judge a doctor's level of experience.

THE WAYS DOCTORS HELP PATIENTS OUTSIDE THEIR PRACTICES

Treating each person individually is the standard way a doctor helps patients get better. But there are additional ways that a doctor can help people—ways in which he can reach out to large groups of people with liver disease and to their loved ones all at once.

If a doctor spends his spare time involved in activities relating to liver disease, such as writing articles, lecturing, making radio or television appearances, creating instructional videos, or running a website devoted to liver disease, it's pretty obvious that this doctor is dedicating his career, as well as his free time and spare energy, to helping people with liver disease. Patients should not hesitate to ask their doctors if they are involved in any of these worthy activities.

Publications

A doctor who writes articles on liver disease can reach a large number of people. The article can be contributed to a local newspaper, a health-related magazine, or the newsletter or brochure of a support group or a nonprofit organization devoted to liver disease, such as the American Liver Foundation (ALF) or Hepatitis Foundation International (HFI). Similarly, many pharmaceutical companies involved in the treatment of liver disease also have literature concerning the disease and its treatment. The patient should find out if the doctor has contributed information to any of these publications. Doctors who have had articles published will often have copies available at their offices that the patient can take home to read.

Lecturing

Does the doctor give voluntary lectures on liver disease, either within the local community or nationally? Lectures are regularly sponsored by nonprofit organizations such as ALF or HFI. The general public is normally invited to attend these lectures, either free of charge or for a very minimal fee. The doctor should be able to inform the patient of the date and location of scheduled lectures in the community or nearby areas. The patient should find out if the doctor is invited to speak at these lectures. A doctor who is involved in lecturing to the public will gladly tell the patient when the next lecture is scheduled, so that the patient may attend if he wishes. Or the doctor will describe to the patient the most recent lecture that he has given.

Media Appearances

The media is a means by which the doctor can reach out to many people with liver disease and their loved ones all at the same time. By communicating to the public through the media, the doctor is able to spread information about liver disease to thousands, if not millions, of people. Health topics are frequently discussed on news programs and even talk shows. Often, local or cable television stations devote entire programs to liver disease, and radio programs often have short segments related to health topics. The patient should find out if the doctor has appeared on television or radio shows concerning liver disease, or if the doctor has participated in the production of any videotapes devoted to liver disease. A doctor who has appeared on television, radio, or videotape will probably be able to provide the patient with a taped copy of the show, or at the very least, provide information about how to obtain a copy.

Internet Websites

There are numerous liver-related websites on the Internet. The patient should find out if the doctor is involved in running one of these websites. The doctor should also be able to direct the patient to other informative, accurate Internet websites. This topic will be discussed in more detail later in this chapter on page 47.

Associations and Foundations

Methods for the diagnosis and treatment of liver disease change rapidly on an ongoing basis. It is important to be treated by a doctor who is familiar with the most up-to-date developments. There are many professional organizations that keep doctors abreast of the most recent information on liver disease. The most prominent of these organizations in the field of liver disease is the American Association for the Study of Liver Disease (AASLD).

A doctor who has been elected to membership in the AASLD is most likely to be actively involved in liver disease. The AASLD is an association of physicians and scientists who are dedicated to the advancement and application of knowledge of liver disease. To be elected to membership, a doctor must pass a rigid set of criteria, including successful completion of specialty training; evidence of at least two publications pertaining to the liver; and nomination by two other members of AASLD. A patient can telephone, e-mail, or write to the AASLD to confirm that his physician is a member. (See Appendix.)

There are also numerous lay (non-professional) organizations that are dedicated to increasing the awareness of liver disease. The American Liver Foundation (ALF) is a voluntary nonprofit organization whose membership consists of doctors, patients, or any other individuals interested in liver disease. ALF's major goals include educating the public about liver disease and fostering the prevention and treatment of liver disease. A doctor may be involved with ALF to varying degrees, ranging from being a member to running a support group to lecturing to the public on a topic pertaining to liver disease. Doctors who have demonstrated exceptional dedication to the cause of helping individuals with liver disease are often invited to serve as a board members of ALF, either at the national or local level. A patient can contact ALF to inquire about a doctor's level of activity in this organization. (See Appendix.)

THE DOCTOR'S OFFICE AND STAFF

Often, the patient can get a baseline impression of the doctor by observing how the office is run. Take note of whether the office staff seems to be knowledgeable about liver disease. A person telephoning the office may not always be able to contact the doctor immediately. Does the doctor have a nurse or medical assistant who can promptly and accurately answer questions in the doctor's absence? What is the availability of the doctor and the doctor's staff? How many days a week is the office open? Are the doctor's hours flexible? Are evening and weekend appointments available? How long must the patient wait to get an appointment?

A doctor may not have an appointment available the same day a patient calls, but no matter how busy the doctor's practice is (even in the busiest of practices), a patient should be able to schedule an appointment within two to three weeks—at most.

How long does the patient have to wait once in the doctor's office? If on every visit, the patient is left waiting for more than two hours in the waiting room, then there is something wrong with the doctor's method of scheduling. But a long wait on occasion should not be cause for concern. Emergencies sometimes arise and can result in delays.

People with liver disease generally need frequent assessment of their blood work. Therefore, it is important to find out whether blood will be drawn at the doctor's office or whether the patient will be sent to a laboratory to have blood drawn. Obviously, it is a great convenience to have blood drawn in the doctor's office at the same time of the visit.

Finally, find out whether there is one or many doctors in the practice and whether the patient will be seeing the same doctor at each visit. It is in the best interest of the patient to establish a relationship with one doctor. This way, the doctor's familiarity with the patient's medical history and special needs will be maximized. This is likely to lead to the highest rate of success in treatment of the patient's liver disease.

INSURANCE AND HMO PLANS

A full discussion of insurance plans, including HMOs and PPO, is beyond the scope of this book. However, the patient should be aware of one very important point concerning insurance plans, which is described in the following scenario: *After Tom's exhausting search, he finally found a specialist that he wanted to consult with. However, when he checked in his insurance book, to his great disappointment, the specialist's name was nowhere to be found! Now what?*

All patients should be aware that most insurance plans will pay for a visit to a doctor who is not included in their plan, *if*—and this is an important if—the doctor offers special or unique services that no other doctor in the plan offers. For example, some liver specialists offer a wealth of experience treating people with liver disease, which greatly exceeds that of any other doctors who are currently listed on the plan, or they are offering treatment options that are not available through any of the other doctors on the plan. In these circumstances, an appeal letter or even a phone call to the appropriate insurance company representative explaining the dilemma often results in the patient being granted coverage for a consultation with the desired specialist. Also, the patient may want to ask the doctor personally if he would consider joining his health plan.

LIVER DISEASE SPECIALISTS AND THE INTERNET

The Internet may be considered a double-edged sword when it comes to liver disease. It is an ocean of both information and misinformation. Surf with caution. The number of Internet websites continues to grow at an explosive rate. Despite the relative newness of the Internet, there are already many Internet websites devoted to liver disease and hepatitis. It can be difficult for the layperson to determine which information is correct and which information is not. It is most important for the patient using the Internet to determine who is sponsoring the website.

Is a pharmaceutical company maintaining the website? For example, Schering-Plough, Amgen, and Smith-Kline Beecham, three major drug companies that manufacture and distribute pharmaceuticals used in the prevention or treatment of liver disease all maintain Internet websites. Each of these websites contains useful information. Is it a well-respected hepatologist who maintains the website? For example, I maintain a regularly updated Internet website, and there are a number of other excellent hepatologists who also maintain websites devoted to liver disease. Does a well-established not-for-profit organization maintain the website? For example, ALF and HFI, in addition to many other groups maintain helpful websites. Is it a knowledgeable patient eager to help others who maintains the site? Or is it a not-so-knowledgeable patient who is giving false and possibly dangerous information? Be careful. (See Appendix for some helpful website addresses.)

Some websites provide referrals to doctors who purportedly specialize in liver disease. Unfortunately, it is often impossible to ascertain what criteria were used in selecting the referred doctors. Some sites merely require a doctor to pay a fee in order to be listed. While it may be difficult to obtain accurate information from searching the Internet, one likelihood may be relied on: If the doctor has a website devoted to liver disease, it is likely his practice is focused on taking care of people with liver disease.

CONSULTING WITH THE SPECIALIST

Now that the patient has located a specialist, there are a few tips to follow, which will help make the appointment as smooth and efficient as possible for both the patient and the doctor. It is normal to be nervous about seeing a specialist. So much new and crucial information will be provided to the patient during this visit. It is, therefore, to be expected that after the initial consultation is over, the patient will not recall a significant amount of what the doctor has said. For this reason, the patient should try to have a relative or close friend along for the consultation. Prior to the visit, the patient should make a list of all of the questions that he wants answered during this visit. The patient should bring this list to the consultation and should not leave the doctor's office until every question has been satisfactorily answered. It's perfectly okay to take short notes while the doctor is talking and to check off each question after the doctor has answered it. If necessary, the patient should request that the doctor write down unfamiliar technical medical terms used during the conversation.

The patient can make the initial consultation more productive for the specialist by bringing all prior records from other doctors to the visit. This will better enable the doctor to promptly and accurately assess the patient's condition on the initial visit. It is especially important to bring the doctor copies of all previously performed blood work, imaging studies, and liver biopsy reports or slides. Doing so will not only assist the doctor, but it can sometimes eliminate the necessity of repeating the tests and/or biopsy.

Remember, all prior records, reports, and slides legally belong to the patient. These records should never be difficult for the patient to obtain. However, most doctors' offices, hospitals, and medical facilities require a written request authorizing the release of the records to another doctor or hospital.

Finally, the patient should always bring the doctor a list of all medications, including over-the-counter medications, vitamins, dietary supplements, and/or herbal remedies, that he may be taking. The more comprehensive information the patient provides to the specialist, the more accurate the specialist's advice will be.

FINDING SECOND OPINIONS

If a patient is not comfortable with the advice he receives from a specialist, it is advisable to seek another opinion. Always make sure that a second opinion is provided by a doctor whose knowledge of liver disease is superior, or at least equal to, that of the first specialist. But patients should keep multiple opinions in perspective. Under no circumstances should patients ever make it their objective to shop around for opinions until they hear the diagnosis or prognosis that they are looking for. A game plan of this nature could only cause a serious illness to be left neglected and untreated. It is natural for anyone to hope to hear that there is nothing wrong and that a liver biopsy and treatment aren't necessary. In some cases, these statements may in fact be accurate; however, if the patient has seen two or three well-respected specialists, all of whom concur that something is wrong, the patient must accept that he has a chronic illness that may require treatment.

CONCLUSION

It should be the goal of every patient to get the best medical care available. While everyone hopes that his specialist is supplying him with the most accurate and up-to-date information, it is the patient's responsibility to do more than just hope. Patients can and should independently research the expertise level and credentials of a doctor prior to making an appointment for the consultation. Although this is time-consuming and requires some effort, there is no question that it is well worth it. Once the "right" specialist has been found, the patient will be proud to have enhanced his prospects for treatment and wellness. The patient can start down the road to recovery by feeling confident in the doctor's abilities and by concentrating on getting better. In the long-run, this is actually the quickest route to follow. Don't wait years to find "Dr. Right." Start your search today! Now that you know what to look for in a doctor, the next chapter will tell you what to expect from a liver biopsy.

5

What the Patient Should Know About Liver Biopsies

After a long search, Tom found a liver specialist about whom he felt confident. This specialist provided Tom with an abundance of additional information about liver disease. After reviewing the results of Tom's blood work and the sonogram of Tom's liver, the specialist recommended a liver biopsy. Tom was relieved that he would soon find out what condition his liver was in, but he was also a little nervous—what was undergoing a liver biopsy all about?

All of the aspects of liver biopsies, including exactly what a liver biopsy is, why a biopsy is often necessary for diagnosing a liver problem, and who should avoid having a biopsy are addressed in this chapter. You will also be taken step-by-step through the actual process of the biopsy and provided with information on what to do before and after the procedure has been performed. Although the risks of having a liver biopsy are very low, this chapter will also describe the potential complications of this procedure.

THE LIVER BIOPSY AND WHY IT'S NECESSARY

A liver biopsy is the removal of a tiny piece of liver tissue using a special needle. The fragment taken out resembles a one-inch piece of string or a tiny worm. Its removal will not disturb the functioning of the rest of the liver. The liver sample is sent to a laboratory, where it is carefully examined by a pathologist under a microscope. Hepatologists also have expertise in examining liver biopsy specimens and will customarily examine this sample in conjunction with the pathologist.

Microscopes have the capability of greatly magnifying the liver cells—allowing abnormalities to be seen that could not otherwise have been detected by the physical examination, the blood tests, or the imaging studies. Because most liver diseases affect the entire organ uniformly, this tiny sample is usually representative of the entire liver and provides a complete story. It is unlikely that this specimen would look better or worse than the rest of the liver, but it can happen—though very rarely. This uncommon occurrence is known as *sampling error.*

The liver biopsy is the only diagnostic procedure that can really take the mystery out of liver disease. A biopsy can determine exactly what's wrong with the liver and exactly how badly the liver has been damaged. This information is crucial in order to outline a course of treatment and to determine a prognosis. The information obtained through a liver biopsy cannot be as accurately obtained through any other method, including imaging studies and extensive blood work.

WHEN A LIVER BIOPSY ISN'T NECESSARY

The doctor and the patient must work together to determine all aspects of the patient's care, including the issue of undergoing a liver biopsy. The potential benefits of the biopsy must outweigh the potential risks. When the risks outweigh the benefits, other approaches to the patient's care are in order. There are two general categories of people who should not have a liver biopsy.

The first group includes those individuals in which the information obtained from the biopsy would lend no additional insight into their treatment or prognosis. For example, a person with acute hepatitis A (see Chapter 8) would receive the same treatment regardless of the liver biopsy results. Or a person with a suspected medication-induced liver disease (see Chapter 24) may benefit from discontinuing the medication first, and then assessing whether or not the liver-related abnormalities normalize. If they don't, a liver biopsy may then become necessary.

The second group includes people who are simply too ill to undergo a biopsy. For example, a patient who has cirrhosis complicated by ascites runs the risk of leakage of ascitic fluid through the liver biopsy incision site, in addition to multiple other complications, such as excessive bleeding. Finally, if the patient is uncooperative (for example, unable to remain still), the biopsy should not be performed.

PREPARING FOR THE LIVER BIOPSY

There are many ways that a person can prepare for the biopsy to maximize the odds that things will go smoothly. Prior to scheduling the biopsy, the patient should make the doctor aware of any drug allergies or of pregnancy or possible pregnancy. Because the liver is packed full of blood vessels, the greatest (although still minimal) risk of complications stems from bleeding. Therefore, as discussed below, all blood-thinning substances should be avoided for at least one week to ten days prior to the biopsy. Also, the patient should ask the doctor for specific instructions on when, in relation to the biopsy, he should stop taking prescribed medications. The patient should also know that more blood work and perhaps a sonogram (if not already done) will be performed.

The doctor will usually request that a patient fast—abstain from eating or drinking—for at least eight hours prior to the biopsy. Some doctors, however, may permit a light breakfast in order to allow the gallbladder to empty.

Drugs and Other Substances to Avoid Prior to the Biopsy

Although it's important to keep in mind that bleeding occurs in only a small percentage of biopsies, it is vital that for at least one week to ten days prior to the biopsy and one week after the biopsy, the patient refrain from taking any drugs that interfere with the body's ability to produce blood clots. This will minimize the danger of excess bleeding. The drugs to be avoided include blood thinners, such as Coumadin; aspirin or any of the nonsteroidal anti-inflammatory drugs (NSAIDs), such as ibuprofen (Advil, Motrin, Pamprin, Nuprin, etc.) and naproxen (Aleve). (Note that medications containing acetaminophen [Tylenol] are permissible in moderation.)

Because vitamin E can enhance the effects of drugs like Coumadin and aspirin, it should also be discontinued a week prior to the biopsy. Multivitamin supplements and preparations usually contain vitamin E and must, therefore, also be avoided. Some herbs, such as *ginkgo biloba,* also have blood-thinning properties and should be avoided.

If the patient has not already done so, the consumption of all alcoholic beverages should be discontinued at least one month prior to the biopsy.

Blood Work and Sonogram

Blood work to assess the risk of bleeding during the procedure—for example, prothrombin time and platelet count—will be performed by the doctor no more than one month prior to the biopsy. If one of these tests is abnormal, a transfusion of fresh frozen plasma (FFP) or platelets may be necessary before proceeding with the biopsy. Alternatively, if the patient has a known bleeding disorder, such as hemophilia, the doctor may suggest having the biopsy done by a special method (see page 55) or avoid the biopsy altogether.

It is standard procedure for the doctor to take a sonogram of the liver to assess the possible presence of any unusual anatomic abnormalities or the presence of any unsuspected liver masses prior to the biopsy. If an abnormality is detected, the doctor may opt to perform the biopsy while visualizing the liver with an imaging study (see page 55).

THE DAY OF THE BIOPSY

The patient will be required to make advance arrangements to be driven home from the hospital the day of the biopsy by a friend or relative. Most biopsies are performed in either a hospital's gastroenterology procedure suite or in its ambulatory (outpatient) unit. On the day of the biopsy, a consent form must be signed by the patient, formally giving permission for the procedure to take place. If the consent form raises any issues that the doctor hasn't already addressed, the patient should ask for clarification right away.

The patient will be asked to remove all clothing from the waist up and to put on a hospital gown. It's a good idea for the patient to use the restroom at this time. This is because he will not be allowed out of bed for four to six hours after the biopsy.

It's normal to feel anxious prior to any procedure. Therefore, the patient should feel free to request a mild sedative. In this case, a small *intravenous* (IV) catheter will be inserted into a vein in the arm. A small amount of sedative medicine, such as Valium or Versed, will be administered to take the edge off. However, it is not advisable to be totally asleep. It's important for the patient to be alert enough to let the doctor know if there is any pain or other symptoms.

After the biopsy is over, the patient is instructed either to lie flat on his back or to lie on his right side for four to six hours. For most people, the hardest part of the biopsy is having to lie still for this length of time. However, it's an important precautionary measure. If anything is going to go wrong (see Complications of a Liver Biopsy on page 56), it is most likely to happen in the first few hours after the procedure has been completed. Fortunately, this waiting period usually turns out to be one long bore—it's a good idea to bring along a book or a personal stereo with earphones to while away the hours. During the waiting period, a nurse will come by regularly to monitor the pulse, blood pressure, breathing, and temperature. Usually, after a few hours have passed, the patient is given a light lunch. Then, four to six hours after the biopsy, it's time to go home.

TECHNIQUES FOR PERFORMING LIVER BIOPSIES

There are many different techniques used in performing a liver biopsy. The actual technique used is dependent upon the patient's overall health, in addition to the expertise and preference of the doctor. These techniques are explained in the following pages.

The "Blind-Stick" Method

The classic technique doctors use to perform a liver biopsy is commonly called the "blind percutaneous stick" method. But don't let this somewhat alarming nickname bother you. Although it's true the doctor cannot see the liver through the layers of skin, muscles, and fat that make up the abdomen, an experienced doctor can locate the liver by using a combination of sound and feel. The word *percutaneous* simply means passage through the skin.

The doctor will begin by asking the patient to lie flat on his back with his hands under his head, and to remain as still as possible. In much the same way that a carpenter might tap a wall to find a hollow area, the doctor will tap the abdomen to determine where the liver is and where it isn't. The next step is to reduce the risk of infection by cleaning the skin with an antiseptic agent and by covering the biopsy site with sterile towels. The antiseptic may feel a bit cool to the touch. Then, the doctor will inject a local anesthetic agent, such as Lidocaine, into this area in order to numb the skin. The injection usually stings a little, but this mild discomfort generally disappears after a few seconds. Once the anesthetic has taken effect, the doctor will make a very tiny nick in the skin about the size of a pinhead over the area where the doctor determined the liver to be. While some doctors instruct the patient to hold his breath at this point, others instruct the patient to just breathe normally.

The biopsy itself involves a quick jab with a special needle through the skin, into the liver, and out again. This jab literally takes no longer than one-tenth of a second. Yes, only one-tenth of a second. The needle will suction out one or two tiny slivers of liver, about one inch to one-and-a-half inches long. The procedure is now over! Remember, with the exception of the skin, the liver is the largest organ in the body; therefore, an experienced specialist should have little difficulty locating it by using the "blind percutaneous stick" method.

Occasionally, the liver sample isn't large enough, and the doctor may have to insert the biopsy needle a second time. This may happen if the liver has become so hardened by cirrhosis that the needle has difficulty penetrating the liver's surface, or in cases where the patient is very obese.

The doctor will now put a bandage over the insertion point and will ask the patient to lie either flat or on the right side for the next four to six hours. At this point, most patients can't believe that the biopsy is over. They wonder what they were so nervous about in the first place. From start to finish, the entire procedure should take no longer than ten minutes.

The Guided Biopsy

A sonogram or a computerized tomography (CT) guided biopsy is used when more precision is required. Such cases arise when the doctor is uncertain about the location of an appropriate site, or when the doctor wants to sample an abnormal growth found in one specific area of the liver. In rare cases, other organs, such as the gallbladder or the intestines, may be in the way of the liver, making it more difficult to find. Or, if the patient is extremely overweight, the liver may be surrounded by so many layers of fat that it can be difficult to locate. Or, if cirrhosis is present, the liver may have shrunk so much that some doctors need extra help in finding it. In any of these scenarios or due to the personal preference of the doctor, the doctor may decide to use a sonogram or a CT scan to guide the biopsy needle to the liver.

Other Biopsy Methods

The other methods used to obtain a liver specimen are somewhat more complicated. In some special cases, a radiologist will be brought in to perform what is called a *transvenous* or *transjugular* liver biopsy. This technique is used if a patient has a problem with blood clotting, known as *coagulopathy,* which is defined as a prolonged prothrombin time to greater than 3 seconds; if the patient has a platelet count of less than 60,000, known as *thrombocytopenia;* or if the patient has ascites, an abnormal accumulation of fluids in the abdomen.

A small tube is first inserted into a vein in the neck (the jugular vein) and then passed into the vein that drains the liver (the hepatic vein). The biopsy needle is passed through this tube into the liver and a sample of liver tissue is retrieved.

Another technique is known as the *laparoscopic* liver biopsy. It is usually performed in the operating room by a surgeon, but some liver specialists are trained in this procedure. It involves the insertion of a thin, lighted tube—a *laparoscope*—into a small incision made in the abdominal wall, in order to directly view the liver. A biopsy needle is inserted into this lighted tube and a sample of liver tissue is retrieved.

Finally, if a patient is undergoing open abdominal surgery for an unrelated reason, a liver sample can be taken by the surgeon at that time.

COMPLICATIONS OF A LIVER BIOPSY

As with any invasive procedure, there are inherent risks involved. The good news is that in the hands of a qualified, experienced doctor, the incidence of problems resulting from a liver biopsy are extraordinarily rare, and if caught in time, can generally be corrected. In fact, complications from a liver biopsy have been reported in less than one percent of all individuals undergoing the procedure. Moreover, the risk of death from a liver biopsy is virtually unheard of—occurring in approximately 0.01 percent of patients, resulting from one of the complications discussed below.

The incidence of complications increases with the number of attempts to obtain a piece of liver. Most complications arising from a liver biopsy are evident within the first few hours after the procedure. This is the reason for the four- to six-hour waiting period after the procedure has been performed. Early recognition is the most important aspect in the treatment of any complications resulting from the biopsy. It's extremely important to contact the doctor in the event that any problems are suspected of having occurred after the biopsy. The following are some potential complications that may occur as a result of this procedure.

Bleeding

Most incidents of bleeding after a liver biopsy are inconsequential and do not require treatment. If massive bleeding does occur, however, it can usually be treated with blood transfusions and close monitoring in the intensive care unit of a hospital. Only rarely will surgical intervention be required. Bleeding usually results from puncturing an enlarged blood vessel within the liver, which sometimes cannot be avoided. Bleeding is usually evident within the first few hours after a liver biopsy.

Puncture of Other Organs

Since the liver is surrounded by so many other organs, sometimes the kidney, colon, or lung may be punctured in error. This rarely results in any serious problems. An exception to this is the uncommon instance of puncturing the gallbladder or its bile ducts, which can result in leakage of bile into the abdomen causing *peritonitis*—an infection of the abdominal fluid. This is usually treated with intravenous antibiotics and admission to the intensive care unit. Since a sterile technique is used, other types of infection are rare, but when they occur, they are usually transient, mild, and easily treated with antibiotics.

Pain

Most people agree that their liver biopsy was relatively painless and much easier than they ever expected it to be. While not actually a complication, pain is the most common complaint after a biopsy. Between 10 and 50 percent of liver biopsy patients state that they felt as if someone had quickly punched them in the side, or they describe a dull, aching sensation in the right shoulder. Pain may also occur around the stomach and over the site of the needle stick, but is typically mild. Any discomfort is best remedied by taking one or two acetaminophen tablets. This discomfort will usually resolve within an hour. Remember, don't take any NSAIDs and aspirin-based products either a week before or after the biopsy, as they can increase the chance of bleeding.

If the patient finds that that he is still in pain more than twenty-four hours after having left the hospital, or that the pain is getting worse, he should call his doctor immediately.

WHAT TO DO AFTER THE BIOPSY

After undergoing a biopsy, the patient should take it easy the first day. He should refrain from doing any heavy lifting or undertaking any strenuous activities. In addition, he should not drive for at least twenty-four hours or undertake any energetic activities, including dancing and sports. After twenty-four hours, he can remove the bandage and take a bath or a shower. If the patient has a physically demanding job, he should plan to stay out of work for at least forty-eight to seventy-two hours. People who have desk jobs may return to work the next day.

It may take as long as a week to obtain the results of the biopsy. It is best for the patient to make a follow-up appointment with the doctor to discuss these findings at length. It is also a good idea for the patient to bring a family member or close friend along to assist in asking questions concerning the results.

CONCLUSION

After reading this chapter, any fears a person has about undergoing a liver biopsy should be significantly, if not totally, alleviated. You should now feel confident that a liver biopsy is a very quick and relatively painless procedure with an extremely low complication rate when performed by an experienced doctor. One purpose of undergoing a biopsy is to determine the degree of scarring that has occurred in the liver. Total scarring of the liver is known as cirrhosis. The next chapter discusses this irreversible condition, which can occur as a result of a number of different liver diseases.

6

A Look at Cirrhosis

Tom's liver biopsy went smoothly. It was much easier than he had expected it to be. He made an appointment for the following week to discuss the results with his specialist. Tom's wife went to the follow-up appointment with him. When the receptionist led them into the doctor's private consultation office, Tom's anxiety level rose. Once the couple was seated, the doctor said, "Tom, the results from the biopsy indicate that you have cirrhosis." "Cirrhosis?!" Tom exclaimed. "What is cirrhosis, and how did I get it?"

In this chapter, you are provided with an in-depth description of cirrhosis—irreversible scarring of the liver. The symptoms and signs associated with this condition are described and the diagnosis of cirrhosis is discussed. This chapter will also address which liver diseases can lead to cirrhosis, and what the potential complications of this condition are.

WHAT IS CIRRHOSIS?

The liver is an incredibly resilient organ, but unfortunately it isn't indestructible. Sometimes the damage that occurs as a result of alcoholism, a virus, or some other chronic disease overwhelms the liver's capacity to function. Healthy liver cells are permanently destroyed, and irreversible scarring occurs. The liver becomes rock hard and nodular (lumpy). This condition is known as cirrhosis.

Cirrhosis is the end product of any one of a number of different liver diseases, which will be discussed briefly on page 60 and in more detail in later chapters. It is important to emphasize the point that cirrhosis is irreversible. Regardless of the cause, the consequences of cirrhosis are the same. Whereas a healthy liver has the potential to repair and regenerate itself when injured (see page 10), once cirrhosis has occurred, the damage cannot be undone. The scars on the liver will never heal. The process of cirrhosis can occasionally be slowed, or even halted, but can never be reversed.

Progress is being made in the control of cirrhosis. This is confirmed by the declines in cirrhosis-related death rates in the United States over the last twenty years. However, cirrhosis continues to be the eighth most common cause of death overall in the United States and the fourth leading cause of death among Americans between the ages of thirty and sixty years old. But being diagnosed with cirrhosis is not necessarily an automatic death sentence. Usually, when cirrhosis is fatal, it is because it has proceeded unchecked and untreated for many years. If, however, it is caught in its early stages, there will often be steps that the patient and doctor can take to control its progression.

Despite having cirrhosis, many people have lived well past the age of ninety. Of course, prevention remains the best medicine; therefore, most of the treatments doctors prescribe, as well as the nutrition and exercise tips discussed in Chapter 23, are aimed at trying to keep the liver from progressing to cirrhosis in the first place.

LIVER DISEASES THAT CAN LEAD TO CIRRHOSIS

Not all liver diseases cause cirrhosis—only those that cause chronic, ongoing damage to the liver can lead to permanent scarring of liver tissue. For example, someone with hepatitis A will usually recover completely after a few weeks, and as such, will not be at risk for developing cirrhosis. But someone who has lived for decades with a chronic liver condition, such as hepatitis C or hemochromatosis, would be a prime candidate for cirrhosis.

Fortunately, in most cases, cirrhosis takes many years to develop. Therefore, just because a person is at risk for cirrhosis, it doesn't necessarily mean that he will definitely develop this condition over the course of a normal life span. Also, the slow pace at which cirrhosis develops allows a person to obtain treatment from a liver specialist *before* cirrhosis occurs.

Alcoholic liver disease and chronic hepatitis C are the two most common causes of cirrhosis in the United States. However, there are other circumstances that can give rise to permanent liver damage. Even some herbal remedies and medications can trigger massive scarring of the liver (see Chapters 21 and 24 respectively). Although a discussion of every condition that has the potential to cause cirrhosis is beyond the scope of this book, some causes include the following:

- Viral hepatitis—hepatitis B, C, and D (see Part Two).

- Autoimmune hepatitis (see Chapter 14).

- Primary biliary cirrhosis (see Chapter 15).

- Fatty liver and nonalcoholic steatohepatitis (see Chapter 16).

- Excess alcohol consumption (see Chapter 17).

- Hemochromatosis (see Chapter 18).

- Excessive intake of vitamins, such as vitamin A (see Chapter 23).

- Certain herbal remedies, such as comfrey (see Chapter 21).

- Certain medications, such as methotrexate, isoniazid, Aldomet (see Chapter 24).

- Primary sclerosing cholangitis (see Chapter 15).

- Vascular anomalies—for example, Budd-Chiari syndrome (see Chapter 21).

- Congestive heart failure (see your doctor for more information).

- Wilson's disease, a genetic disorder of copper overload (see your doctor for more information).

THE SYMPTOMS AND SIGNS OF CIRRHOSIS

The symptoms and physical signs of cirrhosis are virtually the same regardless of the cause of cirrhosis. The silent nature of liver disease, as discussed in Chapter 2, often leaves few obvious clues as to the extent of the damage being done. Some people with cirrhosis feel perfectly normal or may have vague symptoms, such as fatigue, decreased appetite, nausea, and loss of libido. These individuals are known as having *compensated cirrhosis.* People with compensated cirrhosis usually live a normal life span with relatively few health-related consequences due to cirrhosis. However, they remain at risk for developing complications, such as internal bleeding, jaundice, encephalopathy, and/or ascites. When one of these complications develops, it is known as *decompensated cirrhosis.* The potential complications of cirrhosis will be discussed in more detail on page 62.

DIAGNOSING CIRRHOSIS

As discussed in Chapter 2, the doctor may be able to detect signs of cirrhosis on a physical exam. General signs of malnutrition, such as muscle wasting, will be looked for. The doctor will pay close attention to the texture and size of the liver. As opposed to the soft, smooth feel of a healthy liver, a cirrhotic liver feels hard and bumpy. This is because normal liver tissue has now been replaced by scar tissue and nodules. (An astute doctor can feel this through the skin.)

The size of the liver is variable. Despite what most people think, a cirrhotic liver may stay the same size, shrivel up, or enlarge (a condition known as hepatomegaly). As discussed on page 22, the spleen may enlarge—a condition known as splenomegaly—to compensate for the decreased functional abilities of the damaged liver.

A digital rectal exam will be performed to check for signs of internal bleeding. Upper intestinal bleeding, which is known as *melena,* produces distinctive black, foul-smelling stool. A person experiencing such a condition should bring it to his doctor's immediate attention.

Some laboratory test results may suggest cirrhosis. These results include a low albumin level, an abnormally low cholesterol level, an elevated or prolonged prothrombin time, and/or a decreased platelet count. (See Chapter 3 for a discussion of these tests.) Imaging studies of the liver may suggest, but cannot confirm, cirrhosis. Ultimately, the only way to confirm the suspicion of cirrhosis is through a liver biopsy.

There are two basic types of cirrhosis—*macronodular* cirrhosis, in which the cirrhotic nodules in the liver are very large, and *micronodular* cirrhosis, in which the cirrhotic nodules in the liver are very small. In general, cirrhosis—whether it is macronodular or micronodular—due to any liver disease looks pretty much the same. Thus, once cirrhosis has occurred, even a liver biopsy cannot definitively identify which liver disorder caused it.

THE POTENTIAL COMPLICATIONS OF CIRRHOSIS

Chapter 1 discussed the liver's varied and essential functions that are crucial to our daily existence. Cirrhosis interferes with these everyday functions. Although the presence of cirrhosis does not signify that health problems will inevitably develop, a person with cirrhosis should be aware that he is at an increased risk of suffering many serious complications. These complications are discussed in detail below. Treatments for some of these potential complications will be discussed in Chapter 20.

Bleeding Problems

A normally functioning liver makes many factors—known as *coagulation factors*—that help blood clot. When the liver becomes scarred, it can no longer effectively produce these factors. Therefore, some people with cirrhosis have difficulty clotting, which is manifested by a tendency to bleed excessively. This is known as a *coagulopathy.* A person experiencing this complication may find that his daily routine has become a challenge—simple activities, such as brushing his teeth or shaving, may result in a severe bleeding episode.

The doctor can detect coagulopathy by performing a blood test. An elevated or prolonged prothrombin time (see Chapter 3) will indicate the presence, but not the cause, of a coagulopathy. Administration of vitamin K may correct a coagulopathy if it is due to cholestasis. However, simply replenishing vitamin K stores in the body will not help if cirrhosis is the problem, as the liver is too damaged to properly synthesize this vitamin. Transfusions of fresh frozen plasma (FFP) will temporarily stop bleeding and should be given in emergency situations, or prior to undergoing any invasive procedure or surgery.

Another cause of excessive bleeding in people with cirrhosis may be *thrombocytopenia,* a low platelet count (see Chapter 3). Platelets are also intricately involved in helping blood to clot. The spleen plays an important role in the storage of platelets. An enlarged spleen (splenomegaly) often occurs in people with cirrhosis. This indicates that the spleen is working overtime, which often results in a diminished platelet count.

Kidney Problems

Damage to the largest filtering organ, the liver, puts a great deal of stress on the body's other major filtering organs—the kidneys. Many kidney disorders have been associated with cirrhosis. The most common of these is fluid retention, resulting in edema and ascites. This is usually treated with water pills, known as *diuretics,* and a special low-sodium (low-salt) diet.

The most serious complication associated with the kidneys is known as *hepatorenal syndrome* (HRS). HRS is defined as progressive deterioration of kidney function occurring in a person with advanced liver disease. This usually happens in patients who are already in the hospital due to other complications of cirrhosis. HRS can result in death unless a liver transplantation is performed. Since this complication is primarily associated with lack of urination, kidney dialysis may be necessary as a time-gaining measure until liver transplantation can be performed. HRS can be prevented by avoiding the use of medications that can damage the kidneys, such as aminoglycosides (for example, gentamycin) or nonsteroidal anti-inflammatory drugs (NSAIDs), and by avoiding the overuse of diuretics used to treat fluid accumulation. Early recognition and prompt treatment of other complications of cirrhosis, such as infection and internal bleeding, may also prevent this syndrome from occurring.

Osteoporosis (Bone Loss)

Osteoporosis is a condition marked by decreased bone mass and decreased bone density. This leads to a weakening of bones, thereby increasing the risk of bone fractures. People with any chronic liver disease are at increased risk for the development of osteoporosis due to a lack of activity resulting from excessive fatigue, poor nutritional habits, reduced muscle mass, and impaired production of hormones, known as *hypogonadism.*

Certain types of liver disease make a person particularly susceptible to bone disorders. Bone disease occurs more frequently in people with cholestatic liver disease, such as primary biliary cirrhosis (PBC; discussed in Chapter 15), than in those with other chronic liver diseases. This is in part due to PBC-related fat malabsorption, which may lead to calcium and vitamin-D deficiencies. Fat-soluble vitamin absorption is likely to worsen when such a person is being treated for pruritus (itching) with cholestyramine (Questran)—a medication that further inhibits fat-soluble vitamin absorption.

People with alcoholic liver disease (ALD; discussed in Chapter 17) have bone problems not only due to advanced liver disease, but also due to the following: effects of alcohol on the bones; poor dietary habits along with calcium and vitamin-

D deficiencies that typically characterize people with ALD; impaired hormone production (hypogonadism); and a lack of activity.

People with diseases of iron overload, such as hemochromatosis (discussed in Chapter 18), often have hypogonadism due to iron overload in the reproductive organs, which puts these people at increased risk for osteoporosis due to altered hormone levels. People with autoimmune hepatitis (AIH; discussed in Chapter 14) are at increased risk for osteoporosis due to the use of prednisone—a steroid medication commonly used to treat AIH.

There is a very high incidence of bone fractures after liver transplantation—occurring in approximately 24 to 65 percent of people who received liver transplants. In most cases, these people already had weak bones prior to transplantation, and this condition was worsened by post-transplant medications, such as prednisone and cyclosporine.

Other risk factors for osteoporosis, unrelated to liver disease, include cigarette smoking, family history of osteoporosis, female gender, a slender body frame, excessive caffeine intake, and the postmenopausal state.

Hepatocellular Carcinoma (HCC)/Hepatoma (Liver Cancer)

Anyone who has cirrhosis—whether compensated or decompensated—is at risk for developing liver cancer; also known as hepatocellular carcinoma (HCC) or hepatoma. Risk varies with the cause of liver disease. Prognosis (the anticipated course of a disease without treatment) depends upon many factors. Liver cancer will be discussed in detail in Chapter 19; however, you should note that, if a person with cirrhosis has unexplained weight loss or abdominal pain, an extensive search for liver cancer should follow.

Other Cancers

Aside from liver cancer, other types of cancer have been found to occur in people who have cirrhosis with increased frequency compared with the general population. These cancers include cancers of the lungs, larynx, pancreas, kidneys, urinary bladder, pharynx, colon, and breasts.

Some of these cancers have been shown to occur in people who also drink excessive amounts of alcohol and smoke cigarettes. Whether cirrhosis led to an increased risk of cancer or whether an individual's personal habits were the cause is unknown. Most likely, a person's increased chance of getting one of these types of cancers is influenced by a combination of factors. In any case, people who have cirrhosis or who are at risk for cirrhosis are best advised to avoid all use of alcohol and tobacco.

Portal Hypertension and Its Possible Complications

Most people are familiar with the word *hypertension*—the medical term for high blood pressure. But most people do not know that the liver can also suffer from its own type of high blood pressure, which is known as *portal hypertension*. Due to extensive scarring of the liver that occurs in cirrhosis, the vessels associated with blood flow to and from the liver may become obstructed. This, in combination with increased blood flow to the liver, leads to elevated pressure in the portal circulation. While this is perhaps an oversimplification of what actually happens, there are so many factors and theories concerning portal hypertension that a more in-depth explanation is beyond the scope of this book.

The liver—a very resourceful organ—attempts to adapt to the above situation by creating alternative routes that bypass this obstruction. These alternative passageways for blood flow are known as *collateral shunts* or *collaterals*. These shunts now enable blood to be rerouted and circulated to the rest of the body. Unfortunately, the formation of these shunts has its drawbacks, as they can give rise to serious and even life-threatening complications. Therefore, people with any form of portal hypertension should be evaluated for liver transplantation. The following is a discussion of the complications of portal hypertension.

Ascites

Ascites, the most common complication of portal hypertension, is a disorder characterized by massive accumulation of fluid in the *peritoneal cavity*—the space between the abdominal organs and the skin. In addition, the kidneys tend to retain sodium and water in people with portal hypertension, leading to further fluid accumulation. This accumulation results in abdominal swelling and distention. In most cases, the disorder is readily apparent to the doctor on a physical exam. In cases where the diagnosis of ascites is suspected but not obvious, an abdominal sonogram can be used to detect whether small amounts of ascitic fluid have accumulated. A fever in a person with established ascites may indicate that an infection of this fluid is present. This is a serious condition known as *spontaneous bacterial peritonitis* (SBP).

It is estimated that half of the people with compensated cirrhosis will develop ascites within approximately ten years. While the presence of ascites usually stems from cirrhosis, there are other causes of ascites, such as kidney failure or ovarian cancer, that are unrelated to liver disease.

Varices

Varices are enlarged, distended blood vessels that result from the formation of collateral shunts in people with portal hypertension. (Think of varices as varicose veins that occur inside the body.) Between 20 and 70 percent of people with cirrhosis have varices. While varices may occur in many parts of the body, those occurring in the esophagus (food pipe) and upper portion of the stomach are the most likely to burst. Bursting occurs about one-third of the time and usually results in profuse, uncontrollable vomiting of bright red blood. This is known as *hematemesis*. Hematemesis is a life-and-death emergency that requires immediate hospitalization and therapy. An *upper endoscopy* is required for both diagnosis and treatment of bleeding esophageal varices. An upper endoscopy is a procedure in which a thin tube with a light at the end—somewhat like a flexible telescope—is inserted into the patient's mouth and passed into the esophagus, stomach, and duodenum. This simple procedure does not hurt and is usually done after the administration of intravenous *conscious sedation*—which means that the patient is given a mild sedative medication, such as Versed, Valium, and/or Demerol, through an IV. As a result, the patient does not remember or feel the procedure.

Varices also can occur in the rectum, where, in some cases, they may bleed. The bleeding of rectal varices is sometimes mistaken for hemorrhoidal bleeding. Since the treatments are different for these two unrelated conditions, it is important for the doctor to differentiate between them. Usually, bleeding from rectal varices is treated in much the same manner as esophageal variceal bleeding. Therapies for varices will be discussed in greater detail in Chapter 20.

Congestive Gastropathy

Up to 50 percent of people with cirrhosis are likely to bleed due to a buildup of pressure in the stomach known as *portal hypertensive gastropathy* or *congestive gastropathy*. Bleeding in this situation often manifests as *melena*—upper intestinal bleeding, resulting in black stools. This form of bleeding must be distinguished from the other causes of bleeding that can occur in cirrhosis patients. These other causes include peptic ulcer disease and *gastritis*—inflammation of the stomach. These disorders are also diagnosed by an upper endoscopy. Treatment depends on the source of bleeding.

Encephalopathy

Encephalopathy is an altered or impaired mental status, which typically leads to coma, that can occur in people with cirrhosis. Encephalopathy can also be associated with poor coordination, fetor hepaticus (foul-smelling breath), and asterixis (uncontrollable flapping of the hands—see Chapter 2). The exact cause of encephalopathy is not entirely known, but may be due to a combination of factors. Most researchers believe that it has something to do with the ailing liver's inability to clear toxins—primarily *ammonia*—from the body. In fact, elevated blood levels of ammonia are found in approximately 90 percent of people with encephalopathy. When ammonia and other poisons begin to accumulate in the brain, a variety of mental disturbances occur.

In mild cases, a person will develop subtle personality changes, such as irritability, a change in sleeping patterns, or short-term memory loss. Speech may be slurred and the individual may appear confused. People suffering from encephalopathy will commonly lose their tempers over minor incidents or have mood swings for no apparent reason. Or a person may repeatedly enter a room, forgetting what he needed from the room in the first place. Or he may continually misplace common objects, such as reading glasses, only to find that they were on top of his head the whole time! These people may also have an increased incidence of automobile accidents, as their reaction time may be somewhat impaired.

In more severe cases, total confusion, associated with inappropriate behavior, will occur. A person may become outright violent or may be so confused that he cannot properly identify the current year, season, or even his own family members. Sometimes, a person will sleep all day and can only be partially aroused. This, obviously, is a more serious condition and requires hospitalization.

In most cases, encephalopathy is easily detected on a physical examination in a patient with known cirrhosis. Whenever there is a question about the diagnosis, an imaging study, such as CT scan or MRI, of the brain should be performed in order to eliminate other potential causes, such as a brain tumor, blood clot, or *meningitis* (brain infection). Those factors that can precipitate encephalopathy in the cirrhotic patient should be searched for and immediately addressed by the doctor. These factors as well as the treatment of encephalopathy will be discussed in Chapter 20.

CONCLUSION

In this chapter, you learned that cirrhosis is irreversible scarring of the liver. But, fortunately, the process leading to cirrhosis can often be slowed and sometimes even halted. Also, you now have an awareness of some of the potential complications that may occur in people with cirrhosis. Many of the liver diseases that can potentially lead to cirrhosis will be discussed throughout the remainder of this book. Part Two of this book will discuss another term, which is often misused and misunderstood—hepatitis.

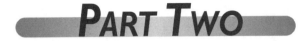

Understanding and Treating Viral Hepatitis

7

An Overall Look at Hepatitis

The results of Tom's liver biopsy revealed that he has cirrhosis. But how did he get it? Tom wanted to know. The doctor told him that his cirrhosis—still in its early stages—was caused by hepatitis. Tom's doctor suggested that he start therapy, in an attempt to halt or slow the progression of his cirrhosis. But Tom was very confused and wondered to himself, "How did I get hepatitis? How can I have both hepatitis and cirrhosis? Did hepatitis lead to cirrhosis? Will I still be able to work? Can I infect my wife and son?" Tom's doctor answered all of his questions, putting his concerns to rest.

This chapter explains the concept of hepatitis—a medical term that is often misunderstood and misused. It outlines the differences between acute, chronic, and fulminant hepatitis, and also discusses the multiple causes of hepatitis. In addition, this chapter helps you to distinguish between *viral* hepatitis and other causes of hepatitis. The symptoms and physical signs associated with hepatitis are discussed, as well as the way in which a doctor arrives at a diagnosis. This includes a discussion of liver function test (LFT) abnormalities and the necessity of imaging studies and/or a liver biopsy. Treatment is briefly discussed, but will be dealt with in greater detail in the respective chapters for each type of hepatitis. This chapter also provides a brief overview of the different types of viral hepatitis, and helps to dispel some common misconceptions about viral hepatitis. Finally, this chapter provides a preview of the immune system—the body's personal army in the fight against viruses—and how it relates to viral hepatitis. The *natural history of a disease* (the course that a disease most likely will take if untreated) and the *prognosis* of a disease (a prediction of the probable outcome of the disease if untreated) are discussed in the corresponding chapters on each type of hepatitis.

WHAT IS HEPATITIS?

Many people mistakenly believe that the medical term *hepatitis* is synonymous with the medical term *viral hepatitis,* and that all forms of hepatitis are contagious. Actually, the word *hepatitis* is a catchall term that refers to any inflammation *(itis)* of the liver *(hepar)* and does not imply a specific cause or connote contagiousness. (*Inflammation* of the liver is defined as an irritation or swelling of liver cells.)

Hepatitis is a term that encompasses many different causes. Only hepatitis caused by a virus (viral hepatitis) is potentially infectious to others. Consequently, hepatitis from causes other than that of viruses cannot be spread through food or by interpersonal or sexual contact.

Hepatitis is generally described using two broad categories. One category refers to how long a person has hepatitis—acute, chronic, or fulminant. The other category refers to what factor caused the hepatitis—viral hepatitis, autoimmune hepatitis, fatty liver hepatitis, alcoholic hepatitis, or toxin-induced hepatitis. For example, a person may be described as having acute hepatitis B or chronic hepatitis C. The next few pages will describe these categories in more detail.

DIFFERENCES BETWEEN ACUTE, CHRONIC, AND FULMINANT HEPATITIS

One way of describing hepatitis is by how long inflammation in the liver lasts. As such, hepatitis is divided into two broad types—acute hepatitis and chronic hepatitis. Another type of hepatitis, fulminant hepatitis, is an especially severe form of acute hepatitis, and thus, may be considered the third type of hepatitis.

Inflammation of the liver that lasts less than six months is known as *acute hepatitis.* Within six months, most people with acute hepatitis, regardless of the cause, are completely healed. However, some people do progress from acute to chronic hepatitis, and some experience a particularly severe, potentially fatal form of acute hepatitis—fulminant hepatitis. In people with acute hepatitis who do not progress to chronic or fulminant hepatitis, the inflammation in the liver totally subsides. All of the symptoms, signs, and LFT abnormalities associated with this condition resolve. The liver typically self-repairs any short-term damage it may have suffered. No permanent damage is done to the liver and the person does not suffer any long-term consequences.

Inflammation of the liver that lasts longer than six months is known as *chronic hepatitis.* People who progress from acute hepatitis to chronic hepatitis are at risk of developing cirrhosis and the complications of cirrhosis. Those with acute hepatitis who progress to chronic hepatitis typically have very mild or no symptoms. However, it is not always possible for the doctor to identify who will progress to chronic hepatitis or suffer from fulminant hepatitis.

The third category of hepatitis is known as *fulminant hepatitis.* Fulminant hepatitis is a particularly serious form of acute hepatitis associated with jaundice, coagulopathy, and encephalopathy. In these people, liver failure occurs abruptly, usually within approximately eight weeks of the onset of symptoms or within approximately two weeks of the onset of jaundice.

THE CAUSES OF HEPATITIS

The other way of describing hepatitis is by its cause. Although hepatitis is most frequently caused by viruses, other causes include autoimmune liver disease, obesity, alcohol, and some medications and herbs. Don't forget, the precise meaning of hepatitis is simply "inflammation of the liver." The following is a brief discussion of these causes, which will be discussed in more detail in later chapters.

Viruses

At least five different viruses specifically attack the liver leading to viral hepatitis. These are known as *hepatitis viruses*. Each type of viral hepatitis is different, and they all have distinct characteristics. They are known by alphabetical names: hepatitis A through hepatitis E. Four other viruses, hepatitis F, hepatitis G, the *transfusion-transmitted virus* (TTV), and S.E.N.-V (S.E.N. are the initials of the person in whom the virus was first isolated; "v" stands for virus) may also specifically attack the liver. When infection with one of these viruses causes inflammation of the liver, the resulting condition is known as *viral hepatitis.* (Other viruses, such as herpes simplex virus and Epstein-Barr virus, can also attack the liver. However, since the liver is not the principal organ damaged by these viruses, they are not considered hepatitis viruses and will not be covered in this book.) A brief description of the different types of viral hepatitis will be discussed on page 78. Hepatitis A, B and D, and C, will be discussed in detail in Chapters 8, 9, and 10, respectively.

Autoimmunity

Autoimmune diseases occur when the body's immune system fails to recognize one of its own organs as belonging to itself. The immune system then attacks that organ in an attempt to remove the "foreign intruder" from the body. When the organ under attack fights back, it becomes inflamed. In the case when the immune system attacks the liver, the liver becomes inflamed as it fights back. This condition is known as *autoimmune hepatitis* and will be discussed in Chapter 14.

Obesity

Many of the health risks of being overweight, such as heart disease, diabetes, and high blood pressure are well known. But few people are aware of the extent to which being overweight can adversely affect the liver. Being overweight can cause excess fat to deposit in the liver, causing inflammation. This is known as *fatty liver hepa-*

titis. Being overweight is just one of the many causes of fatty liver hepatitis, which will be discussed in detail in Chapter 16.

Alcohol

It is common knowledge that alcohol can be harmful to the liver. Drinking too much alcohol can lead to inflammation of the liver. This is known as *alcoholic hepatitis* and will be discussed in Chapter 17. Many additional factors, such as being of the female gender, genetic vulnerability, diet, and infection with the hepatitis B or C virus may worsen the effects of alcohol on the liver. This will also be discussed in Chapter 17.

Medications and Herbs

Certain medications and herbs can cause both acute and chronic inflammation of the liver, in addition to other liver damage. This particular type of hepatitis is known as *drug-induced,* or *toxin-induced, hepatitis.* A substance that is harmful or damaging to the liver is referred to as *hepatotoxic.* In drug-induced, or toxin-induced, hepatitis, withdrawal of the hepatotoxic herb or medication with evidence of subsequent resolution of elevated transaminases (AST and ALT) is often the only means of confirming the diagnosis. Some of these hepatotoxic herbs and medications will be discussed in Chapters 21 and Chapter 24, respectively.

THE SYMPTOMS AND PHYSICAL SIGNS OF HEPATITIS

Due to the overlapping nature of the different types of hepatitis, it is difficult to determine a specific cause based solely on associated symptoms and signs. However, occasionally, symptoms and signs may give clues to whether or not the hepatitis is chronic (chronicity). The following sections discuss the symptoms and signs of hepatitis according to the length of time the hepatitis is present.

Symptoms and Signs of Acute Hepatitis

Symptoms and signs of acute hepatitis may vary greatly. At one extreme, some people are very ill, with jaundice, fever, decreased appetite, abdominal pain, nausea, vomiting, and fatigue. People who are jaundiced typically experience dark urine and light stools. At the other extreme, people with acute hepatitis may be totally asymptomatic, and may never realize that they had hepatitis. Many people with acute hepatitis pass symptoms off as those of a bad flu and never see a doctor. And, some types of acute hepatitis—for example, acute hepatitis B—are sometimes associated with muscle and joint aches, known as *myalgias* and *arthralgias,* in addition to a rash. On a physical exam, the liver may be slightly enlarged and tender and/or jaundice and a rash may be present. Or it is also possible that the exam will be totally normal.

Often, the more severely ill a person is during the acute phase of hepatitis, the better her chances are of totally recovering, and not progressing into the chronic hepatitis. It is mainly those people with acute hepatitis who have no or mild symptoms that are precisely the ones who insidiously progress to chronic hepatitis.

Symptoms and Signs of Chronic Hepatitis

Symptoms and signs of chronic hepatitis may also vary greatly; however, most people with chronic hepatitis are *asymptomatic,* meaning that they have no symptoms. In fact, many never remember ever having had an episode of acute hepatitis. This accounts for why someone may be surprised when she is first told that something is wrong with her liver. Other people with chronic hepatitis have vague, nonspecific symptoms, such as mild fatigue, which they often attribute to their daily agendas. Others have relentless fatigue, which often prompts a visit to the doctor. Similarly, on a physical exam, there may be no clues that a person has chronic hepatitis, and, in fact, the exam may be totally normal. Alternatively, hepatomegaly (an enlarged liver), jaundice, a rash, or even signs suggestive of liver failure may be the initial findings.

Symptoms and Signs of Fulminant Hepatitis

Symptoms of fulminant hepatitis usual begin with vague nonspecific symptoms, such as fatigue and nausea. Within a few weeks, the person becomes jaundiced. Once jaundice develops, encephalopathy follows about two weeks later. This is a particularly ominous form of hepatitis with a high incidence of complications.

DIAGNOSING HEPATITIS

Many possible scenarios may lead to the discovery that a person has hepatitis. Some people are suspected of having hepatitis during a visit to the doctor for an evaluation of symptoms, or sometimes during the course of a routine check-up. Some people first learn that they have hepatitis upon being rejected for a life insurance policy due to a finding of abnormal liver function tests (LFTs). And others have been rejected as blood donors because they were discovered to have an elevated ALT level or they tested positive for hepatitis B or C. Still others first find out they have hepatitis after developing signs of liver failure.

Symptoms, physical signs, and results from routine blood tests commonly overlap among the different types of hepatitis, rarely indicating a specific cause. Though imaging studies may suggest liver inflammation, they are generally normal and are not helpful in the diagnosis of hepatitis. However, an abdominal sonogram is usually obtained in order to make sure that other abnormalities, such as gallstones, are not the cause of elevated LFTs.

In general, the only way to actually determine the type of hepatitis and what caused it is through a combination of serial LFTs, hepatitis-specific blood tests (see the chapters specifically pertaining to each type of hepatitis), and a liver biopsy. This section will briefly explain what a doctor may find on the results of blood tests in people with acute, chronic, and fulminant hepatitis from any cause; and if and when a liver biopsy is necessary. For explanations of the various types of tests, see Chapter 3.

Diagnosing Acute Hepatitis

In people with acute hepatitis, blood work usually shows that transaminases (ALT and AST) are typically very elevated, with levels varying between 500 and 5,000 IU/L. The bilirubin level may be elevated, as well, but it is uncommon for it to exceed 10 mg/dl. As with the symptoms and physical signs of acute hepatitis, these LFT elevations usually resolve within six months—that is, as long as acute hepatitis does not progress to chronic hepatitis.

A liver biopsy is rarely obtained in people with acute hepatitis, as there is the expectation that symptoms, signs, and LFT abnormalities will resolve within six months. When LFTs remain elevated longer than six months, a liver biopsy is generally performed to determine the extent of inflammation and damage that has occurred, to help determine the cause of chronic hepatitis, and to help predict prognosis.

Diagnosing Chronic Hepatitis

In people with chronic hepatitis, blood work shows transaminases that are elevated for greater than six months. The degree of transaminase elevation can range from about 45 to 300 IU/L. However, the elevation may be intermittent and the degree of transaminase elevation may not correlate to how severely inflamed or damaged the liver is. In fact, chronic hepatitis may be present even in cases where transaminases are totally normal. Additional specific blood work is needed to reveal the type of hepatitis present. (See Table 3.1 in Chapter 3.)

A liver biopsy is advised for most people whose LFTs are elevated for longer than six months. A liver biopsy can help determine the cause of chronic hepatitis and can help predict prognosis. Classically, doctors had categorized liver biopsy findings of chronic hepatitis into three groups: chronic persistent hepatitis, chronic lobular hepatitis, and chronic active hepatitis. These designations were thought to indicate progressively more severe stages of liver disease. Since this classification had many limitations, a new, more accurate classification system was adopted. The present classification system takes into account the cause (hepatitis C, for example), the grade (mild, moderate, severe), and the stage (degree of scarring from none to cirrhosis) of chronic hepatitis.

Diagnosing Fulminant Hepatitis

People with fulminant hepatitis have blood test results similar to those with acute hepatitis. However, a coagulopathy is typically present, and the bilirubin level is often quite elevated. A liver biopsy is rarely performed on patients with fulminant hepatitis due to the presence of a coagulopathy (prolonged prothrombin time resulting in a bleeding tendency).

TREATMENT OF HEPATITIS

Treatment of hepatitis will normally be based on the chronicity and the cause of the particular case. Specific treatments will be discussed in the chapters corresponding to specific types of hepatitis. This section discusses general treatments of hepatitis.

Treatment of Acute Hepatitis

Treatment of acute hepatitis is mostly supportive. This means that treatment depends upon the symptoms being experienced. If a person feels fatigued, she will likely be advised to take multiple naps during the day and to stay out of work for a few days. However, if the person is not feeling sick, there is no reason for extra bed rest— although it is important not to overdo activities during this time. The key for individuals with acute hepatitis when it comes to activity is to listen to their bodies. Alcohol and recreational drugs should be avoided altogether. As a person may experience a loss of appetite, several small meals instead of a few large meals each day may be advisable. People with acute hepatitis should stick to a healthy, low-fat diet and drink plenty of water. No medications or shots are necessary. Furthermore, people with acute hepatitis should also avoid taking unnecessary medications, including excessive vitamins and/or herbs.

Treatment of Chronic Hepatitis

Treatment of chronic hepatitis is somewhat more complicated than treatment for acute hepatitis. Therefore, these treatments will be discussed in each type of hepatitis' respective chapters. Beneficial changes that a person can make in respect to diet, exercise, alcohol abstinence, and other lifestyle modifications are covered in Chapters 23 and 24.

Treatment of Fulminant Hepatitis

Treatment of fulminant hepatitis often depends on the cause. In general, anyone suffering from fulminant hepatitis requires close monitoring in an intensive care unit (ICU) of a hospital. If the person does not improve or if her condition worsens, she should be considered for liver transplantation as soon as possible. Liver transplantation will be discussed in Chapter 22.

A CLOSER LOOK AT VIRAL HEPATITIS

Viral hepatitis has a history that dates all the way back to ancient times. However, it was only recently that the different types of viral hepatitis were identified by scientific researchers, and that the names for each type of hepatitis, including hepatitis A, hepatitis B, hepatitis C, were coined. The following pages discuss some of this history. Following this short history lesson, pages 79 to 80 will focus on dispelling several common misconceptions about viral hepatitis. See Chapters 8 to 13 for a more in-depth look at each of the common types of viral hepatitis.

The History of Viral Hepatitis

A *virus* is a tiny microorganism that is much smaller than a bacteria. Its main function consists of reproducing more viruses. A virus is capable of growth and multiplication only once it has entered a living cell. The goal of the hepatitis virus is to enter a liver cell, reproduce more hepatitis viruses, destroy the cell, and move on to attack the next liver cell.

Viral hepatitis can be traced all the way back to ancient times, when it was believed by scientists that some type of virus existed that attacked the liver, resulting in jaundice. From the late 1800s to early 1900s, scientists believed that there were only two forms of viral hepatitis: *infectious* hepatitis and *serum* hepatitis.

In 1963, a major breakthrough in research occurred—the cause of serum hepatitis was identified and the virus was given the name *hepatitis B virus* (HBV). It took an additional ten years for scientists to isolate the cause of infectious hepatitis, and this virus was thereafter given the name *hepatitis A virus* (HAV). It was at that time that scientists realized that other forms of viral hepatitis must exist that were not caused by either HAV or HBV because there were still so many cases of hepatitis that were not the result of one of these two viruses. These viruses were lumped into the category of *non-A non-B* (NANB) hepatitis.

In 1989, the virus that caused the majority of NANB hepatitis was identified through cloning experiments and was named *hepatitis C virus* (HCV). The *hepatitis delta virus* (HDV), which was first isolated in the mid-1970s, was shown to exist only in the presence of HBV. The existence of another hepatitis virus, which is similar to HAV, was suggested throughout the 1980s, but was not successfully cloned until 1990, at which point it was named *hepatitis E virus* (HEV). Evidence of the existence of a *hepatitis F virus* (HFV) is, at present, only anecdotal and needs further confirmation. The *hepatitis G virus* (HGV), which was discovered in 1995, does not appear to be a significant cause of acute or chronic hepatitis. Another possible hepatitis virus, known as the *transfusion-transmitted virus* (TTV), was identified in 1997. However, further studies are being conducted in order to determine if this virus actually causes any inflammation or damage to the liver. Because approximately 10 percent of hepatitis cases still do not have an identified cause, it is suspected that one or more other hepatitis viruses exist. In fact, in July 1999, possibly the final hepatitis virus was identified by a group of Italian researchers. This virus was named S.E.N.-V. Much more research needs to be conducted on this virus to determine if, in fact, it is a significant cause of liver disease and if, in fact, it is the cause of the 10 percent of hepatitis cases without a clearly identified cause.

Misconceptions About Viral Hepatitis

There are many common misconceptions about viral hepatitis. These misconceptions often lead to confusion, needless worry, and unnecessary lifestyle changes. The following six *false* statements and their explanations will help to dispel some of the most common misconceptions concerning viral hepatitis.

FALSE: All types of viral hepatitis can cause both acute and chronic hepatitis.

HAV, HEV, and possibly HFV cause only acute hepatitis. As such, they totally resolve within six months, and do not have a chronic stage. In contrast, HBV, HCV, and HDV can cause both acute and chronic hepatitis. Therefore, these viruses have the potential to lead to cirrhosis and its complications. Not as much is known about HGV; but so far, it is not believed to be a cause of significant liver disease.

FALSE: A person who was previously infected with one form of viral hepatitis can never catch another form.

Having had one type of viral hepatitis will not make a person immune to becoming infected with other kinds of viral hepatitis. For example, a person who had hepatitis A at some point in the past is now immune to HAV. This means that this person can never get hepatitis A again and cannot transmit it to others. However, this does not mean that she is immune to other forms of viral hepatitis. She is, therefore, still at risk for becoming infected with any other type of hepatitis in the future.

FALSE: One type of hepatitis virus can change into another type of hepatitis virus.

One hepatitis virus cannot change into a different hepatitis virus. For example, HBV cannot transform itself into HCV. However, more than one kind of hepatitis virus can exist in the liver at the same time. Thus, an individual may be *coinfected* with both HBV and HCV.

FALSE: If symptoms of viral hepatitis resolve, it means that the viral hepatitis is gone.

Many people are under the misconception that once the symptoms associated with viral hepatitis resolve, the disease is gone. While, in fact, most people recover totally from many types of viral hepatitis, such as hepatitis A, some viruses such as HCV typically progress to chronic liver disease or even cirrhosis and/or liver cancer without causing any symptoms along the way. Because the liver is so resilient, a person may not even realize that, although she is feeling better, hepatitis is still present and may actually be getting worse.

FALSE: Viral hepatitis and the human immunodeficiency virus (HIV) are the same virus.

The viruses that cause hepatitis are very different from HIV (human immunodeficiency virus), the virus that causes AIDS (acquired immune deficiency syndrome).

While some of the hepatitis viruses may be transmitted by routes similar to the transmission routes that apply to HIV, all the hepatitis viruses are very different, both biologically and structurally, from HIV.

FALSE: Viruses can be treated with antibiotics.

Only bacterial infections can be treated with antibiotics. Viruses differ greatly from bacteria. They are smaller and more difficult to treat. They also typically take much longer to treat. While a bacterial infection may require only a week or two of antibiotic therapy, a viral infection may require up to a year, or possibly longer, of antiviral therapy. Viruses are treated with antiviral medications such as interferon, which will be discussed in further detail in later chapters.

HOW HEPATITIS VIRUSES ARE TRANSMITTED

Not all viruses are transmitted by the same route. It is important to understand the different ways that a person may catch a virus and/or spread it to others. Some viruses are introduced into the body by way of the digestive tract, while others are transmitted either through contaminated blood, during sexual contact, or from mother to child during childbirth.

The Transmission of HAV, HEV, and Possibly HFV

HAV, HEV, and possibly HFV are transmitted by the *enteric* or *fecal-oral route.* Enteric means that these viruses are introduced into the body by way of the digestive tract. This means that these viruses are shed in the feces *(fecal)* of the infected person, and are then transmitted to another person via ingesting *(oral)* by mouth a small amount of infected stools. While such an occurrence may sound absurd, it is actually fairly common, especially in areas where poor sanitation is widespread. In fact, probably more than one-third of people in the United States has been exposed to HAV, and in developing countries virtually everyone has at some time been exposed to HAV. HEV is rare in the United States, but is common in Central America, South America, Bangladesh, and India. In these areas, it has been noted that up to 20 percent of pregnant women who become infected with HEV become severely ill with fulminant hepatitis.

The Transmission of HBV, HDV, HCV, HGV, and TTV

HBV, HDV, HCV, HGV, and TTV are transmitted by the *parenteral route.* Parenteral means that these viruses are introduced into the body by any way other than via the intestinal tract. HBV is transmitted either through contaminated blood, during sexual contact, or from mother to child during childbirth. HDV only occurs in individuals who already have hepatitis B. HCV is transmitted primarily by blood-to-blood contact. Sexual transmission, as well as transmission from mother to child, appear to be insignificant modes of transmitting HCV. HGV is probably transmitted in a manner similar to that of HCV. TTV has only been associated with hepatitis in people who have had a blood transfusion. Therefore, it is presumed that blood transfusions are the primary mode of transmission of this virus.

THE IMMUNE SYSTEM AND VIRAL HEPATITIS

Each person has a built-in natural defense system, an army of defenders, known as the *immune system*. The immune system fights against foreign substances that enter the body, which it perceives as dangerous intruders, such as the hepatitis viruses. A person with a weak immune system who has been exposed to a virus is less likely to be able to eliminate the virus from her body, as compared with a person with a well-functioning immune system who is, therefore, less prone to infection.

Two important terms that are frequently used when discussing the immune system are *antigen* (Ag) and *antibody* (Ab). Think of an *antigen* as a foreign substance (such as a hepatitis virus) and of an *antibody* as one of the immune-system soldiers battling the antigen. For example, when an antigen, such as hepatitis B antigen, is present in the body, an antibody—in this case, the hepatitis B antibody—is produced by the immune system. The antibody combines with the antigen with the intent of eliminating it from the body and thereby making the person immune to hepatitis B.

The specific hepatitis antigens and antibodies may be detected by obtaining specific blood tests. These tests may indicate that a person currently has or was at one time exposed to viral hepatitis. This blood work is referred to as *serologic testing* or more specifically as *hepatitis serology*. (See Table 3.1 in Chapter 3.) The hepatitis serology is necessary in order to determine if viral hepatitis is the cause of a patient's liver-related abnormalities and which specific hepatitis virus is actually the culprit.

While the above explanation of antibodies and antigens is perhaps an oversimplification of what actually happens in the body, hopefully it will help the reader to understand the complex terminology used when referring to the hepatitis serology, which is detailed in the corresponding chapters on viral hepatitis (Chapters 8, 9, and 10).

CONCLUSION

After reading this chapter, you now know the correct meaning of the medical term hepatitis. Most important, this chapter distinguished between viral hepatitis and all other forms of hepatitis. The symptoms and physical signs associated with hepatitis should now be more familiar to you. This chapter also gave you a closer look at viral hepatitis and introduced you to the role that the immune system plays in combating this viral disease. The next chapter discusses hepatitis A in greater detail.

8

Understanding and Treating Hepatitis A

Marty, a forty-two-year-old lawyer, had never missed a day from work due to illness. After three days of hearing him complain of excessive fatigue and nausea, Marty's wife, Pam, demanded he call in sick to work. When he began to have uncontrollable loose bowel movements almost every hour, he had no choice but to stay home to be near the bathroom. Finally, when Marty noticed that his urine resembled fresh brewed tea and his stools looked like clay, he agreed to see a doctor. He made an appointment for the end of the week, figuring his problem would clear up way before then.

But over the next few days, Marty's symptoms actually worsened. Pam called an ambulance when Marty began to show signs of mental confusion. At the hospital, Marty was immediately taken to the intensive care unit (ICU). Pam, frightened and confused, listened to the doctor as he told her that something was wrong with Marty's liver and that it could be a form of hepatitis. He also told her that they would need to wait for the blood test results to confirm this. And because Marty was jaundiced and encephalopathic (disoriented), he would need to remain in the ICU.

Then the doctor asked Pam if Marty had a history of intravenous drug use or if he ever had a blood transfusion. She replied no to both questions. Next, the doctor asked if Marty had eaten any seafood recently or if anyone else in the family was ill. Pam recalled that about a month earlier, Marty had taken their five-year-old son Jason to the beach. Afterwards, the pair had stopped at a fish stand for some clams. Jason had developed what appeared to be a mild cold that lasted only a short time. With this added information, the doctor concluded that

Marty probably had hepatitis A. This diagnosis was subsequently confirmed by the results of Marty's blood test.

Marty's condition seemed touch and go for a while, but after one month, Marty was discharged from the hospital. By six months, Marty was totally better and his jaundice totally resolved.

Patricia, a twenty-year-old college senior, went on a two-week expedition to Africa with some of her classmates. As taking the trip was a last-minute decision, Patricia did not see her doctor prior to leaving the country to find out if she needed any special immunizations. But Patricia wasn't worried—she knew she would be staying in a good hotel and planned to drink only bottled water.

The trip went well, but about two weeks after returning home, Patricia came down with flu-like symptoms that included persistent nausea, fatigue, headache, and low-grade fever. She completely lost her appetite. Also, cigarette smoke began to taste odd, leading to her quitting her smoking habit—something she'd been trying to do for several years. After she began to experience itching so severe that it kept her awake at night, Patricia decided to see her family physician.

Patricia's doctor asked her some questions, including whether or not she had obtained the necessary immunizations before going to Africa. He examined her and noted that her eyes were slightly yellow and that her liver was somewhat enlarged. He drew some blood from her arm for testing.

"I believe that you have hepatitis A," the doctor told her. "Despite the precautions you may have taken as to food and beverages, you probably acquired it on your excursion to Africa."

"Hepatitis A?" Patricia exclaimed. "I thought I had the flu!"

Patricia's doctor advised her to stay home and rest until she felt healthy enough to go back to school. The blood test results confirmed the doctor's diagnosis of hepatitis A. She stayed at home for the next two days and rested. By the third day, Patricia awoke feeling energetic and felt healthy enough to return to school. By the following week, all of her symptoms had resolved.

This chapter discusses the hepatitis A virus (HAV). You will learn the routes by which HAV is transmitted to others, as well as which people are at particularly high risks of becoming infected. In addition, the symptoms and physical signs associated with hepatitis A and the manner in which a person is diagnosed are explained in this chapter. The treatment of hepatitis A and the prognosis for those infected are also covered.

WHAT IS HEPATITIS A?

Hepatitis A is inflammation of the liver due to a virus called the hepatitis A virus (HAV). Prior to its identification in 1973, it was known as *infectious hepatitis,* due to the fact that HAV is so contagious. HAV only causes acute hepatitis. See an explanation of acute hepatitis in Chapter 7. In the United States, HAV is the most common cause of acute viral hepatitis. Each year, approximately 134,000 people in the United States are infected with HAV. In fact, around 33 percent of all people in the United States have, at some point, been infected with HAV, and approximately 74 percent of adults over fifty years old have evidence of exposure to this virus.

HAV is usually thought of as the least serious of all the hepatitis viruses. This is due to the fact that—unlike the hepatitis B and C viruses—HAV does not cause chronic liver disease, and therefore the disease lasts no longer than six months. Cirrhosis and its complications can never result. Moreover, hepatitis A will not result in liver cancer. However, each year, hepatitis A causes a substantial number of people to get very ill. Some of these people require hospitalization. Many others, although not needing hospitalization, still lose a significant amount of time from their jobs.

Though it is typically not fatal, hepatitis A accounts for approximately 100 deaths each year in the United States. Furthermore, it has been shown that when a person with another liver disease, such as chronic hepatitis C, becomes infected with HAV, she may experience a particularly serious and potentially life-threatening form of hepatitis. Fortunately, hepatitis A is the most common vaccine-preventable disease in the entire world. See Chapter 24 for information on prevention and vaccination.

HOW HAV IS TRANSMITTED

As discussed in Chapter 7, HAV is transmitted by the enteric or fecal-oral route. In short, this means that transmission occurs when HAV embedded in the feces of an infected person enters the digestive tract of the another person. More precisely, the virus enters through the mouth, passes from the stomach into the small intestine, and then gains entry into the liver.

The liver is the major site of HAV replication. After the virus is finished multiplying and infecting the liver, it leaves the liver via the bile ducts and is excreted into the bile. As discussed in Chapter 1, the bile ducts enter into the small intestine. So HAV goes back into the small intestine, which directly connects with the large intestine, and is mixed in with the stool and eliminated from the body through the rectum. HAV is now ready to infect the next unsuspecting victim. HAV transmission is likely to occur through person-to-person contact, from consumption of contaminated food or water, or by other routes, all of which will be discussed on the following pages.

Person-to-Person Contact

Person-to-person transmission via close personal contact is perhaps the most common means of acquiring HAV. People living in the same household as an infected person are at increased risk of becoming infected themselves. People who live in communities where sanitation standards are poor and people living in crowded conditions are also are at increased risk for infection.

A person with hepatitis A is at her most infectious during the two-week time period preceding and the one-week period following the development of any symptoms or signs of infection. Many people, especially young children infected with HAV, have no symptoms at all. Thus, young children are often a major route of transmission of HAV, as they commonly harbor the virus unknowingly. Furthermore, their hygiene habits tend to be less meticulous than those of adults. Children are more likely to spread the virus to others, as they tend to play in close contact with other children and are closely handled and cared for by adults. Therefore, a common source of hepatitis A outbreaks has been day-care centers—primarily day-care centers that provide care to children who wear diapers. Another common source of outbreaks has been institutions for the mentally disabled, since many living in these facilities often have poor personal hygiene and live in crowded conditions. Note, however, that outbreaks have been less frequent since conditions in institutions have improved.

A person is no longer infectious to others approximately a week or two after symptoms and signs of hepatitis A have begun. There is no evidence that sexual transmission plays a role in spreading HAV, other than anal-oral sex. HAV is not transmitted to the fetus during pregnancy or childbirth.

Contaminated Food and Water

Ingestion of contaminated food and beverages is another important route of HAV transmission. Foods that have been reported to transmit HAV have included milk, strawberries, pastries, hamburger meat, and salads. In these instances, the food was either uncooked or was handled after cooking by an HAV-infected person who did not properly wash her hands after defecating.

Shellfish often live in bodies of water that may be polluted with HAV. Thus, they appear to have a particularly high incidence of transmitting HAV when eaten raw or incompletely cooked—as is often the case with clams, oysters, and mussels. There have been few incidents of transmission of HAV by water—either by drinking contaminated water or by swimming in HAV infested water. (Don't forget, bottled water containing non-bottled ice cubes is also a risk.)

Other Routes

While there are a few incidents where blood transfusions are believed to be the source of a hepatitis A infection, the blood supply is considered safe and transfusions are not considered to pose a risk for HAV transmission. While intravenous drug users (IVDUs) are at a somewhat increased risk of acquiring HAV as compared with the general population, it does not appear that intravenous drug use is a very significant mode of HAV transmission. Other factors, such as poor hygiene and unsanitary living conditions, may explain the increased incidence of hepatitis A among IVDUs. In general, it appears that blood-to-blood transmission of HAV occurs infrequently. HAV has occasionally been detected in other body fluids, such as saliva and urine. However, it is believed that these are not routes of HAV transmission.

THOSE AT AN INCREASED RISK FOR HEPATITIS A

Hepatitis A is the most common vaccine-preventable disease in the entire world. Aside from vaccination, there are other measures that a person can take to minimize her chances of acquiring HAV. In addition, many precautions may be taken by a person infected with HAV so as to reduce the likelihood of transmitting this virus to others. Prevention of hepatitis A will be discussed in Chapter 24. The following people are at increased risk for contracting HAV.

- People who travel to developing countries, including tourists, military personnel, Peace Corps workers, and missionaries.

- Men who have sex with men.

- People who practice oral-anal sex.

- Intravenous drug users.

- People who have contact with sewage (this appears to be an insignificant mode of transmission in the United States).

- Employees and children (particularly those in diapers) at day-care centers.

- Employees and patients in institutions for the mentally disabled (incidence has greatly decreased since sanitary conditions have improved).

- People who work with non-human primates, such as apes and monkeys, which can also transmit HAV.

- People who live in crowded conditions with poor sanitation.

THE INCUBATION PERIOD OF HEPATITIS A

After entering the body, HAV incubates. The *incubation period*—the time between the entrance of the virus into the body and the initial appearance of symptoms and signs of the disease—of HAV is about one month, but may be as short as two weeks or as long as almost two months. The length of the incubation period is inversely related to the quantity of HAV that enters the body. This means that if a large amount of HAV enters the body, the incubation period is shorter than if only a small amount is ingested. As noted above, a person is most infectious during the two-week period prior to and the one-week period after exhibiting any symptoms or signs of hepatitis A. This helps explain why hepatitis A is so contagious. People are not aware that they harbor the virus, which prevents them from taking the necessary precautions to insure that they do not pass it on to others.

THE SYMPTOMS AND SIGNS OF HEPATITIS A

The development of symptoms is directly related to the age of the person. The younger the person, the more likely the infection will be asymptomatic—without symptoms. In fact, approximately 90 percent of HAV-infected children who are younger than five years old are asymptomatic. Thus, children silently pass the virus in their stools, and it is their parents, exposed unknowingly to HAV, who are the ones most likely to suffer with symptoms due to infection.

The degree of symptoms among people with hepatitis A varies greatly. Some people have no symptoms at all and are surprised to learn that they were ever exposed to the virus. Others may have nonspecific symptoms such as fatigue or symptoms that may be confused with a very bad cold or flu—chills, loss of appetite (especially for fatty foods), and a headache. Often symptoms include a sudden fever, abdominal pain, diarrhea, nausea, and vomiting. Many adults become jaundiced and seek the attention of a doctor when they notice their urine is dark or tea-colored and/or their stools are light or clay-colored. These people often have pruritus (intense itching). Usually, a week prior to becoming jaundiced, these people experience some nonspecific symptoms such as malaise and weight loss. Some HAV-infected individuals state that cigarettes taste distasteful to them, and they actually stop smoking during this time. When adults become very ill, studies have shown that approximately one month is typically lost from work. In fact, 11 to 22 percent of people with hepatitis A become so ill that they require hospitalization.

Some people occasionally develop symptoms and signs of hepatitis that are unrelated to the liver. These are known as *extrahepatic*—outside or unrelated to the liver—manifestations of hepatitis A. These manifestations may include arthritis (inflammation of the joints); vasculitis (inflammation of the blood vessels), often associated with a rash; cryoglobulinemia (abnormal proteins in the blood); kidney failure; diabetes (elevated blood sugar levels); and gallbladder disease.

In very rare instances, people with hepatitis A develop a particularly severe form of acute hepatitis known as fulminant hepatitis A, which is discussed in Chapter 7. These people become extremely ill, developing severe jaundice, encephalopathy (mental disorientation or coma), and coagulopathy (bleeding tendency noted by a prolonged prothrombin time). Liver failure develops abruptly—usually within eight weeks from the onset of symptoms, or within two weeks from the onset of jaundice. All people with fulminant hepatitis A require immediate hospitalization into an intensive care unit (ICU) and prompt referral for a liver transplant. Liver transplantation is discussed in detail in Chapter 22.

People with hepatitis A will usually appear to be in good or normal health during a physical exam. Occasionally, the physical exam may reveal an enlarged, tender liver or jaundice. Though not a frequent occurrence, a person may have a rash.

Symptoms and signs usually last a month or two. Once jaundice appears, symptoms often begin to resolve. Jaundice, accompanied by urine and stool discoloration, typically begins to resolve within a few weeks. About 10 to 15 percent of people with hepatitis A may experience a prolonged course or a relapse (relapsing hepatitis A). During the period of relapse, symptoms and signs return after a previous resolution. Blood work again becomes abnormal and the person is again infectious. In any scenario, by six months all symptoms and signs of hepatitis A will resolve.

DIAGNOSING HEPATITIS A

Neither symptoms, signs, nor LFT abnormalities can definitively confirm that a person has hepatitis A, nor can these manifestations distinguish hepatitis A from other forms of hepatitis.

The only way of definitely diagnosing that a person is infected with HAV is by obtaining specific blood tests known as the *hepatitis A serology*. The standard hepatitis A serology includes both the immunoglobulin M (IgM) antibody to HAV and the immunoglobulin G (IgG) antibody to HAV. The other liver function tests, which were discussed in Chapter 3, are routinely performed when any type of liver disease is suspected.

HAV Antibody Immunoglobulin M (IgM) (HAV Ab IgM)

When a person tests positive for the existence of immunoglobulin M (IgM) antibody to HAV (HAV Ab IgM), it indicates that the person is currently infected with HAV or has been infected recently. HAV Ab IgM becomes positive approximately one week after a person has been exposed to HAV, and may remain positive for up to six months thereafter. This antibody then becomes undetectable in the blood; thus HAV Ab IgM will be negative on blood test results after six months.

HAV Antibody Immunoglobulin G (IgG) (HAV Ab IgG)

When a person tests positive for the existence of immunoglobulin G (IgG) antibody to HAV (HAV Ab IgG)—in cases where HAV Ab IgM is no longer detected—it indicates that the person was exposed to HAV at some point in the past, but no longer has an active infection. (Note, however, that in the acute phase, HAV Ab IgG will be positive.) These people can never become infected with HAV again and are no longer infectious to others. Though these people are protected against future HAV infections, they are not protected against other hepatitis infections, such as B and C. The HAV Ab IgG remains positive lifelong and will always be detected in blood tests (HAV Ab IgG positive) when a test for HAV Ab IgG is specifically ordered by a doctor.

AST and ALT (Transaminases)

People with hepatitis A may have very elevated transaminases (ALT and AST) around 500 IU/L to 2,000 IU/L. The degree of elevation of the transaminases does not correlate with the severity of symptoms, nor is it predictive of the outcome of the disease. In most people, transaminases return to normal in about one month. In virtually everyone with hepatitis A, they return to normal by six months. Thus, if transaminases remain abnormal after six months time, another cause for these elevated liver tests must be searched for. For example, on rare occasions, HAV may trigger the onset of a liver disease known as autoimmune hepatitis, which will be discussed in Chapter 14.

Bilirubin

An elevated bilirubin level occurs in approximately 70 percent of adults with hepatitis A. In contrast, only 20 percent of children younger than two years old are jaundiced. The bilirubin level usually does not rise greater than 10 mg/dl, and usually returns to normal within eight weeks. In cases where the bilirubin level remains elevated for ten weeks or more, the person is known as having cholestatic hepatitis. In people with cholestatic hepatitis, the bilirubin can reach levels as high as 20 mg/dl, and is often associated with pruritus (itching). In any case, the bilirubin level always returns to normal by six months' time.

Imaging Studies and Liver Biopsy

Imaging studies are usually normal for people with hepatitis A and will not provide a basis for a diagnosis. It is especially important to perform imaging studies in jaundiced individuals in order to eliminate the possibility that a disorder other than hepatitis A, such as gallstones, is responsible for the abnormal LFTs. A liver biopsy is not needed to establish a diagnosis of hepatitis A. Therefore, liver biopsies are infrequently performed when hepatitis A is suspected.

TREATMENT OF HEPATITIS A

There are no specific medications used to treat hepatitis A. Treatment decisions are usually based on the symptoms experienced by the patient. Bed rest and decreased physical activity are not necessarily required. Each person should, on her own, determine a comfortable level of activity based on how she feels. If a person feels well, she may go to work. If she feels fatigued, a decreased level of activity or a midday nap is in order. It is always recommended that a person with hepatitis A consume plenty of fluids so as to avoid dehydration. This is especially important if diarrhea is one of the symptoms. All alcohol should be avoided during this time, as alcohol may provoke a relapse of the disease.

People who have fulminant hepatitis A need to be immediately admitted to the intensive care unit of a hospital for close management. These people have a high incidence of doing poorly. Thus, patients who are not improving should be considered for liver transplantation. Approximately 30 percent of people with fulminant hepatitis A are at risk of death without a transplant. Patients with fulminant hepatitis A who undergo transplantation generally do very well, with approximately an 80-percent chance of surviving. Transplantation will be discussed in Chapter 22.

THE LONG-TERM PROGNOSIS FOR THOSE WITH HEPATITIS A

People with hepatitis A do not suffer any long-term consequences from the infection and are not chronically infectious to others. Within six months of contracting hepatitis A, symptoms, signs, and LFT abnormalities related to hepatitis A totally resolve. Chronic liver disease does not occur. Therefore, contracting HAV does not put one at risk for cirrhosis and/or liver cancer.

Approximately 0.2 percent of people infected with HAV develop fulminant hepatitis A. Each year approximately 100 people either die or require a liver transplant as a result of fulminant hepatitis due to HAV. Older people and people with underlying liver disease are more likely to develop fulminant hepatitis A and are more likely to have a poor outcome from fulminant hepatitis A.

CONCLUSION

Increasingly healthier and cleaner living conditions—such as improved sewage disposal and more sanitary water and food supplies—have contributed to a decline in the incidence of hepatitis A in the United States over the past several decades. However, outbreaks continue to occur. While outbreaks are typically without consequences for most people, a small yet significant percentage of people become severely ill, requiring time out of work, hospitalization, and possibly liver transplantation. People especially at risk for a particularly debilitating course of hepatitis A are elderly individuals and those already suffering from some other chronic liver disease, such as chronic hepatitis C. Infection with HAV is 100-percent preventable. This prevention is discussed in Chapter 24. The next chapter will discuss another preventable type of viral hepatitis—hepatitis B. While the acute symptoms and signs of hepatitis B may resemble those of hepatitis A, the major distinguishing point between these two hepatitis viruses is that, unlike hepatitis A, hepatitis B can lead to chronic liver disease, cirrhosis, and liver cancer. Also discussed in the next chapter is hepatitis D, a hepatitis virus that cannot survive without HBV.

9

Understanding Hepatitis B and D

Charlie, a twenty-seven-year-old construction worker, had recently begun a new relationship. His new girlfriend didn't tell him that she had acquired hepatitis B from the prior use of intravenous drugs. A few weeks after an episode of unprotected sex, Charlie felt so fatigued that he could not get out of bed. His joints hurt, he was nauseous, and he had a pain in the location of his liver. When his girlfriend told him that his eyes looked yellow, Charlie immediately went to the emergency room. The doctor suspected gallstones and admitted Charlie as an inpatient. Charlie's sonogram didn't show evidence of gallstones, but his blood work revealed that he had acute hepatitis B.

Woo, a fifty-seven-year-old woman, noticed that her feet and abdomen were becoming progressively more swollen over a period of several weeks. One day, while brushing her teeth, she discovered blood on her toothbrush. After trying some home remedies for the bleeding and swelling, none of which seemed to correct the problem, Woo went to her family doctor. While telling the doctor about her background, Woo mentioned that she had moved to the United States from Taiwan as a child and that her mother had died at the age of fifty of some kind of liver disease. Woo did not smoke or drink alcohol and had never been hospitalized. The doctor examined Woo. Her eyes were yellow, her abdomen was distended with fluid, and her legs were swollen. Her liver and spleen were enlarged. Blood tests were taken, and the results, which came back about a week later, revealed evidence of chronic infectious hepatitis B. Woo's platelet count was low and her prothrombin time was prolonged. The doctor concluded that Woo had decompensated cirrho-

sis due to chronic hepatitis B—a virus she undoubtedly acquired at birth from her mother.

n this chapter, you'll learn about the hepatitis B virus (HBV) and hepatitis delta virus (HDV) and how these viruses are transmitted to others. This chapter also covers who is at risk for contracting these viruses and how people typically discover that they are infected. The differences between acute, chronic, and fulminant hepatitis B are addressed. In addition, factors that determine which individuals are most likely to progress from acute to chronic hepatitis B are discussed. This chapter also explains the blood tests used to diagnose hepatitis B, known as the hepatitis B serology. Also covered are the ways in which people with hepatitis B can become infected with HDV. Finally, the long-term prognosis of people infected with HBV or HBV and HDV is discussed. See Chapter 12 for treatment options for hepatitis B and hepatitis D and Chapter 24 for ways to prevent contracting these viruses.

WHAT IS HEPATITIS B?

Hepatitis B is inflammation of the liver due to a virus called the hepatitis B virus (HBV). Infection with HBV was originally known as *serum hepatitis*. In 1963, the structure of the virus was identified and named the hepatitis B virus. In fact, HBV was actually the very first hepatitis virus to be identified. Almost 400 million people worldwide, including 1.25 million people in the United States have hepatitis B. Hepatitis B is endemic (a disease prevailing continually in a restricted region) in Southeast Asia, China, and Africa. In these areas of the world, more than 50 percent of the population has been exposed to HBV at some point in their lives. Fortunately, the virus has a relatively low prevalence in North America, Western Europe, and Australia.

In most cases, infection with HBV will not prevent a person from leading a normal, productive life. Yet, hepatitis B is not entirely harmless. A long-term infection can lead to cirrhosis and liver cancer. As a result, approximately 1 million people die each year from the complications of hepatitis B. Hepatitis B can present itself in a variety of ways.

WHAT IS HEPATITIS D?

Hepatitis D is inflammation of the liver due to a virus called the hepatitis delta virus (HDV). HDV is a virus that can only live in people with hepatitis B. Approximately 70,000 people in the United States are infected with this virus. Although HDV only accounts for a small percentage of cases of chronic viral hepatitis, it tends to be a particularly severe infection with significant long-term consequences. In fact, chronic hepatitis D causes more than 1,000 deaths each year. See page 105 for more information on hepatitis D.

HOW HBV IS TRANSMITTED

Approximately 200,000 new HBV infections occur annually in the United States. How are these people acquiring this virus? Well, HBV is an extremely hardy virus. It has been detected in blood, sweat, tears, saliva, semen, vaginal secretions, menstrual blood, and breast milk. HBV is much harder to catch than the virus that causes a cold or the flu, but a lot easier to catch than HIV—the virus that causes AIDS.

As discussed in Chapter 7, HBV is transmitted to others *parenterally*. Thus, a person cannot get hepatitis B from eating food prepared by an infected person, by hugging or holding hands with an infected person, or by visiting an infected person. Instead, HBV is transmitted in three different ways: through blood or blood products, through sexual contact, or from mother to child during pregnancy and childbirth.

Only a small percentage of adults in the United States harbor infectious hepatitis B viral particles that can be transmitted to others. Therefore, simply having hepatitis B does not mean that a person is automatically infectious to others. See page 103 to find out how a person can determine if she is infectious. The following is a discussion of how HBV is transmitted.

Blood or Blood Products

Prior to 1975, many people developed hepatitis B after having received a contaminated blood or a contaminated blood product, such as fresh frozen plasma (FFP) or platelets, during a transfusion. But since 1975, the blood supply in the United States has been carefully screened to eliminate HBV. Consequently, few people nowadays contract hepatitis B in this manner. Still, there are a lot of other ways a person can come into contact with infected blood, such as through the sharing of toothbrushes, razors, or nail clippers—each of which can carry and transmit infectious hepatitis B viral particles. Therefore, people living in the same household as someone with hepatitis B need to take special precautions. Intravenous drug abusers, even if needles are shared only once, can transmit the virus among themselves. If not sterilized properly, needles used for tattooing, ear-piercing, body-piercing, and acupuncture may be tainted with flecks of infected blood. Thus, these practices also involve some risk of transmitting HBV. Even barbers and manicurists can transmit the virus if their equipment is contaminated with infected blood. Straws, dollar bills, or other instruments shared when "snorting" drugs, such as cocaine, can transmit small amounts of HBV infected blood from broken blood vessels in the nose from one person to another. And since being accidentally stuck with a needle or other sharp instrument is an occupational hazard of the medical and dental professions, health-care workers are particularly vulnerable to developing hepatitis B. Other people at risk include those with kidney failure undergoing *hemodialysis*—a procedure that helps filter blood—or those receiving a transplanted organ infected with HBV.

Sexual Contact

HBV has been found in vaginal secretions, saliva, and semen. Therefore, it doesn't matter if a person's sexual partner is of the same or opposite gender. If one partner has hepatitis B, the other one can get it. Deep kissing, oral sex, and anal sex are all possible ways of transmitting the virus. In addition, the likelihood of becoming infected with HBV grows with the number of sexual partners a person has. Thus, promiscuous individuals are more likely to get HBV.

Childbirth

An infected mother can transmit HBV to her child during childbirth. This mode of transmission is known as *perinatal transmission.* It accounts for the high rates of infection in Asian and African countries, as asymptomatic mothers, unaware that they carry the virus, invariably transmit it to their newborn infants at childbirth.

In the United States, all pregnant women are screened for the presence of HBV, and all babies born to infected mothers immediately receive immunization. In fact, in the United States, it is now common practice that, regardless of the mother's HBV status, all infants are vaccinated against this virus. In this way, there is hope that this infection can become a disease of the past. For more information on vaccinations, see Chapter 24. New mothers are also advised to avoid breast-feeding if they are infectious, even though this mode of transmission has not been considered very significant.

THOSE AT AN INCREASED RISK FOR HEPATITIS B

Hepatitis B is a disease that is totally preventable through vaccination. Aside from vaccination, there are other measures that a person can take to minimize her chances of acquiring HBV. In addition, many precautions may be taken by a person infected with HBV so as to reduce the likelihood of transmitting this virus to others. Prevention of hepatitis B will be discussed in Chapter 24. Meanwhile, take note of the following people who are at increased risk for contracting HBV:

- People who received blood or a blood-product transfusion prior to 1975.

- Hospital or other health-care facility workers.

- Live-in family members and roommates of an infected person.

- Intravenous drugs users or former users.

- People who have acquired a tattoo or had body piercing with an infected needle.

- Sex partners of infected people.

- Travelers to countries where HBV is endemic.

- People who were born to a mother infected with HBV.

- Transplant-organ recipients who received an infected organ.

WHAT IS ACUTE HEPATITIS B?

Acute hepatitis B is defined as inflammation of the liver lasting six months or less due to the hepatitis B virus. This section discusses the symptoms and signs associated with acute hepatitis B. It also discusses how acute hepatitis B is diagnosed and how it is determined if acute hepatitis B has resolved or progressed to chronic hepatitis B.

The Symptoms and Signs of Acute Hepatitis B

The symptoms of acute hepatitis B are usually similar to those of acute hepatitis due to any cause, which was discussed in Chapter 7. Furthermore, acute hepatitis B can be silent or easily mistaken for something else. For example, a person with acute hepatitis B may, based on symptoms, incorrectly assume that she is merely suffering from a really bad case of the flu. This is one of the reasons why HBV has spread so widely throughout the world. People usually don't know that they have the virus when they pass it on to other people. In fact, the acute phase of a hepatitis B is usually detected in only a small percentage of people who are infected. If symptoms do appear, they generally occur after the virus has incubated in the body for about two to three months (a range of 15 to 180 days). The physical exam is usually normal, but it may reveal an enlarged liver, a rash, and/or rarely jaundice.

Symptoms can include decreased appetite, nausea and vomiting, a low fever, abdominal discomfort, and altered sense of taste and smell. (Some smokers with acute HBV claim that cigarettes taste odd.) All of these symptoms may last for about a week or two. If jaundice occurs, it usually develops after these symptoms disappear, and infrequently lasts more than a month or two.

Other people with acute hepatitis B have symptoms and signs related to *extrahepatic* (outside of, or unrelated to, the liver) manifestations of hepatitis B. This is partly due to the fact that some of the other parts of the body are caught in the crossfire when the immune system fights back against HBV. These are known as immune-complex mediated diseases, and include a type of *vasculitis* (inflammation of vessels) known as *polyarteritis nodosa* (PAN), and a kidney disease known as *glomerulonephritis* (inflammation of the kidneys). Symptoms may include a rash, muscle and joint aches, fever, and excessive protein in the urine. Up to 20 percent of people with acute hepatitis B may suffer from severe joint stiffness and pain. In fact, it is often the rheumatologist, a doctor that specializes in the treatment of diseases of the joints and muscles, who initially discovers that a person is infected with HBV. These extrahepatic manifestations of hepatitis B are discussed further in the section on chronic hepatitis B on page 100.

Diagnosing Acute Hepatitis B

The *incubation period*—the time between the entrance of the virus into the body and the initial appearance of symptoms and signs of the disease—of hepatitis B is about two to three months, but may be as short as two weeks or as long as almost six months. As symptoms may be rather vague, most people never seek evaluation from a doctor during the acute stage of disease, and therefore many people never realize that they were infected with this virus. However, if a person does see the doctor for the evaluation of symptoms or signs of jaundice, acute hepatitis B is usually first detected by abnormal results from blood work. See Chapter 3 for information on the specific blood tests.

Transaminases (AST and ALT) are often quite elevated initially, and levels in the thousands can occur. As the disease progresses, transaminases typically decrease. Resolution of acute hepatitis B is usually indicated by the normalization of transaminase levels by six months time. If transaminases remain elevated—usually around two to three times above normal—at six month's time, this usually indicates progression to chronic hepatitis B (see page 99).

The cholestatic liver enzymes (AP and GGTP) are usually only mildly elevated during acute hepatitis B—around two to three times above normal—and bilirubin levels are usually normal. If bilirubin levels are elevated, they are rarely above 10 mg/dl.

There are specific blood tests that the doctor will perform once she detects that the LFTs are abnormal. This is known as hepatitis B serology (see Table 9.1 on page 101). From the results of these tests, the doctor will be able to determine if the LFT abnormalities are in fact due to hepatitis B. Furthermore, the doctor will be able to gather a great deal of information about the status of the HBV infection. This includes determining if a patient is actively infectious to others, if the acute infection has resolved, and/or if the patient has progressed into a chronic hepatitis B infection.

Typically, imaging studies are normal. Occasionally, an enlarged liver will be detected. In most cases, imaging studies are performed to eliminate other possible causes of elevated LFTs, such as gallstones. A liver biopsy is usually not performed during the acute stages of a hepatitis B infection.

Determining if Acute Hepatitis B Has Resolved Entirely

The doctor will probably want to see a patient several times over the next few months after the diagnosis of acute hepatitis B has been made in order to check on the status of the infection. Six months after the patient has been infected, the doctor will determine if the body has shaken off hepatitis B entirely. Most adults have a strong enough immune system to battle the virus and completely eliminate it from the body. When this occurs, LFT elevations completely normalize, and symptoms, if they were present, totally resolve. Protective antibodies will be formed against HBV. Congratulations are in order. These fortunate people will never have to worry about HBV again, as they are now immune to this virus. They can never get it again or give it to others. However, immunity against HBV won't protect against other hepatitis viruses, such as hepatitis A virus (HAV) or hepatitis C virus (HCV). Also, these people will never again be allowed to donate blood, as they will always have the antibody—hepatitis B core antibody (HBcAb)—for HBV present in their blood (see Table 9.1 on page 101 for clarification).

WHAT IS FULMINANT HEPATITIS B?

Fulminant hepatitis B is a very rare, but very severe form of acute hepatitis B. It is characterized by sudden liver failure; coagulopathy, a bleeding disorder; jaundice; and encephalopathy (coma). Patients with fulminant hepatitis B are severely ill and develop a rapidly progressive downhill course. Approximately 85 percent of these patients are likely to die unless they undergo immediate liver transplantation. Therefore, the treatment of people with fulminant hepatitis B requires immediate hospitalization and notification of a transplant center. Fortunately, this complication of acute hepatitis B occurs in less than 1 percent of patients with hepatitis B.

WHAT IS CHRONIC HEPATITIS B?

Chronic hepatitis B is defined as inflammation of the liver due to HBV that continues for more than six months. These people have failed to clear HBV from their bodies. Once a person is chronically infected with this virus, the potential exists for liver damage and cirrhosis along with its complications, including liver cancer. This section discusses the progression from acute to chronic hepatitis B and the symptoms and signs associated with chronic hepatitis B, as well as its diagnosis.

Determining the Progression From Acute to Chronic Hepatitis B

In the United States, approximately 200,000 people contract HBV each year. However, only 10,000 to 15,000 of these people develop a chronic hepatitis B infection. Why do some people clear the virus from their bodies, while others progress to chronic disease? It appears that the immune system is the most important factor in determining whether a person can rid herself of this virus rather than develop a persistent infection.

The immune system is relatively immature early in life. Therefore, the younger a person is when HBV is contracted, the greater the likelihood that the infected person will become a chronic carrier of the disease. If an adult is infected, her probability of developing chronic disease is very low—approximately 1 to 5 percent. If a person contracts the infection in infancy, there is as much as a 90- to 95-percent chance that her immune system will be unable to eliminate this virus from her body. Children fall somewhere in between, having approximately a 25 to 35 percent chance of going on to chronic disease.

Men are six times more likely than women to become chronic carriers of HBV. The reason for this has not been determined. Also, people with poor immune systems—such as those infected with HIV, organ recipients, and those undergoing chemotherapy—have a much lower success rate of eliminating the virus from their bodies. Surprisingly, patients who are the sickest during their acute illness, especially those who develop jaundice or who survive fulminant hepatitis, have the highest likelihood of totally recovering, and thus not progressing to a chronic disease.

The Symptoms and Signs of Chronic Hepatitis B

As is true with liver disease in general, the symptoms of chronic hepatitis B are usually silent or nonspecific. Often, people don't know that they have the virus when they pass it on to others. Symptoms may include generalized fatigue and weakness. People who have already progressed to cirrhosis may have symptoms and signs related to the complications of cirrhosis, such as jaundice, encephalopathy, and ascites.

Extrahepatic (outside the liver) immune-mediated manifestations of chronic hepatitis B, such as polyarteritis nodosa (PAN), glomerulonephritis, or cryoglobulinemia (excess proteins in the blood), may also be present. Symptoms may include pronounced weakness of the muscles, joint aches, rashes, numbness in the arms and legs, high blood pressure (hypertension), abdominal pain, fever, and infrequently, kidney failure. There is no correlation between the severity of these diseases and the severity of the hepatitis. In fact, some people with severe vasculitis often have a very mild hepatitis. These extrahepatic manifestations of chronic hepatitis B are very uncommon, but may be quite serious. For example, some studies have reported that between 30 to 50 percent of people may succumb to the consequences of vasculitis.

Diagnosing Chronic Hepatitis B

Most people usually find out that they have chronic hepatitis B almost by accident. It may have been discovered that they have slight LFT elevations on blood work done as part of a routine physical exam. Or they may have been turned down for life insurance because of abnormal LFTs. Or their blood may have been rejected for donation because they tested positive for either the hepatitis B antibody or antigen. Of course, some people with chronic hepatitis B had already been under a doctor's care after having been diagnosed with acute hepatitis B. Others have found out about this condition after complaining of general feelings of fatigue to their doctors. Finally, some people with hepatitis B are brought to their doctors' attention only after having already progressed silently to cirrhosis. For these unfortunate people, the first sign of hepatitis B may be a complication of cirrhosis, such as variceal bleeding, ascites, encephalopathy, or liver cancer. (See Chapter 6 for more information on cirrhosis.)

Blood Tests

In people with chronic hepatitis B, transaminases (AST and ALT) are usually mildly elevated (two to three times abnormal). AP and GGTP are usually normal or minimally elevated. These tests do not correlate to the severity of liver disease caused by HBV. The bilirubin is generally normal, unless advanced stages of cirrhosis are present. See Chapter 3 for more information on the specific tests.

The hepatitis B serology is necessary to obtain an accurate diagnosis of hepatitis B. A lot of crucial information may be gleaned from these specific blood tests, such as the chronicity of HBV, immunity to HBV, and/or infectiousness of HBV to others. The hepatitis B serology is quite complicated and is detailed in Table 9.1 below.

Imaging Studies

Usually the doctor will want to obtain at least one imaging study (usually a sonogram) at some point during the diagnostic evaluation of chronic hepatitis B, espe-

Table 9.1. Understanding Hepatitis B Serology

Serological Test	Significance of Serological Test
Hepatitis B Core Antibody IgM (HBcAb IgM) if HBsAg negative	Acute infection with HBV
Hepatitis B Core Antibody IgG (HBcAb IgG) if HBsAg positive	Chronic infection with HBV
Hepatitis B Core Antibody IgG (HBcAb IgG)	A lifelong marker of past infection with HBV that has been successfully cleared from the body (if HBsAg is absent)
Hepatitis B Surface Antibody (HBsAb)	Immunity to HBV or a successful response to the HBV vaccination
Hepatitis B Surface Antigen (HBsAg) if HBcAb IgM positive	Acute hepatitis B infection
Hepatitis B Surface Antigen (HBsAg) if HBcAb IgG positive	Chronic hepatitis B carrier
Hepatitis B "E" Antibody (HBeAb)	Resolved acute hepatitis B infection or inactive (nonreplicating) chronic disease
Hepatitis B "E" Antigen (HBeAg)	Active viral replication—high level of infectivity; seen in both acute hepatitis B and actively replicating chronic hepatitis B
Hepatitis B Viral Deoxyribonucleic Acid (HBV DNA)	Most sensitive marker for HBV replication usually occurs in the presence of HBeAg positivity; when occurs with HBeAg negativity indicates a mutant strain of infectious hepatitis B; disappearance corresponds to resolution of severe infectivity
Hepatitis D Antibody IgM (HDV IgM)	Acute infection with HDV
Hepatitis D Antibody IgG (HDV IgG)	Chronic infection with HDV

cially when LFTs are elevated. While an enlarged liver or spleen may be detected on occasion, in general, imaging studies are usually normal—even in advanced stages of disease. If liver cancer (hepatoma) is present, a mass may be revealed. See Chapter 19 for more information on liver tumors. However, just because the liver looks normal on an imaging study, this does not mean that the liver is normal. That is why a liver biopsy is necessary when more information about the condition of the liver is needed.

Liver Biopsy

As with all liver diseases, even if a person feels fine, that's no guarantee that her liver is doing fine, too. The only way to determine the degree to which a liver is injured is by examining a sample of the liver under the microscope. Therefore, in addition to obtaining a battery of blood tests, including LFTs and the hepatitis B serology, the doctor will need to perform a liver biopsy to determine the full extent of the damage done to the liver by the virus and to determine if treatment is necessary. A liver biopsy is the only reliable means of determining the presence or absence of cirrhosis. Furthermore, some studies have demonstrated that the findings on liver biopsy at initial presentation (when the patient first sees her doctor) predict the patient's future prognosis. This is important especially in light of the fact that the level of LFT elevation and/or a person's symptoms often do not correlate with the extent of inflammation and damage found on a liver biopsy specimen.

The Different Types of Chronic Hepatitis B

People with chronic hepatitis B may be divided into three categories. These are healthy chronic carrier of hepatitis B, chronic infectious hepatitis B, and chronic mutant hepatitis B. Everyone with chronic hepatitis B is, by definition, both HBsAg and HBcAb positive. (Refer to Table 9.1 on page 101 for some clarification of these and similar terms.) This means that both the hepatitis B surface antigen and core antibody are detectable in their blood.

Healthy Chronic Carriers of Hepatitis B

The first type of chronic hepatitis B is found in a person who carries HBV (HBsAg and HBcAb are positive) but has normal LFTs, a normal physical exam, and is asymptomatic. Such a person is sometimes referred to as a *healthy chronic carrier* of HBV. HBeAg and HBV DNA are negative, indicating that this person is not infectious to others. Healthy chronic carriers of HBV usually have minimal, if any, liver inflammation or damage. They usually live a normal life without any complications due to their liver disease; however, compared with the general population, these people are at a somewhat higher risk for cirrhosis and liver cancer. Therefore, regular observation—in the form of yearly visits to the doctor for a physical exam and blood tests—is necessary to check for early signs of disease progression.

In addition, these people are at risk for reactivation of the virus if their immune systems become suppressed. Such an occurrence may happen during treatment with immunosuppressive drugs, such as steroids (prednisone, for example), or during a severe illness, such as AIDS or cancer. The chance of reactivation into the active infectious state is not known.

In some instances, a person can become HBsAg negative. However, this is very uncommon and only occurs at a rate of approximately 1 percent each year. If this does happen, it's great news. The individual will no longer be considered to have chronic hepatitis B.

Chronic Infectious Hepatitis B

The second type of chronic hepatitis B is found in a person who, in addition to carrying the HBsAg, also carries the markers indicating that she is highly contagious or infectious to others. In this person, HBeAg and HBV DNA are positive. People with chronic infectious hepatitis B are actively replicating HBV. They have elevated LFTs and typically have very inflamed and damaged livers. Symptoms bear no correlation with the extent of damage found on a liver biopsy. Some people may be asymptomatic, some may have vague symptoms (such as fatigue), and some may be severely ill. People with chronic infectious hepatitis are more likely to have a progressive disease leading to cirrhosis.

Without treatment, these people have only a 5- to 10-percent probability each year of becoming negative for HBeAg and HBV DNA. This is known as a spontaneous remission. When this happens, a brief, temporary gross elevation in transaminases (AST and ALT) is observed, followed by a rapid return to normal levels. Antibodies (HBeAb) are formed. These people are no longer highly contagious to others and further liver damage is minimal, if it occurs at all. Unfortunately, reactivation to the infectious state can occur in some of these people. Thus, these people must be observed carefully. It is not clear which factors play a role in causing some people to relapse into an infectious state. Certainly, excessive alcohol intake may have a harmful effect on people with chronic hepatitis B. And it has been demonstrated that excessive iron intake may promote persistent HBV replication in some people. (Excessive iron in itself is damaging to the liver potentially leading to cirrhosis and liver cancer. This is discussed in more detail in Chapters 18 and 23.) Therefore, people with chronic hepatitis B are advised to refrain from alcohol intake and should avoid excess iron supplementation.

Furthermore, people whose immune systems subsequently become compromised are at risk for a relapse. Immune-system function can become impaired by a number of factors, including infection with the human immunodeficiency virus (HIV), treatment with chemotherapeutic agents for cancer, or use of corticosteroids, such as prednisone, for various reasons.

Chronic Mutant Hepatitis B

The last category of people with chronic hepatitis B are those who have a *mutant* strain of HBV. A mutation is a permanent alteration of the hepatitis B virus's genetic makeup. In this case, the genetic mutation is characterized by the failure of the virus to make the hepatitis B "E" antigen (HbeAg). This mutation does not affect the virus's ability to replicate. Therefore, on blood tests, these people are negative for HBeAg, but positive for HBV DNA. Mutant hepatitis B has been responsible for several cases of unsuspected transmission of disease to others, as these people are highly infectious. This strain of hepatitis B, believed to be genetically superior and more resistant to treatment, is capable of causing severe liver damage.

The Long-Term Prognosis for Those With Chronic Hepatitis B

The probability each year that a person with chronic hepatitis B will develop cirrhosis is about 2 percent. However, different studies have reported rates varying from 0.1 to 10 percent per year. The cumulative probability of progression to cirrhosis over five years is approximately 15 to 20 percent. After the development of cirrhosis, the probability of developing serious complications, such as decompensated cirrhosis, is about 2 to 10 percent each year. The five-year survival rate after cirrhosis has developed varies from 52 to 80 percent. However, if a person has decompensated cirrhosis, the five-year survival rate decreases to between 14 to 35 percent.

So, why is it that some people can live a long healthy life with hepatitis B and others experience complications? Well, it has been demonstrated that there are many factors that influence the progression from a mild, innocuous illness to a grave outcome. These factors include advanced age and general poor health (for example, depressed immune status); the presence of advanced damage found on samples from liver biopsy; and the presence of markers of chronicity and of active infectiousness, especially HBV DNA. Similarly, people with HBeAg tend to have a more aggressive course than those who are HBeAg-negative. In fact, in some studies it has been shown that people without HBeAg rarely progress to cirrhosis. People who are also infected with the hepatitis delta virus (HDV) (see page 105), and possibly those additionally infected with the hepatitis C virus (see Chapter 10), also have poorer prognoses. In addition, it has been shown that the outcome of a person infected with HBV is highly dependent upon the stage at which she first obtained medical attention. Those people who have more advanced disease on initial evaluation by a doctor have a shorter survival time. Lastly, it has been demonstrated that people infected with HBV are more susceptible to the toxic effects of alcohol on the liver than are those without HBV. It is, therefore, important for people with chronic hepatitis B to avoid all intake of alcohol, as alcohol may worsen the course and accelerate the progression of the disease. See Chapter 17 for more information on alcohol's effects on the liver.

Chronic Hepatitis B and Long-term Liver Cancer Risk

People with chronic hepatitis B are at increased risk of developing liver cancer. The exact risk is unknown, but in some studies, people with chronic hepatitis B were 200 times more likely to develop liver cancer compared with people without this disease. Cancer usually occurs in those who have developed cirrhosis. However, cancer can also occur in chronic HBV carriers without cirrhosis. In fact, in some parts of the world where hepatitis B is endemic, such as Africa, up to 30 percent of people with chronic hepatitis B develop liver cancer without underlying cirrhosis.

Liver cancer generally takes about twenty to thirty years to develop from the time a person becomes infected with HBV. Thus, people who were infected at birth can develop liver cancer as early as twenty years old. It appears that being infected with both HBV and HCV and drinking excessive alcohol can predispose a person to an even greater likelihood of developing liver cancer. See Chapter 19 for more information on liver cancer.

THE HEPATITIS DELTA VIRUS (HDV)

The hepatitis delta virus (HDV) is a virus that infects only people with hepatitis B. When this occurs, a person is known as having hepatitis D. HDV needs HBV in order to live, and therefore cannot cause infection on its own. This is why it has been referred to as a "passenger virus." HDV infection may be silent or may cause the same kind of fatigue and other symptoms associated with other forms of hepatitis. However, up to 20 percent of hepatitis D patients develop fulminant hepatitis, a particularly serious condition that requires hospitalization. See Chapter 7 for a discussion on fulminant hepatitis.

HDV is transmitted through the same blood, sexual, and perinatal routes as HBV, which were discussed on page 96. There are two ways in which a person infected with HBV may become infected with HDV: coinfection and superinfection. When HBV and HDV are acquired at the same time, it is known as *coinfection*. In 90 to 95 percent of cases, such people will be able to eliminate the viruses completely from their bodies. This means that only approximately 5 to 10 percent of coinfected individuals go on to develop chronic hepatitis B and D. HDV can also be acquired in someone who already has chronic hepatitis B. This is known as *superinfection*. In contrast to people infected with both viruses simultaneously, approximately 70 to 95 percent of people who become infected in this two-step fashion progress to chronic hepatitis D.

LONG-TERM PROGNOSIS FOR THOSE WITH CHRONIC HEPATITIS B AND HEPATITIS D

Compared with people who have chronic hepatitis B alone, those with chronic infections of both HBV and HDV are more likely to have a poor outcome. These people tend to develop cirrhosis more frequently and more rapidly. Approximately 60 to 70 percent of all people with chronic hepatitis D develop cirrhosis, and 15 percent of them may develop cirrhosis as little as two years from the time of initial infection. This is much more frequent, and more rapid, than for any other form of chronic viral hepatitis. People with both chronic hepatitis B and chronic hepatitis D are also more likely to develop complications, such as liver failure, and are more likely to require a liver transplant.

While progression of disease is more rapid in people with both hepatitis B and hepatitis D, it is not clear whether these people who are doubly infected have a greater risk of developing liver cancer than those infected with HBV alone. In fact, some researchers believe that HDV may actually suppress the replication of HBV as some studies have noted a reduced incidence of liver cancer in those who are doubly infected. More research needs to be done in this area before definitive conclusions about the interaction between these viruses can be drawn.

CONCLUSION

In this chapter, you learned about two hepatitis viruses that can damage the liver: hepatitis B virus (HBV) and hepatitis delta virus (HDV). These viruses lead to the liver diseases hepatitis B and hepatitis D, respectively. The treatment of hepatitis B and D will be discussed in Chapter 12 and prevention will be discussed in Chapter 24. In cases where treatment fails, a person may be a candidate for liver transplantation. This surgical procedure will be discussed in Chapter 22. Meanwhile, the next chapter discusses another viral infection—the hepatitis C virus (HCV). This virus can cause both acute and chronic hepatitis C. Though HCV has some similarities to HBV and HDV, it also has many important differences.

10

Understanding Hepatitis C

After feeling rundown for about a year, Sue, a thirty-six-year-old office manager and mother of three, finally went to see her family doctor. After examining her and drawing some blood, the doctor said, "Sue, you look fine. You probably just need to slow down a little." Sue went home feeling relieved. She was going to start planning a vacation for herself. But when the doctor called a week later to inform her that her blood tests revealed a problem with her liver, she was shocked. And even more so when subsequent blood tests revealed that she had chronic hepatitis C. "How could I have contracted hepatitis C?" Sue wondered. "Could it have been that summer when I experimented a few times with intravenous drugs? But how could that be? That was twenty years ago and it only happened a few times!" Sue's doctor advised her to see a specialist.

For many years, Jack, a fifty-year-old accountant with long work hours, had donated blood annually at his local Red Cross chapter. Somewhere around 1990, he stopped for a few years, for no specific reason, then decided to start again. About a week after donating two pints of blood, Jack received a letter from the blood bank stating that they could no longer accept his blood for donation—he had tested positive for the hepatitis C antibody (HCV Ab). Jack could not believe what he was reading. He was in great physical shape! Moreover, he'd never experimented with recreational drugs of any kind and only drank alcohol at social gatherings. He'd been in the same monogamous relationship ever since his senior year of high school. He'd never been jaundiced and never received a blood transfusion. In fact, with the exception of minor

colds, he had never really been sick. The letter was a mistake, Jack con-
cluded, but made an appointment to see his doctor anyway.

During his exam, Jack's doctor told him that his past blood work
never revealed any kind of problem with his liver. He would need to run
additional blood tests to confirm the diagnosis of hepatitis C. The tests
were performed, but the results would take two weeks to return.

The waiting period was difficult for Jack and his wife. During that
time, they researched hepatitis C on the Internet. The more information
they read, the more worried they became. Two weeks later, Jack's doc-
tor told him that he had tested positive for the hepatitis C antibody, so
it appeared that at some point in the past he'd been exposed to the hep-
atitis C virus (HCV). (But from the information Jack provided, they
couldn't figure out when or how.) There was good news, however:
Jack's hepatitis C virus load was non-detectable. It appeared that he
was among the approximately 15 percent of the population who had
been exposed to HCV, but had not developed a chronic infection.

This chapter discusses the hepatitis C virus (HCV)—how it is transmitted and who is at risk for contracting it. It clarifies the difference between the acute and chronic forms of the disease and the reason why such a high percentage of people who are exposed to HCV become chronically infected. In addition, this chapter covers the various ways that an HCV infection is diagnosed and what signs and symptoms are common to this virus. Also, the diagnostic blood tests related to HCV are explained. Towards the end of this.chapter, the probable long-term outcome of chronic hepatitis C and some risk factors that promote disease progression will be covered. (See Chapter 13 for a detailed discussion of the treatment of hepatitis C.)

WHAT IS HEPATITIS C?

Hepatitis C is inflammation of the liver due to a virus called the hepatitis C virus (HCV). After the discovery of hepatitis A virus in 1973 and hepatitis B virus in 1963, the remaining hepatitis viruses were lumped into the category of *non-A non-B (NANB) hepatitis*. Any cases of acute or chronic hepatitis or cirrhosis without identifiable causes were suspected to be a result of the NANB hepatitis viruses. In 1989, a major breakthrough regarding this mysterious and intriguing disease occurred—the hepatitis C virus was identified. Now, HCV is believed to be the virus responsible for about 90 percent of all cases of NANB hepatitis.

HCV is the most common cause of chronic liver disease in the United States. Over 4 million Americans (approximately 2 percent of the United States population) and more than 1 percent of the world's population are infected with HCV. The Centers for Disease Control (CDC) estimate that only a small percentage (probably around 5 percent) of infected individuals are even aware that they harbor this virus in their bodies. While the incidence of people becoming acutely infected with HCV is decreasing, approximately 8,000 to 12,000 deaths are attributed to hepatitis C each year. Moreover, it is estimated that this number will triple within the next two decades. In fact, chronic hepatitis C is the most common reason that a person will need to undergo a liver transplant in the United States.

HOW HCV IS TRANSMITTED

Most people are surprised to learn they have hepatitis C. Many people believe they were never at risk for acquiring this virus. They, therefore, cannot imagine how they contracted it. Other people have a definable risk factor, such as a history of intravenous drug use, but feel that it occurred such a long time ago that it has no relevance. And some people know exactly how they contracted it.

There are, in fact, many ways that a person can contract HCV. The most efficient mode of transmission is via blood-to-blood contact. This means that blood from an infected person gets into the bloodstream of another person. HCV can only enter the bloodstream by first getting through the protective covering of skin. This is known as the *percutaneous route.* Read on for more information about all these routes of transmission.

Blood and Blood Product Transfusions

It has been estimated by the Centers for Disease Control (CDC) that almost 300,000 Americans have contracted HCV (prior to the advent of screening of donated blood and blood products for HCV) as a result of receiving HCV-infected blood—packed red blood cells (PRBC) or blood products, such as platelets, fresh frozen plasma (FFP), or immune globulin. In addition, it has been estimated that almost 1 percent of all potential blood donors are infected with HCV. Fortunately, blood banks have been screening all potential donors for HCV since 1990. And since 1992, these screening techniques have been exceptionally accurate.

Today, the incidence of obtaining this virus by receiving a blood transfusion is approximately 1 in 200,000 units of blood transfused (the risk of infection is 0.001 percent per unit of blood transfused). In essence, the likelihood of contracting HCV from a blood transfusion has been minuscule since 1992. The reason that this small risk still exists is that when a person initially becomes infected with HCV for a short period of time, known as *the window period,* the HCV antibody (HCV Ab) is not detectable in the blood. If this person donates blood during the window period, her blood will carry HCV, but it will not be detectable.

It is recommended that anyone who received a blood transfusion prior to 1992 be tested for HCV. In fact, in 1998, the United States Surgeon General recommended putting into action a "look-back" program, aimed at identifying and notifying people who had a blood transfusion prior to 1992 from a HCV-positive blood donor.

Please note: Once somebody has tested positive for HCV, she should refrain from donating blood or organs.

Intravenous Drug Use

Currently, intravenous drug use (IVDU) is the most common way of transmitting HCV, and it accounts for approximately 60 percent of all new HCV infections. HCV has been found in approximately 85 to 100 percent of IV drug users—this compares to a finding of HIV, the virus that causes AIDS, in approximately 30 percent of IV drug users. The longer a person uses IV drugs, the greater the likelihood she has of becoming infected with HCV. HCV is transmitted from one person to another through the sharing of needles and/or other drug paraphernalia. Even a speck of blood so small that it is undetectable to the human eye can carry a great deal of hepatitis C viral particles. Therefore, drug paraphernalia that appears to be adequately cleaned may still contain HCV.

The decades of the 1960s and 1970s were characterized by considerable experimentation and rebellion. Intravenous drug use was sometimes a part of the culture that prevailed during this era. Though many users were aware that IV drug use was illegal, they were not aware that it had the potential to transmit a serious viral infection (that had not even as yet been identified) into their livers. For some, IV drug use was a daily occurrence. Others may have tried it only once or twice. But even a one-time occurrence long ago still has relevance. Remember, HCV can reside in the body for many years, clandestinely doing damage to the liver even though the person feels fine.

Intranasal Drug Use

Intranasal drug use, or "snorting" drugs, is also a potential route of virus transmission. Small blood vessels in the nose may break open and bleed when an instrument such as a straw or a rolled-up dollar bill is used to snort a drug, such as cocaine. Most of the time, the amount of blood on the instrument is so small that it is undetectable. When these instruments are shared, HCV can pass from one person to the other. Once again, engaging in this activity even only once may be sufficient to cause a person to contract HCV.

Health-Care and Occupational Exposure

Anyone who works in a health-care facility, including a hospital, doctor's office, dentist's office, or a laboratory that handles blood specimens, and emergency medical technicians, are at risk of contracting HCV. Public safety workers, such as firemen and correction officers, may also be exposed to blood due to the nature of their jobs and, therefore, are also at risk for becoming infected with HCV. The virus may be transmitted through a needle stick injury, a blood spill, or through pricking oneself with a contaminated sharp instrument. The larger the amount of contaminated blood that enters a person's body, the higher the likelihood she will become infected. After a single incident of accidental exposure to HCV, the risk of contracting HCV is approximately 2 percent—although this probability has been reported to range between 0 and 16 percent. (For comparison, the probability of contracting HBV by this route is 15 to 30 percent and for contracting HIV it is 0.3 percent.) Even with the potential risk to health-care workers due to the nature of their profession, the prevalence of HCV infection among this group of professionals is actually about the same as that of the general population, which is 1 to 2 percent.

Medical Procedures

Medical knowledge of appropriate hygiene practices has advanced considerably over the past several decades. In the past, unsterile medical practices, such as reusing needles, was common. This may partly explain the discovery of chronic hepatitis C in older individuals who have no other definable risk factor. Similarly, people who received vaccinations prior to the widespread use of disposable needles may have acquired the virus through this means. And, while transmission of HCV from infected health-care workers to patients, such as during cardiovascular surgery, has been reported, these incidences are extremely rare, and the risk of this mode of transmission is not considered significant.

A more significant risk is found in people with kidney failure. These people are often treated by *hemodialysis*—a medical procedure that involves removing the blood through an artery, cleaning it, and then returning it to the person through her vein. People undergoing hemodialysis have been found to have an increased risk of acquiring HCV. In fact, it is estimated that in the United States, approximately 20 to 30 percent of hemodialysis patients are infected with HCV. This is due to a combination of receiving frequent blood transfusions prior to 1992, possible inadequate sterilization of equipment used during the hemodialysis procedure, and the possible sharing of supplies among patients. Fortunately, the incidence of chronic hepatitis C in this group of people is decreasing due to the use of universal precautions in dialysis units and improved methods of screening transfused blood.

Another medical procedure that puts people at risk of contracting HCV is undergoing organ transplants. People may become infected with HCV by receiving an organ, such as a kidney, an eye, a heart, and even a liver from a person infected with HCV. If an organ donor is infected with HCV, there is approximately a 50-percent chance that she will transmit the virus to the transplant recipient. Since there is a shortage of liver donors, some transplant centers will utilize the liver of a hepatitis-C-positive organ donor for transplant to a person with hepatitis C who requires a new liver. Unfortunately, prior infection with HCV will not protect the transplant recipient from developing another HCV infection with a different HCV genotype. (See page 124 for a discussion of HCV genotypes.)

Tattooing and Body Piercing

Tattooing and body piercing, including piercing the ears, are practices that involve breaking the skin with a needle. In the course of these procedures, a small amount of bleeding can occur. If the needles, ink, or other equipment that are used during these practices are not sterile, HCV may be transmitted as one customer's HCV-infected blood makes its way into the bloodstream of a subsequent customer. However, this mode of HCV transmission has not been documented as a significant form of transmission in the United States.

Sexual Contact

Sexual contact, whether it is genital, oral, or anal, appears to be an extremely inefficient means of HCV transmission. In fact, many studies evaluating this route of transmission have failed to detect the presence of HCV in either the saliva, semen, or urine of HCV-infected people—except when these body fluids have been contaminated by the person's blood. However, it is important to emphasize that HCV has the potential to be transmitted through intimate contact if there are breaks in the skin or in the lining of the mouth, vagina, or anus. This may occur for a variety of reasons including the presence of active, bleeding herpes sores; an inflamed and infected prostate gland, known as prostatitis; or as a result of traumatic or rough sex, especially anal intercourse.

HCV has been detected with greater-than-average frequency among people who have a history of sexual promiscuity. While there is no exact definition for sexual promiscuity, one study published in the *New England Journal of Medicine* defines it as a "history of a sexually transmitted disease, sex with a prostitute, more than five sexual partners per year, or a combination of these." Of interest is that it appears to be easier for a man to transmit HCV to a woman than vice versa.

A person who is in a long-term monogamous relationship with an HCV-infected person rarely contracts this virus. Only approximately 2 percent (a range of 0 to 6 percent) of sexual partners of HCV-infected people also test positive for HCV. However, it is important to note that this statistic is based on indirect evidence only. Therefore, whether these people became infected through a sexual act or by another route is unclear. For example, people in long-standing relationships generally care for one another in times of illness or injury. During such times, HCV may be transmitted to the spouse or partner as blood-barrier precautions may not always be taken into consideration—even among the most cautious of couples.

Household Contact

Transmission of HCV among family members or other people living together may occur. This potentially can happen through the sharing of razors, toothbrushes, or any sharp instruments that carry HCV-infected blood. Therefore, it is crucial to keep all personal items, such as toothbrushes, in a separate part of the bathroom or specifically labeled. In this manner, the accidental use of a potentially HCV-infected household item will be decreased. The incidence of contracting HCV from accidental household contact in the United States is unknown. However, data from other countries indicate that it is low—approximately 4 percent.

Childbirth

Of great concern to pregnant women infected with HCV and to women with chronic hepatitis C who are contemplating pregnancy is the likelihood of transmitting the virus to their babies. If this occurs during pregnancy, it is known as *vertical transmission,* and if it occurs around the time of birth, it is known as *perinatal transmission.* However, the risk for either of these types of transmission is very low— occurring only approximately 3 to 5 percent of the time. Transmission to the newborn has been found to occur only in HCV-infected women who had high viral loads (the amount of HCV viral particles per milliliter of blood) of at least 1 million. It has also been noted that women who are doubly infected with HIV and HCV appear to have a higher probability of transmitting HCV to their children than women who are not infected with HIV.

Breast-feeding is not considered a means of transmitting HCV. Therefore, it is believed that an HCV-infected mother may safely breast-feed her child. In fact, studies comparing the incidence of HCV in breast-fed versus bottle-fed infants whose mothers were infected with HCV showed a fairly equal incidence of HCV in each group of infants—approximately 4 percent.

Sporadic Hepatitis C

Some people who have hepatitis C state that they cannot identify a risk factor to account for their HCV infection. This group of people has been classified as having *sporadic hepatitis C.* In some studies, sporadic hepatitis C accounts for up to 40 percent of cases of chronic hepatitis C. Note, however, that some people who have sporadic hepatitis C probably do have an identifiable risk factor, but may be concealing it for personal reasons. They may have a fear of a lack of confidentiality on the part of their doctors, they may have a fear of being judged as having done something bad in the past, or they may have a fear of being rejected for life or medical insurance. Others do not consider a certain behavior to count as a risk—behaviors such as having a body part pierced or an isolated occurrence of intravenous or intranasal drug use—and therefore deny it when questioned. In fact, in one study, many former IV drug users with hepatitis C who attempted to donate blood, denied their IV drug use when screened at the time of blood donation, as they felt that their former habit was such an insignificant event that it would not affect the purity of their blood. Others feel that an episode that happened long ago doesn't count anymore, and, therefore, they don't disclose it to their doctors. Finally, some people simply do not recall the incident that caused the infection.

Other Routes of Transmission

Though the reasons are not entirely clear, some population groups, such as in certain parts of Africa and Japan have been found to have a particularly high incidence of hepatitis C. Some indigenous healing or folk-medicine practices common to these regions, which involve skin-piercing (often with unsterilized instruments), are suspected to account for the increased transmission of the virus. In other countries, mass immunization programs are suspected to be a method of transmission—such as the immunization in Egypt against the parasitic worm called *schistosomiasis.*

Another potential, yet unlikely, route of transmission involves insects. Theoretically, transmission by insects can only occur if an insect first bites an HCV-infected person then immediately bites someone else. In this way, the HCV-tainted blood could enter the second person. Viruses other than HCV, such as yellow fever and dengue, have been shown to spread by this route. One study conducted in New Jersey concluded that mosquitoes are unlikely agents of transmission of HCV. Therefore, while not believed to be a significant source of HCV transmission, further investigation into the area of insect transmission is needed.

In some societies, cults and fraternity members mix their blood together as part of a ritual or in order to be inaugurated. Sometimes, people will mix their blood with that of a close friend in a process by which they become "blood brothers." This potential mode of HCV transmission also warrants further investigation.

Finally, even going to the barber or to a manicurist may be a risk factor. If instruments are not properly cleansed, they can potentially carry a small amount of HCV. Similarly, people undergoing acupuncture or electrolysis are at risk of becoming infected with HCV if the needles and other equipment being used have not been properly sterilized.

THOSE AT INCREASED RISK FOR HEPATITIS C

Unlike hepatitis A and B, hepatitis C is not preventable through vaccination. However, there are other measures that a person can take to minimize her chances of acquiring HCV. In addition, many precautions may be taken by an HCV-infected person so as to reduce the likelihood of transmitting this virus to others. Prevention of HCV will be discussed in Chapter 24. Meanwhile, take note of the following individuals who are at increased risk for contracting HCV:

- People who have received blood or a blood-product transfusion prior to 1992 and especially prior to 1990.

- Intravenous-drug users, past and present.

- Household members of an infected person.

- Hospital and other health-care facility workers.

- Public-safety workers.

- People who have acquired a tattoo or who have had a body part pierced.

- People who have had multiple sexual partners, especially where there is a history of a sexually transmitted disease.

- People who have been born to a mother infected with HCV, especially if the mother has a high viral load.

- Organ transplant recipients of an HCV-infected organ.

- Hemodialysis patients.

WHAT IS ACUTE HEPATITIS C?

Acute hepatitis C is defined as inflammation of the liver due to HCV, lasting six months or less. The number of people who become acutely infected with HCV has been steadily decreasing over the years. For example, in 1984 approximately 180,000 to 230,000 new acute infections were estimated to have occurred, compared with only 28,000 to 35,000 new acute infections estimated in 1996. The reason for the declining incidence of newly acquired infections is not entirely known, but it has been associated with a decrease in acute hepatitis C among IV drug users. Increased knowledge and publicity about HIV, the virus that causes AIDS, has probably contributed to a decrease in the sharing of drug paraphernalia among IV drug users, thereby resulting in a decreased incidence in HCV transmission. Increased knowledge and awareness about HCV transmission and prevention, as well as improved diagnostic testing for the screening of blood and organ donors may have contributed to this decline. As knowledge of hepatitis C continues to grow, the number of people who become infected with HCV will likely diminish even further.

The Symptoms and Signs of Acute Hepatitis C

The *incubation period*—the time between the entrance of the virus into the body and the initial appearance of symptoms and signs of the disease—of HCV is about six to eight weeks; however, it may be as short as two weeks or even as long as about five months.

The symptoms of acute hepatitis C are usually similar to those that commonly occur in a person suffering from acute hepatitis regardless of the cause (see page 74). However, most people with acute hepatitis C experience no symptoms. Only about 25 to 35 percent of the individuals with hepatitis C manifest any symptoms at all. Usually, these symptoms are nonspecific and may easily be mistaken as stemming from something unconnected to hepatitis C, such as the flu. Symptoms, if they do occur, may include fatigue, decreased appetite, and weakness. Occasionally, a person may experience a skin rash and/or muscle and joint aches. People with acute hepatitis C become jaundiced approximately 25 percent of the time. It has been shown that people with another liver disease, such as hepatitis B, who become additionally infected with acute hepatitis C, are particularly likely to experience a severe course of acute hepatitis C. Usually, the physical exam of a person with acute hepatitis C appears normal. Occasionally, a physical exam will reveal an enlarged tender liver, jaundice, and/or a rash.

Diagnosing Acute Hepatitis C

As mentioned previously, approximately 28,000 to 35,000 new acute hepatitis C infections are estimated to occur each year. However, it is also estimated that only 25 to 30 percent of these newly acquired infections are actually diagnosed. The most likely explanation for this low percentage is that most people with acute hepatitis C are either asymptomatic or have very vague symptoms. Therefore, evaluation by a doctor during the acute stage of this disease is a rare occurrence. As such, the majority of people with hepatitis C do not discover that they harbor this virus until years or, often, decades later. Therefore, there are probably thousands of people who currently have hepatitis C and have no idea that they are infected. However, if a person sees her doctor for an evaluation of symptoms, acute hepatitis C is usually detected from abnormal blood test results.

Transaminases (AST and ALT) are often quite elevated initially. Levels of approximately 200 to 600 IU/L can occur. (The normal range is approximately 0 to 45 IU/L.) Elevations in transaminases usually occur approximately six to eight weeks after infection with HCV (or within a range of two to twenty-six weeks). As the disease progresses, transaminases typically decrease. Transaminase levels often fluctuate between normal, or near normal, and elevated before permanently returning to normal. This fluctuation is a typical characteristic of hepatitis C. Persistent normalization of transaminases by six months usually indicates that acute hepatitis C has resolved. This occurs 15 percent of the time. If transaminases remain elevated (usually around two to three times normal) after this period or if the ALT levels elevate after a period of normalization, it usually indicates progression to chronic hepatitis C (see page 117), which occurs approximately 85 percent of the time. Progression to chronic disease is always accompanied by an elevated HCV viral load.

Cholestatic liver enzymes (AP and GGTP) are usually only mildly elevated during acute hepatitis C—around two to three times normal—and bilirubin levels are usually normal. Around one-fourth of all people with acute hepatitis C become jaundiced. Even among these people, bilirubin levels usually normalize rapidly, usually within about one month.

None of these blood test abnormalities are diagnostic of acute hepatitis C. But once the doctor detects abnormal LFTs, additional blood work specific for hepatitis C, known as the hepatitis C serology, will be performed (see page 122). From the results of these tests, which detect antibodies to the hepatitis C virus and the hepatitis C viral load, the doctor will be able to determine if the LFT abnormalities are due to hepatitis C.

Imaging studies are typically normal and are not needed to make a diagnosis of hepatitis C. If performed, imaging studies are generally done in order to eliminate other possible causes of elevated LFTs, such as gallstones. A liver biopsy is usually not performed during the acute stage of a hepatitis C infection.

Determining Whether Acute Hepatitis C Has Resolved

After the diagnosis of acute hepatitis C has been made, the doctor will probably want to see the patient several times over the next few months in order to check on the status of the infection. Six months after the patient has been infected, the doctor will determine whether the patient has shaken off HCV entirely or whether she has progressed to chronic hepatitis C.

Hepatitis C is limited to acute infection in only around 15 percent of all people (like Jack in the story at the beginning of this chapter). These fortunate people have a total resolution of symptoms, physical signs, and any LFT abnormalities due to infection with HCV. Also, their HCV RNA by PCR will permanently return to normal (see page 123 for clarification of these terms). These people do not develop chronic infection and, therefore, are not at risk for the long-term consequences of hepatitis C. Furthermore, they are now immune to hepatitis C. They can never get it again nor can they transmit it to others. However, immunity against HCV does not protect a person from other hepatitis viruses, such as hepatitis A or B. Also, these people will never be allowed to donate blood, as they will always have the antibody for hepatitis C present in their blood.

WHAT IS FULMINANT HEPATITIS C?

Fulminant hepatitis C is a very rare but severe form of acute hepatitis C. It is characterized by the sudden onset of liver failure, coagulopathy, jaundice, and encephalopathy. Patients become severely ill and develop a rapidly progressive downhill course. Approximately 85 percent of these people are likely to die unless immediate liver transplantation is undertaken. Fortunately, this complication of acute hepatitis C is a very rare occurrence.

WHAT IS CHRONIC HEPATITIS C?

Chronic hepatitis C is defined as inflammation of the liver caused by HCV that continues for more than six months. In people with chronic hepatitis C, the immune system has failed to clear the virus from the body. Therefore, all individuals with chronic hepatitis C will have an elevated HCV RNA. Once a person is chronically infected with HCV, the potential exists for liver damage and cirrhosis along with its complications, including liver failure and liver cancer. (The treatment of chronic hepatitis C will be discussed in Chapter 13.)

The Reason So Many Cases of Acute Hepatitis C Become Chronic

When a person becomes infected with HCV, it is very difficult for her to clear the virus from her body. Once most people become infected with HCV (acute hepatitis C), they develop chronic disease (chronic hepatitis C). In fact, approximately 85 percent of infected people develop chronic hepatitis C. This is in stark contrast to the incidence of progression from acute to chronic in other forms of viral hepatitis. For example, hepatitis B progresses to chronic disease only about 5 percent of the time when the infection is acquired as an adult. And hepatitis A never leads to chronic disease. It appears that the immune system is not very efficient in clearing HCV. So, what makes HCV so formidable?

The genes that make up HCV can vary slightly from one HCV to another. These different genetic variations of HCV are known as *hepatitis C mutants*, or *quasispecies*. The entire hepatitis C viral population that is present in a person infected with HCV is made up of a conglomerate of related, yet slightly different, HCV species. This virus population usually consists of one HCV mutant group that is stronger and dominant and numerous other HCV mutants that are weaker. These mutants are all similar in structure but differ slightly from one another. These slight variations in structure account for the fact that some HCV mutants are stronger and thus better equipped to fight the immune system than other HCV mutants. This is analogous to Darwin's theory of evolution: the survival of the fittest.

The fact that HCV is such a clever and conniving virus probably accounts for why most people progress to chronic disease. When HCV is being attacked by the immune system during the acute infection, HCV can mutate into a stronger quasispecies variant. In this manner, HCV is able to outwit the body's immune system and fail any attempt to eradicate it. Thus, HCV tricks the bodies' immune surveillance and escapes eradication, allowing for progression to chronic disease. This explains why long-term response rates to therapy with interferon (see Chapter 13) have been somewhat disappointing. It also may explain why it is so difficult to create a vaccination against HCV (see Chapter 24).

Risk factors determining which people are most likely to progress to chronic disease have not yet been identified. Excessive alcohol consumption is probably one risk factor, but this requires further study to say for sure.

The Symptoms and Signs of Chronic Hepatitis C

Most people with chronic hepatitis C are surprised to find out that they harbor this virus. This is because even at advanced stages of the disease, symptoms are usually absent. This is true even in some people who have progressed to cirrhosis. And, as with many other liver diseases, if symptoms are present, they are usually nonspecific. Only approximately 20 percent of people with chronic hepatitis C experience symptoms—most commonly fatigue and generalized weakness. Some people complain of vague abdominal discomfort, often in the area over the liver. Still others suffer with a decreased appetite, weight loss, and depression. The severity or lack of symptoms is not a good indicator of the amount of liver inflammation and damage.

Physical findings are often normal in people with chronic hepatitis C. An enlarged, tender liver is rarely detected. Other physical findings, such as an enlarged spleen (splenomegaly) or jaundice, may be indicative of cirrhosis. In general, symptoms and signs of chronic hepatitis C will not provide the basis for its diagnosis.

People with chronic hepatitis C often have symptoms and signs of infection that are manifested in organs other than the liver, known as *extrahepatic* manifestations. This is partly due to the fact that other parts of the body are often caught in the crossfire when the immune system fights against an HCV infection. These extrahepatic symptoms are known as immune-complex mediated diseases. The following is a brief discussion of some of the extrahepatic manifestations of chronic hepatitis C.

Skin Diseases

Vasculitis—inflammation of blood vessels—may present (show up during a doctor's initial examination of a patient) as a raised, purplish skin discoloration, known as *purpura,* which is most commonly located on the legs. This discoloration is due to the leakage of blood under the skin.

Porphyria cutanea tarda (PCT) is a skin abnormality that may present as easy bruising of the skin, in addition to blisters that are sensitive to the sun and bleed easily. Areas of increased or decreased skin pigmentation and increased hair growth, known as *hirsuitism,* may also be associated with PCT. In addition to HCV, alcohol, excessive iron, and estrogens are believed to precipitate the manifestations of PCT in predisposed people.

Lichen planus is a raised, itchy skin rash that often occurs in the mouth, hair, and nails.

Several other skin changes have been noted to occur in association with chronic hepatitis C, but further study needs to be conducted to clarify their significance.

Hematological (Blood-Related) Diseases

Cryoglobulinemia (excess proteins in the blood) presents with purpura, joint aches (known as *arthralgias),* and weakness. Cryoglobulinemia may also affect the kidneys, brain, and nerves. Although cryoglobulinemia has been found in approximately 40 percent of all individuals with chronic hepatitis C, only about half of these people experience symptoms related to cryoglobulinemia.

Lymphoma is a malignant tumor of the lymphoid tissue (cells related to the immune system) that has infrequently been found in people with chronic hepatitis C.

Idiopathic thrombocytopenic purpura (ITP) is a disease characterized by an abnormally low platelet count of unclear origin and is generally manifested in the form of a rash. It is believed to be caused by an immune attack on platelets. A consequence of ITP may be a bleeding disorder, as the function of platelets is to facilitate the clotting of blood.

Endocrine Disorders

Thyroid disorders, both *hypothyroid* (an overly slow thyroid) and *hyperthyroid* (an overly fast thyroid) have been noted to occur in approximately 5 percent of the individuals with chronic hepatitis C. These disorders often worsen once therapy with interferon (see Chapter 13) has been initiated.

Diabetes—elevated blood sugar (glucose) levels—has been found to be present in many people with chronic hepatitis C in some studies, but further study is needed to confirm this association.

Eye Disorders

Although multiple eye disorders have been found in some people with chronic hepatitis C, a direct association has not been proven. However, all of the following have been reported to have occurred in people with chronic hepatitis C: ulcers in the cornea of the eye, known as *Mooren's corneal ulcers; uveitis,* which is inflammation of the uvea (the middle layer of the eye); *Behcet's syndrome*—a syndrome associated with uveitis and ulcers of the mouth and genitalia; and *Sjögren's syndrome* (dry eyes and dry mouth) have all been reported to occur in people with chronic hepatitis C.

Kidney Disorders

Inflammation of the kidney, known as *glomerulonephritis,* has been associated with chronic hepatitis C. Occasionally, people with this kidney disorder have either blood or excess protein in their urine.

Musculoskeletal Disorders

Muscle weakness and joint pain have been noted to occur in people with chronic hepatitis C. These people often also have associated cryoglobulinemia. Further study needs to be conducted to confirm these associations.

Other Problems

Other rare, unsubstantiated associations found in people with chronic hepatitis C include *pulmonary fibrosis* (lung scarring); a type of vasculitis known as *polyarteritis nodosa* (PAN); and *vitiligo,* a loss of skin pigmentation. Further studies will need to be conducted in order to confirm that these disorders are associated with chronic hepatitis C.

DIAGNOSING CHRONIC HEPATITIS C

Most people find out that they have chronic hepatitis C purely by accident. Since the majority of people either have vague symptoms or no symptoms at all, an evaluation for hepatitis C is usually prompted by the discovery of abnormal LFTs—most commonly and characteristically ALT. (See Chapter 3 for more information on LFTs.) These abnormalities may be found during a routine annual physical, during a physical for a life insurance application, or during a medical evaluation for an unrelated problem. Others discover that they have chronic hepatitis C in the course of seeing their family doctors for the evaluation of one of the nonspecific symptoms associated with chronic hepatitis C, such as fatigue or loss of appetite.

Sometimes a specialist, rather than the family doctor, will discover that a person has chronic hepatitis C—perhaps during an evaluation of one of the extrahepatic manifestations of hepatitis C discussed on page 119. Others seek medical evaluation for ascites or jaundice and, therefore, find out that they have chronic hepatitis C when the disease is already far advanced.

Some people learn that they have chronic hepatitis C when they are rejected for blood donation due to testing positive for the hepatitis C antibody. The hepatitis C test that is used for blood-donor screening is known as the ELISA, which stands for enzyme-linked immunosorbent assay (see page 122). Approximately 40 percent (a range of 30 to 70 percent) of people who test positive for HCV by this screening blood test actually do not have hepatitis C. This is known as a *false-positive test*. Therefore, if a person tests positive by the ELISA method of HCV detection, it is imperative that she be tested again, using a more accurate method known as RIBA (recombinant immunoblot assay). The following is a discussion of the diagnostic tests used to diagnose chronic hepatitis C.

Liver Function Tests (LFTs)

Transaminases (ALT and AST) are elevated in approximately 70 percent of all individuals with chronic hepatitis C. The ALT value is more likely to be elevated and it is more characteristic of a hepatitis C infection than an AST elevation. In fact, the ALT level is often used as a marker of HCV inflammation, even though it is not an accurate indicator of the extent of inflammation in the liver. In people with chronic hepatitis C, ALT and AST levels usually range from approximately 80 to 180 IU/L. This is around two to four times the upper limit of normal (normal value being approximately 0 to 45 IU/L). But the person may have values as high as 450 IU/L or as low as 46 IU/L and still have chronic hepatitis C.

There are two important characteristics that apply to the transaminase levels in people with chronic hepatitis C. First, transaminase levels in people with chronic hepatitis C typically fluctuate. Some days, transaminase levels are very abnormal and other days, transaminase levels will be near normal, or even normal. But the fact that transaminases have decreased or normalized does not indicate that chronic hepatitis C has improved or has gone away. By the next day, week, or year, the transaminase levels may be elevated again. Second, the level of elevation of transaminases usually bears little correlation with the severity of liver disease caused by HCV, and, furthermore, the level of elevation rarely predicts the outcome of disease.

Regardless of the degree of transaminase elevation, the findings on liver biopsy specimens may range anywhere from mild inflammation to advanced cirrhosis. However, some studies have found that elevations persistently greater than ten times the normal value are a predictor of excessive liver scarring.

Approximately one-third of people with chronic hepatitis C have transaminase levels that are persistently normal. This means that transaminase levels have never been elevated. Despite normal transaminase levels, these people have an elevated HCV RNA. Thus, these people are often referred to by some experts as "healthy chronic carriers" of HCV. However, further research is needed to confirm the validity of this designation. Approximately 80 percent of these people never experience any significant consequences due to chronic hepatitis C. However, it is thought that up to 20 percent of hepatitis-C patients with persistently normal transaminase levels will worsen and suffer from severe liver disease. Also, there does not appear to be any concrete factors that can predict which of these people will experience progressive disease and which ones will continue to remain stable with no long-term consequences due to HCV.

In summary, transaminase elevations provide little significant information about the nature of the liver disease caused by chronic hepatitis C. If levels are very elevated, they may predict severe damage of the liver in some people. In general, however, they merely provide a clue that something is wrong with the liver. Finally, transaminase levels do have some significance when used to monitor a person's response to therapy (see Chapter 13).

In people with chronic hepatitis C, bilirubin levels are usually normal unless the person has advanced liver disease. GGTP is often mildly abnormal. Immunoglobulin G is usually elevated, but has no value in determining a prognosis. Iron studies (iron, ferritin, and transferrin saturation), which will be discussed in Chapter 18, are often elevated in people with chronic hepatitis C and are generally associated with increased inflammation and damage of the liver.

Hepatitis C Antibody Tests

Blood tests to determine the presence of the hepatitis C antibody (HCV Ab) in the body are necessary in order to make a diagnosis of hepatitis C. These tests determine whether the immune system is producing antibodies against one or more of the hepatitis C antigens (see page 81 for a brief explanation of antigens and antibodies). The presence of the antibody to HCV may indicate that a person was previously exposed to hepatitis C, or, alternatively, it may indicate that a person is currently infected with HCV. It is not possible to determine which scenario applies in a given case from the mere presence of the antibody alone. Therefore, the presence of the HCV Ab does not mean that a person is either immune to, or in any way protected against HCV. Nor are these tests capable of distinguishing between acute and chronic hepatitis C. There are currently two blood tests readily available in the United States that can detect hepatitis C antibody in the blood. In fact, these tests are currently the only tests approved by the FDA for the diagnosis of hepatitis C. These tests are known as ELISA (enzyme-linked immunosorbent assay) and RIBA (recombinant immunoblot assay).

The ELISA I blood test was the first available screening test to detect the HCV Ab. Made commercially available in May 1990, this test detects the antibody against one of the hepatitis C antigens. ELISA I is capable of detecting HCV Ab approximately sixteen weeks after exposure to HCV. Therefore, since 1990, this test was available to all doctors to determine whether the cause of a person's elevated LFTs was in fact due to hepatitis C. This test was supplanted by the ELISA II in May 1992. ELISA II detects the antibody against four of the hepatitis C antigens, and is, therefore, significantly more accurate than the ELISA I test. ELISA II is capable of detecting HCV Ab in the blood approximately nine to ten weeks after exposure to HCV. ELISA III is the test used since May 1996 to screen blood products in the United States for HCV. This test detects the antibody against five of the hepatitis C antigens and is, therefore, more accurate than ELISA II. This blood test can detect the HCV Ab approximately six to eight weeks after exposure to HCV. All ELISA tests are typically reported as being positive or negative.

RIBA 2.0, made commercially available in June 1993, is supposed to be used as a supplemental blood test necessary in certain people once they have tested positive for HCV Ab by ELISA II who are at a low-risk for infection with HCV. These people include blood donors and individuals without an apparent risk factor such as intravenous drug use. RIBA 2.0 is a more accurate test than ELISA II, as it detects the exact HCV antigens that the HCV antibodies are reacting against. Therefore, it is typically the test most often ordered by the doctor to determine if her patient has HCV Ab. This test may be reported as being either positive, negative, or indeterminate. An indeterminate result must be carefully evaluated by a specialist to conclude if the result is really positive or negative. Additional, even more accurate tests for hepatitis C, such as RIBA 3.0, are currently being used in parts of Europe and are under investigation for use in the United States.

In 1999, the first over-the-counter home test was made available to the public to diagnose hepatitis C. This home test, called the "Hepatitis C Check," allows people to collect a sample of blood on their own at home and mail it to the appropriate laboratory for hepatitis C antibody testing. The results are available by phone within a week or two and are strictly confidential.

Hepatitis C Viral RNA

There are currently two tests commercially available since 1995 that can actually detect the amount of the HCV ribonucleic acid (HCV RNA—the genetic material of HCV) in the blood. They are HCV RNA RT-PCR and HCV bDNA. While neither the RT-PCR nor the bDNA test for HCV is currently FDA-approved, they are both routinely ordered by doctors to determine their patients' HCV RNA load. These tests can detect HCV in the blood approximately three days to two weeks after exposure to the virus.

HCV RNA RT-PCR measures HCV RNA by a technique known as reverse transcription-polymerase chain reaction (RT-PCR). Reverse transcriptase is an enzyme capable of copying deoxyribonucleic acid (DNA). PCR is a technique that allows the amplification (augmentation) of a small amount of the copied viral DNA to generate a large amount. This can then be readily detected via a routine blood sample.

This test is very sensitive as it is capable of detecting as little as 100 hepatitis C viral particles (viral genome copies) per milliliter of blood. However, the lowest level of detection typically depends upon the laboratory conducting the test and can range from 100 to 2,000 viral particles per milliliter of blood.

The other technique for determining HCV RNA is known as branched-chain DNA (bDNA). This test is not as sensitive as the RT-PCR test, as it is not capable of detecting less than 200,000 viral particles per milliliter of blood.

Both of these tests are capable of determining the presence—positive or negative (qualitative)—and/or the actual amount, also known as the viral load (quantitative), of HCV in the blood. These tests are used both to confirm that a person is infected with HCV and to monitor and predict response to antiviral treatment (see Chapter 13). A positive test also confirms that the person is infectious to others.

It is important to understand that the viral load usually does not correlate with the severity of liver disease. Therefore, a very high viral load (5 million viral particles/mL) does not automatically indicate that a person has more liver inflammation and damage than a person with a viral load of 500 viral particles/ml. Furthermore, the viral load typically fluctuates and does not correlate with the degree of elevation of the transaminases (AST and ALT).

Hepatitis C Antigen

Development of a blood test for the HCV antigen is currently under way. The preliminary results regarding its usefulness in the diagnosis of hepatitis C and in determining the response of hepatitis C to therapy appear to be very encouraging.

HCV Genotype

The term *HCV genotype* refers to the genetic makeup of the different HCV mutants in the hepatitis C viral population of a single person. There have been six different HCV genotypes clearly identified: genotypes 1 through 6. (However, some researchers believe that genotypes 7 through 11 also exist and that these genotypes may be common in parts of Asia.) The HCV genotype can be determined through a blood test—although not all insurance companies will cover the cost of this test.

One HCV genotype may differ genetically from another by as much as 35 percent. To further complicate matters, within each genotype, there exist at least two or three subtypes that may differ genetically from one another by about 15 percent. These subtypes are classified alphabetically as "a, b, and c." Different HCV genotypes are found in different areas of the world and among different groups of people. For example, in the United States, genotype 1a and 1b are the predominant HCV variants. And genotype 3a is believed to be the predominant HCV genotype among intravenous drug users in Europe.

What is the significance of HCV genotypes? First, some researchers have suggested that certain genotypes respond less favorably than others to interferon treatment (see Chapter 13). Specifically, studies have found that people with genotype 1, especially 1b, were less likely to have a long-lasting response to treatment with interferon as compared with people who have other HCV genotypes. However, many other factors, including viral diversity, viral load, immune status, age, gender, alcohol intake, and extent of liver damage, need to be taken into consideration when making treatment decisions. Second, some investigators believe that there is a correlation between genotype and the long-term outcome of people with chronic hepatitis C. A number of studies have shown that people with genotype 1b have a disproportionately more severe and aggressive course of disease. In these studies, people with HCV genotype 1b have been shown to develop cirrhosis and liver cancer more quickly and in a greater percentage of cases as compared with those who have other genotypes. However, other studies have concluded that there is insufficient proof of a relationship between genotype and the outcome of the disease.

Clearly, further investigation concerning HCV genotypes need to be conducted before any definitive conclusions concerning their significance can be drawn.

Imaging Studies

Usually the doctor will want to obtain at least one imaging study—typically a sonogram—as part of the diagnostic evaluation of chronic hepatitis C, especially when transaminases are elevated. While an enlarged liver or spleen may occasionally be detected, imaging studies are usually normal, even in advanced stages of disease. If liver cancer (hepatoma) is present, a mass may show up on the sonogram or other imaging study (see Chapter 19). Note, however, that just because the liver looks normal on an imaging study, it doesn't mean it actually is normal. In order to provide maximum information about the condition of the liver, a liver biopsy is necessary.

Liver Biopsy

As with all liver diseases, even if a person feels fine, that's no guarantee that her liver is fine. Furthermore, physical findings, LFT abnormalities, HCV RNA viral load, HCV genotype, and imaging studies cannot accurately determine the extent of liver inflammation and damage caused by HCV.

The only way to determine the degree to which a liver is inflamed and injured is by examining a sample of the liver under the microscope. A liver biopsy is the only reliable means of determining the presence or absence of cirrhosis. Thus, a liver biopsy is necessary in order to assess the amount of liver inflammation due to the virus—known as the *grade* of hepatitis C. It determines the amount of scarring or fibrosis on the liver—known as the *stage* of disease. The results obtained from a liver biopsy provide crucial information that is used to guide treatment decisions and to assess a person's long-term prognosis. See Chapter 5 for more information on liver biopsies.

THE LONG-TERM PROGNOSIS FOR THOSE WITH CHRONIC HEPATITIS C

Chronic hepatitis C progresses at a very slow pace. That means that most people will not develop significant liver inflammation or damage until at least fifteen to twenty years after becoming infected with the virus. Some may even take as long as forty to fifty years. And others may never develop serious liver disease.

It appears that cirrhosis develops in about 20 to 30 percent of all individuals with chronic hepatitis C within approximately twenty years after they are infected; however, percentages as high as 50 percent have been cited. Moreover, possibly more than half will develop cirrhosis approximately thirty or forty years after they are infected. Even after cirrhosis has developed, most people live long, healthy lives with chronic hepatitis C. However, once a person has developed one of the complications of cirrhosis, such as variceal bleeding or ascites, which is known as decompensated cirrhosis (see Chapter 6), she has a 50-percent chance of dying within the next five years. In a given year, decompensated cirrhosis occurs in approximately 4 percent of people with compensated cirrhosis.

From these statistics, it is apparent that some people with chronic hepatitis C have a relatively innocuous course of disease, while others have a more progressive and more serious course of disease. So the question is why do some people with chronic hepatitis C fare so much better than others? Unfortunately, no one knows the complete answer to this question, but there may be many contributing factors that can accelerate the rate of disease progression. Read on for a discussion of some of these factors.

Prognosis Based on Viral Characteristics

Viral characteristics are believed by some researchers to play a role in determining disease progression. However, results from studies on some of these parameters, such as viral load and transaminase elevation, have been inconsistent, and therefore, no definitive conclusion can be drawn. On the other hand, other parameters such as liver biopsy results appear to predict prognosis quite well. The following sets forth some of these factors.

Viral Load and Genotype

While some studies have pointed out that high viral loads exist in a disproportionately high percentage of people with advanced disease, other studies have concluded that the viral load does not affect disease progression.

While some studies have found that people with genotype 1, especially genotype 1b, have a particularly progressive disease course as compared with people who have other HCV genotypes, other studies have been unable to document any correlation between genotype and disease outcome. Therefore, the viral load and viral genotype appear to be unpredictable measures of prognosis.

Viral Diversity

Some researchers have found that the more diverse the population of HCV quasi-species is in a given person, the more likely it is that the person will progress to advanced disease. Further study needs to be conducted on HCV quasispecies before definitive conclusions can be drawn.

Transaminase Levels (ALT and AST)

As noted previously, the level of transaminase elevation correlates poorly with chronic hepatitis C disease progression or the development of advanced liver disease. Furthermore, some people with chronic hepatitis C have persistently normal transaminases. In fact, approximately one-third (1.3 million Americans) of all individuals with chronic hepatitis C have never had abnormal transaminase levels. It is believed by some experts that these people with persistently normal transaminase levels are possibly "healthy chronic carriers" of HCV, and thus, will have neither an aggressive course nor a poor outcome of disease.

One study demonstrated that liver disease progression in people with persistently normal ALT levels is at least twice as slow as in people with elevated ALT levels. And another study suggested that in people with persistently normal ALT levels, it may take about eighty years for cirrhosis to develop, especially if people refrain from drinking alcohol. By contrast, a few studies have shown significant damage associated with people with chronic hepatitis C who have normal ALT levels. Clearly, more research needs to be conducted on this group of people.

Liver Biopsy Results

As stressed in Chapter 5, the only real way to determine the extent of inflammation and damage in the liver is by sampling a piece of liver tissue. It has been shown that the amount of inflammation and scarring found in liver biopsy samples may determine a person's rate of progression to cirrhosis. For example, people found to have severe inflammation and scarring on a liver biopsy sample have been shown to progress to cirrhosis rapidly—in approximately ten years. Those with only mild inflammation and no scarring progress very slowly and are estimated to take many decades to advance to cirrhosis.

Prognosis Based on a Patient's Characteristics

Certain individual patient characteristics have been noted to have an impact on the course of the disease. These include age, gender, duration of infection, genetic predilection, immune status, and route of transmission.

Age and Gender

Some studies have found that people who become infected with HCV after the age of fifty-five appeared to have a more progressive course compared with people who became infected under the age of fifty-five. Also, some studies have found that men are as much as four times more likely to develop liver cancer due to HCV than women.

Duration of Infection

Some experts believe that since hepatitis C is a progressive disease, the longer a person is infected with the virus, the greater her chance of developing the possible complications of chronic hepatitis C, including cirrhosis, liver failure, and liver cancer.

Genetic Predilection

Some studies have suggested that some people infected with chronic hepatitis C may possess a genetic predilection that protects them from developing the complications that may arise from the disease. Similarly, it is possible that some people possess genetic characteristics that promote progression of liver disease due to HCV. Further studies need to be conducted to confirm these findings.

Route of Transmission

In people with chronic hepatitis C, the route by which the person became infected with HCV probably influences the course of the disease. Several studies have demonstrated that people who acquire HCV by a blood transfusion have a greater chance of developing significant liver disease than those who acquired HCV through other routes. This could be due to the fact that a large amount of hepatitis C viral particles may potentially be transmitted to a person in the course of a blood transfusion, whereas the sharing of a needle through illicit drug use (for example) provides the opportunity for a comparatively small amount of HCV to be transmitted. Fortunately, the application of accurate screening tests for HCV for all potential blood donors has made the transmission of HCV via blood transfusion an event of the past.

Immune Status

The immune status of a person with chronic hepatitis C may influence the rate of progression to liver disease. Some people with poor immune systems, who are known as being *immunosuppressed* or *immunocompromised*—such as those with AIDS, those who are on immunosuppressive medications (such as tacrolimus) after receiving an organ transplant, and those undergoing cancer chemotherapy—often have a severe and aggressive course of liver disease due to chronic hepatitis C when compared with people who have chronic hepatitis C but have functioning immune systems. However, this finding is not universal and is subject to variables. In fact, some immunosuppressed people, including some with chronic kidney disease and some with HIV infection, have experienced a particularly mild course of liver disease due to infection with HCV. And the course of HCV infection in cases where a person has reinfected her newly transplanted liver with HCV is also variable. Some studies have noted an aggressive course of disease, with cirrhosis developing within a year due to HCV reinfection, while other studies have shown that infection with HCV caused virtually no damage to the new liver. It is clear that many factors come into play in the case of immunosuppression and how it affects the rate of progression of chronic hepatitis C. Issues pertaining to liver transplantation will be discussed further in Chapter 22.

By reducing the body's immune defenses, immunosuppressive medications, such as the steroid prednisone and the antirejection drug cyclosporine, promote a surge of viral replication (manifested by an increased HCV RNA viral load) by reducing the body's immune defenses. Therefore, immunosuppressive medications may have the effect of accelerating the progression of chronic hepatitis C. Thus, people with chronic hepatitis C are advised to avoid the use of such medications, unless these medications are absolutely warranted.

Prognosis Based on Other Characteristics

Other factors that may independently cause liver disease may coexist in people with chronic hepatitis C. When combined together, a particularly aggressive course of liver disease with a poor outcome often results.

HCV and Alcohol

Alcohol is a strong toxin to the liver and can lead to cirrhosis and liver cancer. People with chronic hepatitis C who drink excessive amounts of alcohol are at an especially high risk for a particularly accelerated course of liver disease to advanced stages. This has been found to apply even to former excessive alcohol users who currently abstain and even to some people who consider themselves to be social drinkers. It appears that alcohol actually promotes replication of HCV. You may accurately visualize alcohol as a potent fuel that HCV utilizes to multiply and prosper in the body. People with chronic hepatitis C who drink alcohol are more frequently found to have cirrhosis and liver cancer and are more likely to die at an earlier age than people who do not subject their livers to this additional insult. Therefore, it would be prudent for all people with chronic hepatitis C to minimize their alcohol intake. In fact, the best advice for these people is to totally abstain from all alcohol. See Chapter 17 for more information on alcohol and the liver.

HCV and Cigarette Smoking

Cigarette smoking has been cited as a possible factor in promoting disease progression in people with chronic hepatitis C. However, further study is needed to confirm this possible association. Other forms of tobacco, such as from a pipe or cigar, have not been linked to promoting the progression of hepatitis C. This may be due to the fact that these forms of tobacco have never been specifically evaluated in this context. However, it can most likely be concluded that all forms of tobacco are not healthy for the liver.

HCV and Other Hepatitis Viruses

It is not infrequent for people with chronic hepatitis C to be additionally infected with another hepatitis virus. It has been noted by some researchers that fulminant hepatitis (see Chapter 7) and even death can occur in people with chronic hepatitis C who become infected with the hepatitis A virus (HAV). Some studies have found that people infected with both HCV and HBV have a very aggressive course of disease and are at increased risk of developing cirrhosis and decompensated liver disease. Therefore, everyone with chronic hepatitis C who has not been exposed to HAV or HBV is urged to obtain the vaccinations against these other hepatitis viruses. Vaccinations will be discussed in Chapter 24.

Coinfection of HCV with the hepatitis G virus (HGV) is not believed to influence the outcome of liver disease due to HCV.

HCV and Autoimmune Hepatitis

A form of autoimmune hepatitis (AIH) may occur in people with chronic hepatitis C. It has been shown that the coexistence of these two liver disorders does not lead to a poorer outcome of disease in a person with chronic hepatitis C. However, the coexistence of these two liver disorders may cause some treatment dilemmas. This is discussed in more detail in Chapters 13 and 14.

HCV and Herbs

There has been a boom of interest in the use of herbal remedies for the treatment of chronic hepatitis C. However, many herbs are in and of themselves toxic to the liver. Due to the lack of FDA regulation regarding marketing and labeling, it is quite possible that many people are unknowingly ingesting herbs that are actually toxic to their livers in the mistaken belief that what they are ingesting will improve the health of their livers. Herbal remedies and how they may affect the progression of chronic hepatitis C is an area that warrants further investigation. See Chapter 21 for information on which herbs to avoid and which herbs may be safe.

HCV and Iron Overload

Excessive iron can be harmful to the liver and can lead to liver damage and cirrhosis. Chapter 18 is devoted to this topic. Many people with chronic hepatitis C (especially men) have increased iron levels in their blood—iron, ferritin, and transferrin saturation. This may be due to iron being released into the bloodstream by dying liver cells. Some of these people may carry a gene for hereditary iron overload. It is possible that iron may promote the replication of HCV. Some studies have noted that people with chronic hepatitis C who have high iron levels respond poorly to treatment with interferon (see Chapter 13). This is why iron reduction therapy in the form of phlebotomy (removal of blood through a vein) has been proposed by some researchers as a possible treatment or adjunctive treatment option for people with chronic hepatitis C who have high iron levels. In any case, it is probably wise for people with chronic hepatitis C, especially those with high iron studies and also those with cirrhosis, to avoid iron supplementation or foods fortified with iron. Nutrition for people with chronic hepatitis C will be discussed in Chapter 23.

HCV and Environmental Factors

Environmental toxins, such as toxic fumes and pollutants from work sites, polluted air, waste, paints, and other sources, may potentially promote acceleration of disease in people with chronic hepatitis C. This association remains largely unexplored. However, since everything that we are exposed to, including what we breathe and absorb through the skin, is filtered through the liver to be detoxified, it makes sense that certain environmental factors may also contribute to a worsening course of liver disease.

Chronic Hepatitis C and Liver Cancer Risk

Among people in whom cirrhosis develops, approximately 1 percent per year are at risk for liver cancer, also known as hepatocellular carcinoma (HCC) or hepatoma. It has been estimated that approximately 15 percent of people with cirrhosis due to HCV develop liver cancer within approximately ten years of the time cirrhosis occurred. In contrast to hepatitis-B-associated liver cancer, cirrhosis is present in all cases of hepatitis-C-associated liver cancer.

In people with chronic hepatitis C, drinking alcohol excessively appears to increase the risk of developing liver cancer, thereby underscoring the importance of abstinence in people with hepatitis C. As stated above, it appears that coinfection with both HBV and HCV also greatly increases a person's chances of developing liver cancer. As such, it is important for people with chronic hepatitis C who are not already infected with hepatitis B to obtain the hepatitis B vaccination. (See Chapter 24 for more information on vaccinations). It usually takes more than thirty years for liver cancer to develop from the time of initial infection with HCV. Males and people older than fifty-five years appear to develop liver cancer more frequently than females and younger individuals. It has been demonstrated that treatment with the antiviral drug interferon (see Chapters 11, 12, and 13), prior to the development of liver cancer may actually lower the incidence of liver cancer in some people with chronic hepatitis C (see Chapters 13 and 19). This underscores the importance of early detection and aggressive treatment of chronic hepatitis C prior to the development of advanced liver disease.

CONCLUSION

Perhaps the most frightening aspect of chronic hepatitis C is its clandestine and progressive nature. Most people harbor the virus for ten, twenty, or even thirty years, not knowing it's in their bodies and oblivious to the liver damage it has caused. However, there are some encouraging aspects of this disease—the most common cause of liver disease in the United States. The number of new HCV infections has declined significantly. There is greater awareness and knowledge about HCV transmission and prevention. With the application of improved diagnostic blood tests to screen prospective blood donors, which have been in use since 1992, acquisition of HCV by blood transfusion is now virtually impossible. This is of tremendous significance, as studies have shown that those people who have acquired HCV via this route are the most likely to develop progressive disease. Some controllable risk factors that can accelerate progression of disease, such as alcohol consumption and co-infection with other hepatitis viruses, have been pinpointed. Thus, a person can, on her own initiative, take measures that will help diminish her risk of disease progression. As the knowledge of HCV continues to grow, the number of people becoming infected with HCV, and the number of people having a poor outcome due to HCV will surely diminish even further.

The next chapter is an overview of the treatment of chronic viral hepatitis. As such, interferon, the first effective treatment for both chronic hepatitis B and C will be discussed in detail.

Treating Chronic Viral Hepatitis— An Overview

When diagnosed with an illness, one of the first questions that a person typically asks her doctor is *"How is this disease treated?"* Prior to 1991, when it came to chronic hepatitis B or C, the answer to this question would have been *"There is no proven effective treatment."* Fortunately, this is not the same answer that a person asking this question hears today. While current therapies do not work for everyone, people with chronic hepatitis B and C should consider themselves fortunate. Not only are effective medications available to treat these diseases, but there is a variety of treatment regimens from which a person can choose. Even those people who have carried the virus for several decades can often be successfully treated.

This chapter discusses important issues that a person with chronic hepatitis B or C should consider as she decides which treatment option will be best for her. These issues include the difference between FDA-approved and experimental drug therapy; the advantages versus the disadvantages of participating in a clinical research trial of a promising new drug; and what to look for when evaluating a clinical research study. Also included is a general overview of interferon—the first therapy to be proven effective for treating chronic viral hepatitis B and C. This overview includes the history of interferon, its potential side effects, and how best to deal with the side effects if they occur. Also, some financial issues regarding interferon are addressed. (More specific information on interferon therapy is covered in Chapters 12 and 13.)

WHAT ARE INVESTIGATIONAL DRUGS?

There are many drugs available to treat chronic hepatitis B and C. Some drugs have already been approved by the United States Food and Drug Administration (FDA) and are available by prescription to anyone requiring treatment. However, before a drug is made available to the general public, it must undergo years of rigorous scrutiny by its manufacturer and the FDA. During this stage, the experimental drug is known as an *investigational* drug, and is only available to people who voluntarily enter clinical drug trials. A clinical drug trial involves the evaluation of a new drug's effectiveness in treating a disease as well as its potential adverse side effects. As discussed in Chapter 4, a clinical trial may be conducted in an academic institution or the office of a private practitioner (hepatologist).

Even before a drug becomes available through clinical trials, it is first tested on laboratory animals and/or human cells in a test tube. This precautionary step helps researchers determine whether the investigational drug is safe enough to try on humans. If this initial stage of drug testing is deemed successful by the drug manufacturer, it provides its findings to the FDA in order to obtain the green light to start a clinical trial on humans. Thereafter, the process of evaluating an investigational drug progresses through three phases.

Phase I Testing

Phase I studies involve an initial evaluation of the drug for safety in treatment with humans. This experimental phase involves approximately fifty people who are usually paid for their participation in the study. The length of the investigation will vary depending upon the drug, but typically does not last more than one year. Investigators will look for serious adverse events that will halt further investigation of the drug.

Phase II Testing

Once researchers have demonstrated that the drug is safe on humans, Phase II testing begins. This phase involves evaluating the drug to determine proper dosage as well as potential side effects. This phase usually involves several hundred people. Phase II trials are usually conducted in a manner of investigation known as a *randomized, double-blinded, controlled study*. This means that people in the study are randomly selected to receive either the investigational drug or a placebo—an inert, harmless substance that has no actual effect on a person's illness, but is identical in appearance to the medication under investigation. Placebos are sometimes called "dummy" pills. Neither the study participants nor the investigators know who is receiving which substance. This *double-blinded* method eliminates any potential for bias when the results are evaluated.

Phase III Testing

Phase III studies involve anywhere from several hundred to several thousand subjects. By using this many people, the manufacturer and the FDA have the opportunity to evaluate the investigational drug for how effective and beneficial it is on the disease under study on a large group of people. Furthermore, a wide range of potential side effects of the drug can be evaluated.

FDA Approval

All these phases of testing may sound like a lot of hoops to go through, but what is gained from this rigorous process is the confidence that allows researchers to say that a particular drug truly does work. It also allows the FDA to look at the data and determine whether the conclusions of the investigators of the drug are justified. Assuming all is in order, the manufacturer and the FDA then decide what information should appear on the drug's label, as well as what instructions should be given to physicians, pharmacists, and patients. The drug is then approved and made available for prescription.

THE PROS AND CONS OF PARTICIPATING IN A CLINICAL TRIAL

As with all important life decisions, the decision to participate in a clinical trial involves weighing the potential positives against the potential negatives.

There are many advantages to participating in a clinical drug trial. First, the participant will gain access to a potentially effective drug years before it is available to the general public. Second, the trial may enable the participant to obtain top-notch medical care at a reduced fee or possibly free of charge. Finally, the participant will be contributing to the advancement of science and the medical profession.

There are also downsides to participating in a clinical drug trial. First, all of the possible side effects associated with the investigational drug may not be totally known yet. Therefore, there is the possibility that an unforeseen adverse reaction to the drug may occur. Second, it is quite possible that the participant may not even receive the real drug at all and may instead be receiving a placebo. (The potential for receiving a placebo should appear on the consent form, which is discussed below.) Finally, the participant must be willing to adhere to a strict set of protocol guidelines. These guidelines may include adhering to a specific schedule of office or clinic appointments, having blood drawn on specific days and at specific hours, and having special testing done—for example, a heart or an eye evaluation prior to beginning the study.

THE CONSENT FORM

A written consent form explaining the details of the study and the subject's requirements must be signed by the potential participant prior to entering a clinical trial. This consent form should clearly spell out all issues concerning the study and the investigational drug. The consent form should not be signed unless all of the significant issues are included in the form. These are outlined in the inset "Items on a Consent Form" on page 136. Moreover, the consent form should not be signed until the doctor, nurse, and/or study coordinator has satisfactorily answered all the patient's questions. A witness—other than the doctor running the study—must always cosign the consent form.

Whether everyone in the study will be receiving the investigational drug or

Items on a Consent Form

A patient should not sign a consent form for participation in a clinical study on an experimental drug unless all of the following components are included on the form:

❏ Title of study.

❏ Name, address, and telephone number of the doctor in charge of the study.

❏ The purpose of the study.

❏ The subject's obligations under the study—for example, must she adhere to a regular schedule of appointments with his or her doctor for the duration of the study? Must she refrain from all alcohol use during the study? Must she use a form of birth control during and for a specific amount of time after the study?

❏ Individual's qualifications to participate in the study—for example, must she be age eighteen to seventy? Must she not be pregnant? Must she not be on any other antiviral medications?

❏ Risks and discomforts potentially associated with the study drug.

❏ Benefits from participating in the study.

❏ Potential costs incurred to the subject during the study.

❏ Alternative treatments available (does not have to be very detailed as the subject will have discussed these with her doctor).

❏ Assurance of confidentiality of the subject's records.

❏ The names and telephone numbers of the people to contact in case of an emergency.

❏ The names and telephone numbers of the people that the subject may contact while participating in the research study if she has questions regarding her rights.

❏ The subject's right to leave the study.

❏ Potential reasons for study termination.

❏ Place for the subject and witness to sign.

❏ Official stamp from the physician's ethical or institutional review board indicating that the study has been reviewed by the board and is considered safe and ethical.

It is a good idea for all participants in a clinical study to keep a copy of the signed consent form for their personal files.

whether some people will be randomly chosen to receive a placebo should be clearly understood and discussed prior to entering the study. Remember, not all studies include placebos. In addition, the potential participant should inquire as to whether or not the results of blood work or other testing performed during the study will be revealed to her while the study is ongoing or only once the study is over. Finally, all other available treatment options must be discussed with the doctor before the patient decides to go ahead with the study.

WHAT IS ANTIVIRAL THERAPY?

Antiviral therapy is the use of any drug or other agent acting or directed against a virus. The immediate goal of antiviral therapy is to interfere with the replication of the virus. The ultimate goal of antiviral therapy is to totally eradicate the virus from the body. Viruses are much more difficult to treat than bacteria. Bacteria are treated with agents called antibacterials, otherwise commonly known as antibiotics. Antibiotics have no action against viruses. Many different antivirals have been used to treat hepatitis B and C. Chapters 12 and 13 detail these treatments. The remainder of this chapter discusses interferon—the first antiviral therapy proven to be effective for some people with hepatitis B and C.

WHAT ARE INTERFERONS?

Interferons (IFNs) are a family of proteins made naturally by the body. In 1957, it was discovered that when a virus attacks the body, interferon is produced by special cells in the body in an effort to *interfere* with further viral replication and damage and to protect other cells in the body that were not already infected from becoming infected. Thus, interferons were found to have the ability to fight viruses, which is known as *antiviral activity.* It was also discovered that interferons play an important role in fighting cancers, which is known as *antitumor activity,* and in regulating the immune system, which is known as *immunomodulatory activity.*

Sometimes the body does not produce enough natural interferon to fight infections, cancers, and immune disorders. It has been shown that supplementing the interferon made in the body with synthetically manufactured interferon given by injection provides benefit to many people. In addition to being used to treat the viruses that cause chronic hepatitis—HBV and HCV—interferons have been used to treat a variety of diseases, including hairy cell leukemia, a rare blood disorder; Kaposi's sarcoma, a type of skin cancer that occurs in elderly people and in people with AIDS; and condyloma acuminatum, a warty growth on the genitals

Interferon, independent of the type, is administered by injection only. It is most commonly injected by what is known as the subcutaneous route (beneath the skin), but can also be injected intramuscularly (into the muscle). Patients are typically injected by a doctor or nurse, or they are taught to inject themselves at home. (Patients are often given an instructional video to supplement the office lesson.) Unfortunately, interferon is not effective if taken orally and, therefore, no pill form is available.

The Classes of Interferon

There are three different classes of interferon: alfa (also spelled alpha), beta, and gamma. Alfa and beta interferons are known as type I interferons, whereas gamma interferon is known as type II interferon. While there is only one form of beta and gamma interferon, it was discovered that there were numerous forms of alfa interferon. The different types of alfa interferon are closely related in structure, but differ slightly from one another, and therefore each is classified as a different *subtype*. The slight variations among the subtypes of alfa interferon make up the basis for the differences in the three FDA-approved synthetically manufactured alfa interferons currently available.

Interferon and FDA Approval

The first interferon was approved by the FDA in 1991 for the treatment of chronic hepatitis C. It is known as Intron A (IFN alfa 2b) and is manufactured by Schering-Plough Corporation. Intron A was FDA approved for the treatment of chronic hepatitis B in 1992 and is currently the only type of interferon approved for the treatment of hepatitis B. In 1996, IFN alfa 2a (commercially marketed as Roferon A and manufactured by Roche Pharmaceuticals) was approved for the treatment of chronic hepatitis C. Both Intron A and Roferon are identical to the corresponding natural alfa interferon that occurs in humans.

The first bioengineered non-naturally occurring interferon for the treatment of chronic hepatitis C was approved by the FDA in 1997. It is manufactured by Amgen and is marketed under the trade name Infergen (also known as IFN alfacon-1 or consensus interferon). Infergen represents an effort to create a type of interferon that is superior to those produced naturally by the body.

There are many other alfa interferons for which pharmaceutical companies are seeking FDA approval for the use in the treatment of chronic hepatitis C and/or hepatitis B. Examples include Wellferon (IFN alfa n1; manufactured by Glaxo-Wellcome) and Alferon N (IFN alfa n3; manufactured by Interferon Sciences).

Also, experimental studies are underway that involve variations on the standard type of alfa interferon, such as pegylated interferon—an interferon requiring only a once a week administration as opposed to three times a week (manufactured by Schering-Plough and Roche Pharmaceuticals). Finally, other interferons, such as Rebif, a type of beta interferon, are being tested for effectiveness.

A BRIEF DISCUSSION OF THE SIDE EFFECTS OF MEDICATION

All drugs have potential side effects. To realize this, you need only to read the informational insert that accompanies any medicine—whether prescribed or over-the-counter. (By the way, if such information is not included, you can ask the pharmacist to provide you with it.) For any given medication, there is a list of many potential side effects that may occur as a consequence of taking the drug. This is true even for the most commonly used over-the-counter medications, such as an aspirin or an antacid.

The reason for this extensive list of potential adverse reactions is that when a drug is being evaluated for FDA approval, every symptom that a person experiences while taking that drug must be reported. Some of the listed side effects may have occurred in only a very small percentage of people and some of the listed side effects may not even have been due to the drug at all.

SIDE EFFECTS AND INTERFERON THERAPY

There are some important points to keep in mind when evaluating the risks versus benefits of taking a medication, such as interferon. Side effects associated with any drug, including interferon, vary from person to person. This means that not everyone will experience a particular potential side effect. While some people feel quite ill while undergoing interferon therapy, others experience few, if any, side effects. (A discussion of the specific side effects associated with interferon therapy begins on page 140.) And there are some people who actually feel better while on interferon. That's right! This point bears repeating. It is possibile that a person will have minimal to no side effects or will even feel better than usual while on interferon. And those who do experience adverse side effects usually do not experience them all the time. In fact, studies have shown that only approximately 2 to 5 percent of people find the side effects of interferon so debilitating that the discontinuation of therapy is necessary.

Side effects are usually the worst during the first few weeks of therapy. So it is important to try to stick with therapy for at least a month or two. Some people schedule time off from work for when they plan to start interferon therapy. Others plan to begin therapy when their work schedule or personal responsibilities are light, thereby making it is easier to get through the initial period. Side effects associated with interferon are usually dose related, meaning that the higher the dose of interferon, the greater the side effects. Sometimes a reduction in dosage may satisfactorily mitigate the side effects.

It has been demonstrated that people with advanced liver disease and cirrhosis are the ones most likely to experience side effects. However, people with cirrhosis may have less side effects if they commence treatment with a relatively low dose of interferon. The importance of treatment in the early stages of the disease, when people are strongest and healthiest and best able to tolerate interferon, cannot be overstated. Finally, the side effects due to interferon will totally abate after interferon therapy has been discontinued.

If people can adopt strategies to cope with the side effects, then interferon therapy need not interfere with their daily lives. One positive aspect to interferon therapy is that unlike insulin injections for diabetes, which continue throughout the patient's life, interferon shots for chronic hepatitis B and chronic hepatitis C do not last forever. This is important to keep in mind for people who are experiencing difficulty dealing with the side effects of interferon—it's just for a limited amount of time.

Discontinuation of Interferon Therapy Due to Side Effects

All side effects experienced while taking interferon must be reported to the doctor. If the side effects of interferon become too difficult to manage, it is possible that she may suggest discontinuation. Such a determination will depend on many factors. That is why a liver biopsy is so important to obtain prior to starting interferon therapy. For example, if the liver biopsy findings from a person with chronic hepatitis C reveal little scarring and/or inflammation, the doctor may recommend discontinuing interferon if the side effects are too overwhelming. Since chronic hepatitis C progresses so slowly, such a person may benefit from deferring treatment until the trial of a promising new drug becomes available (see page 133).

On the other hand, if the liver biopsy findings on a person with chronic hepatitis reveals extensive scarring and inflammation, the doctor may recommend that this person attempt to continue therapy, despite the side effects.

Specific Potential Side Effects of Interferon Therapy

The following is a discussion of the potential side effects associated with interferon therapy and some tips on how to best manage them.

Flu-Like Symptoms

Flu-like symptoms are the most common side effects experienced while taking interferon. Flu-like symptoms typically include a low-grade fever, chills, headache, muscle and joint aches, fatigue, and weakness. These side effects may occur throughout treatment, but tend to be most pronounced during the first month of treatment and to diminish as treatment progresses. They are best managed by taking acetaminophen (Tylenol) about a half hour prior to the interferon injection. Aspirin and other nonsteroidal anti-inflammatories (NSAIDs), such as Motrin and Naprosyn, should be avoided (see Chapter 24 for more information). Also, injecting immediately prior to going to bed is helpful, since this will limit the side effects primarily to the sleeping hours. However, if the side effects from interferon either cause or contribute to insomnia, then changing the injection time to the morning is advisable. Some people find that it is easiest to handle the side effects of interferon if they are busy working as this deflects their attention from their symptoms.

Amantadine (Symmetrel) is an antiviral medication used to treat people with influenza A (the flu) as well as people with Parkinson's disease, a neurological disorder. Although one study has demonstrated that amantadine is an effective treatment for people with chronic hepatitis C, this finding has not been duplicated in other studies. However, amantadine, which is easy to take and has few side effects of its own, may be helpful in combating some of the flu-like symptoms that are associated with interferon therapy. Therefore, amantadine may be useful adjunctive therapy with interferon to control some interferon-associated side effects.

Fatigue

Fatigue may be caused by interferon or by chronic hepatitis itself. Unfortunately, there is no pill or other quick fix one can take to eliminate fatigue. However, there are some helpful things that one can do to boost energy levels. A healthy, well-rounded diet, low in fat, accompanied by lots of water (at least eight to twelve eight-ounce glasses per day) is important. And, it's best not to eat a large meals. After consuming a large meal, it is common to become tired. Therefore, multiple small meals throughout the day should become a habit.

If at all possible, a fifteen- to twenty-minute nap once or twice a day will provide a quick "pick-me-up." Everyone with chronic hepatitis, especially those on treatment, should get plenty of sleep—at least seven to eight hours a day.

Exercise is crucial. It may seem like a catch-22—the person is too tired to exercise, yet exercise will provide her with a boost of energy. The solution is to start slow. Even if only ten minutes a day is all the person can manage, by the end of the week, she will have exercised an entire hour, which, of course, is better than nothing. With time, most people are able to build up their stamina to the point where they can exercise for at least twenty minutes to a half hour each day. (See Chapter 23 for more tips on exercise.)

It goes without saying, but bears repeating anyway—alcoholic beverages should be totally avoided. Also, many people have reported feeling more energetic as a result of totally eliminating caffeine intake. Finally, cannabis (marijuana) has been shown to decrease the effectiveness of interferon. Since smoking marijuana may also contribute to fatigue, it is advised to avoid this habit totally.

Psychiatric Symptoms

Any chronic illness, especially liver disease, may cause a person to become depressed. Furthermore, interferon itself may also cause depression or worsen underlying depression. Interferon therapy has additionally been associated with causing irritability, confusion, emotional instability, insomnia, and a lack or concentration.

People who already suffer from severe depression associated with suicidal thoughts or suicide attempts, or other psychiatric disorders should avoid interferon therapy until their underlying psychiatric problems have stabilized or abated. People who do not have severe psychiatric problems, but who are prone to depression, emotional instability, or other related symptoms, may benefit from beginning an antidepressant or antianxiety medication prior to commencing interferon therapy.

All drugs are metabolized at least to some extent through the liver. While people with a chronic liver disease should avoid any non-essential medications so as not to subject their livers to additional stress, this directive may be outweighed by the great benefit to be obtained by treatment with an antidepressant or an antianxiety medication while on interferon therapy. Probably the safest antidepressants are the selective serotonin reuptake inhibitors (SSRI), such as Paxil (manufactured by SmithKline Beecham), Zoloft (manufactured by Pfizer) or Prozac (manufatured by Dista/Eli Lilly), and a good antianxiety medication is BuSpar (manufactured by Bristol-Myers Squibb). If depression or any other psychiatric problem becomes severe, a reduction in the dose of interferon is advised. People who develop any psychiatric side effects while on interferon are best managed jointly by a liver specialist and a psychiatrist.

Interferon may also cause thyroid abnormalities, symptoms of which may mimic psychiatric disorders. Those on interferon must have their thyroid profile periodically checked via blood tests, especially when any of the above symptoms develop on therapy. Thyroid abnormalities are discussed below.

Thyroid Abnormalities

Thyroid abnormalities may occur while on interferon therapy. People who are prone to autoimmune disorders are more likely to develop a thyroid disorder than people without this propensity. A person may develop either a slow-functioning thyroid (hypothyroidism) or a fast-functioning thyroid (hyperthyroidism). Symptoms associated with hypothyroidism include fatigue, weakness, hair loss, dry skin, memory impairment, and psychosis. Symptoms associated with hyperthyroidism include nervousness, heat intolerance, palpitations, weight loss, weakness, shortness of breath, poor concentration, emotional instability, and depression.

As noted above, symptoms of thyroid disorders are similar to those of psychiatric disorders. Thyroid disorders are readily diagnosed by obtaining a thyroid profile from blood tests. Both hypothyroidism and hyperthyroidism are easily treatable with thyroid medication. Thyroid abnormalities that developed while a person is on interferon commonly resolve after interferon is discontinued.

Weight Loss

Weight loss in the range of ten to twenty pounds may occur while a person is on interferon therapy. This is another reason why exercise, especially weight-bearing exercise—which increases muscle and bone mass—is important in people with chronic hepatitis. Interferon may cause loss of appetite, altered taste sensation, nausea, abdominal discomfort, flatulence, and diarrhea, thereby leading to weight loss. Eating multiple small, healthy, low-fat meals throughout the day and consuming plenty of water will help maintain a steady weight while on interferon. Large meals should be avoided. Flatulence and diarrhea may be lessened by adhering to a lactose-free (dairy-free) diet and avoiding raw vegetables and fruits. Vegetables may be eaten if well-cooked and fruits may be eaten if peeled. (See Chapter 23 for more information on nutrition.)

Decreased Blood Counts

People on interferon may develop decreased red and white blood cell counts in addition to decreased platelet counts. This is most common in people who have cirrhosis. These reductions are usually not significant and resolve promptly upon reducing the dosage of interferon. Occasionally, blood counts become dangerously low, thereby necessitating the discontinuation of interferon.

Injection-Related Symptoms

Some people may experience occasional mild pain, redness, and swelling at the site of injection. Most of the time this is normal. If pain, swelling, and redness worsen or do not abate, it should immediately be reported to the doctor or nurse, as it may be a sign of infection. If an infection is discovered to be present at the injection site, antibiotics need to be started immediately. The infected site should not be used again, until totally healed. It is of crucial importance to assure that the injection site is clean in order to avoid this complication. A person should always clean the site with alcohol or an antiseptic, such as Betadine, prior to injecting. Also, it is important to change the site of injection. For example, the right thigh, the left thigh, and the stomach may each be used in rotation as injection sites.

The person can also request that the needle size be changed to a thinner one. Thinner needles, such as an insulin-type needle (a 28 or 29 gauge needle), are virtually painless. Schering-Plough and Amgen both manufacture a multi-dose pen that many people find to be a convenient method of injection since it does not require a mixing of medication. Finally, it is important to keep the injection site covered from direct sunlight, as sunlight may exacerbate redness and irritation. So, it's knee-length shorts in the summer! Also try to avoid tanning salons, as this too may worsen any rashes that occur while on treatment.

Hair Loss

Hair loss while on interferon therapy occurs, yet is infrequent, very mild, and usually unnoticeable to others. It is not the type of baldness experienced by people on cancer chemotherapy. Hair loss appears to be more frequent in Caucasians with black hair and in Asians. People should refrain from using hair dye or bleach while on interferon therapy, which may exacerbate the problem. Some have found some help by using the vitamin biotin (see Chapter 23 for more information). Fortunately, hair loss induced by interferon therapy is temporary and regrowth is noted within three months of discontinuation of the drug.

Other Effects

People can develop a rash and/or itching while on therapy. These symptoms are usually mild and can be relieved with the use of diphenhydramine (Benadryl). Other side effects that can occur during interferon therapy include an elevated triglyceride level and decreased libido. These side effects are infrequent, and they abate once interferon is discontinued.

FINANCIAL ISSUES CONCERNING INTERFERON

There are three financial issues that people must consider prior to beginning interferon or any other treatment regimen: the cost of the drug, the cost of the doctor visits, and the cost of the blood tests. This section will discuss each of these financial issues.

The Cost of the Drug

The FDA has approved interferon as a treatment for chronic hepatitis C on a schedule of three times a week lasting for one year, and for chronic hepatitis B daily for four months. As noted on page 138, three types of alfa interferon have been approved by the FDA for chronic hepatitis C, and one type has been approved for chronic hepatitis B. Experimental treatment regimens vary regarding the duration of treatment (for example, six months to two years) and number of injections administered per week (for example, once a week to daily). Therefore, the actual cost for a full course of interferon therapy varies widely depending upon many variables. However, the two most important cost variables are usually the pharmacy the person is using and the type of insurance she has.

Without discussing the actual cost, the bottom line is that it can be very expensive to treat chronic hepatitis B and chronic hepatitis C with interferon. However, the treatment is well worth the expense, as interferon can increase life expectancy and decrease the likelihood of liver-related complications. The cost of the FDA-approved alfa interferons is covered by most insurance plans, including most managed-care plans. On occasion, an insurance company will be unwilling to pay for treatment. In this situation, the patient's doctor must telephone or write to the insurance company to explain the necessity of the treatment. This letter is known as a letter of medical necessity. When this is done, the insurance company will typically reverse the decision and agree to coverage.

If the person is unable to obtain coverage for treatment or if she does not have any insurance coverage, the pharmaceutical company that manufactures the drugs may be able to assist with the cost. However, the person may be required to supply her latest tax return. And, not everyone in this situation will qualify for financial assistance. (See the Resource Groups listed in the Appendix for the telephone numbers of pharmaceutical companies to call when seeking pharmaceutical financial assistance.)

Medicare will cover the cost of interferon therapy, but with one restriction—the interferon injection must be administered by a doctor or the doctor's staff in her office or clinic or by a Medicare-approved nurse at the patient's home. (Non-Medicare patients may administer their injections to themselves, in their own homes.)

Finally, if the person is still having difficulty covering the cost of the treatment, she should search for an experimental trial to enter. Often, but not always, the medications in an experimental trial are provided free of charge.

The Cost of the Doctor Visits

A person with chronic hepatitis B or chronic hepatitis C who is starting therapy will require frequent visits to the doctor's office; and she should, therefore, make sure that the doctor accepts her particular insurance or managed care plan. If the doctor accepts the plan, then the visits are covered by the insurance company. With some managed care plans, the doctor will need to write a letter to the insurance company, and/or to the patient's primary care physician, explaining the need for multiple long-term visits.

If the doctor does not accept the plan, then it may be necessary to arrange a payment schedule with the doctor's office. Usually, a reduced fee can be arranged in view of the fact that multiple visits will be required. Remember, the doctor is there to help the patient get better and will usually be willing to work out some kind of reasonable reduced-fee payment plan—especially if discussed in advance. Also, as discussed in Chapter 4, even if the doctor does not belong to a particular managed-care program, reimbursement for the doctor visits may still be arranged through the insurance company. Usually this requires a telephone call or a letter from the patient to the insurance company explaining the necessity for seeing that particular specialist. Once again, this is why it is important to be under the care of a hepatologist. The insurance companies will commonly reimburse a hepatologist if she presents evidence that she has training in liver disease not offered by any of the other specialists on the insurance plan.

For people enrolled in an experimental study, the visits to the doctor are often free of charge or at a reduced fee. The person should always inquire whether her doctor is conducting any clinical trials or is aware of any nearby trials that will cover the costs of treatment.

The Cost of the Blood Tests

As with medications and doctor visits, the cost of blood tests is usually covered by the insurance plan or managed-care plan. Managed-care plans typically contract with specific laboratories to process blood work. It is important that the doctor is aware of which laboratory is contracted by the insurance company to insure that all blood work is covered.

If a person does not have insurance, either she or the doctor's office staff should personally contact the supervisor of the laboratory to inquire about payment arrangements. Usually a reduced-fee payment schedule to cover the costs of blood work can be arranged.

If the patient is enrolled in a clinical trial, the blood work is often sent to a centralized laboratory. In such cases, the costs are usually, but not always, covered by the sponsor of the trial.

CONCLUSION

This chapter discussed some important issues concerning treatment of chronic viral hepatitis. Hopefully the information contained in this chapter will assist a person with chronic viral hepatitis in making a decision about treatment, whether she should stick with a time-tested, FDA-approved medication or enter a clinical trial of a promising new medication. As interferon is often an effective treatment for chronic viral hepatitis, most people with chronic hepatitis B and/or chronic hepatitis C will need to consider it as a treatment option at some point. Therefore, this chapter also provided some helpful tips to assist a person who is experiencing side effects from interferon. Financial issues are the last thing that a person wants to worry about when she is sick. Therefore, this chapter also provided some tips that will hopefully lessen money worries, with the ultimate objective being to help concentrate on the more important issue—getting better!

Now that the groundwork has been laid on treatment issues of chronic hepatitis B and chronic hepatitis C, the next two chapters will deal with specific treatment options for people with these diseases.

12

Treating Hepatitis B and Hepatitis D

Hepatitis B is one of the most common infections in the world. Almost 400 million people worldwide, including 1.25 million people in the United States, have hepatitis B. Chronic infection with this virus can lead to cirrhosis and liver cancer. As a result, approximately 1 million people die each year from the complications of hepatitis B. However, early medical intervention can prevent many of these deaths. People with chronic hepatitis B must attempt to eradicate the hepatitis B virus (HBV) from their bodies before long-term complications develop and before the disease can be transmitted to others. The ultimate goal of therapy, therefore, is to eliminate HBV from the body. If this cannot be achieved, an alternative goal is to suppress the replication of HBV. The less HBV replicates, the less damage will be done to the liver and the less infectious the person will be to others. Hepatitis delta virus (HDV) is a virus that can only live in a person infected with HBV. Approximately 70,000 people in the United States are infected with HDV. Hepatitis D tends to be a particularly severe infection with significant long-term consequences, causing greater than 1,000 deaths each year. Therefore, treatment of people infected with HDV is crucial.

This chapter focuses on the medical treatment of people who have progressed to chronic hepatitis B and analyzes which individuals will benefit most from therapy. It also discusses the circumstances under which people do or do not require treatment. Interferon, the first treatment for chronic hepatitis B to be approved by the FDA, is discussed in detail. While eradication of HBV can occur with interferon, not everyone responds to this therapy. Therefore, other medications for chronic hepatitis B, specifically lamivudine, are also discussed. In fact, most specialists believe that lamivudine, instead of interferon, is the first line of treatment for these people. Since there are many other therapies currently under investigation, this chapter also discusses some promising treatment options for chronic hepatitis B. In addition, the treatment of people infected with HDV is addressed. Finally, appropriate monitoring of people who are not undergoing treatment is covered.

TREATMENT OF ACUTE HEPATITIS B

Fortunately, only a small percentage of adults with acute hepatitis B progress to chronic hepatitis B. Most adults have an immune system that is strong enough to battle the virus and completely eliminate it from their bodies during the acute stages of disease, without the help of any medical treatment. Consequently, people with acute hepatitis B are not treated with antiviral medications, such as interferon or lamivudine. There is no pill, vitamin, or vaccination necessary during the acute stage of disease. Most people are managed conservatively, at home, based on how they are feeling. Home therapy involves drinking plenty of fluids and bed rest, if necessary. A person's level of activity should be judged on an individual basis. While some people are very fatigued and require long periods of inactivity and bed rest, others feel perfectly normal and are able to return to work and daily activities immediately. Therefore, bed rest is not a requirement for everyone. Many people report an aversion to cigarette smoking during this time, which is better off avoided in any case. Finally, people should avoid alcohol and eat a healthy, well-balanced diet. See Chapter 23 for more information on diet, nutrition, and exercise.

APPROVAL OF MEDICATION FOR CHRONIC HEPATITIS B

The first medication found to be effective for chronic hepatitis B, Interferon alfa 2a (Intron A; manufactured by Schering-Plough Corporation) was approved by the FDA in July 1992. Lamivudine (Epivir-HBV; manufactured by GlaxoWellcome) was approved by the FDA in December 1998 for use in the treatment of chronic hepatitis B. Other antiviral medications for chronic hepatitis B are in the process of investigation and FDA approval.

MONITORING A PERSON BEFORE AND WHILE ON THERAPY

Prior to starting therapy, a complete physical exam and several blood tests are necessary. These blood tests should include a complete blood count (CBC), which includes a platelet count; thyroid profile, including thyroid stimulating hormone (TSH); alpha-feto-protein (AFP); human immunodeficiency virus (HIV); and complete blood chemistries, including a liver profile (total bilirubin, transaminases, and GGTP), prothrombin time (PT), and antinuclear antibody (ANA). (See Chapter 3 for an explanation of most of these tests.) A liver biopsy is typically performed in order to determine the severity of disease. (See Chapter 5 for a complete discussion of liver biopsies.)

While the patient is on therapy, the doctor will re-examine her and re-run blood tests approximately once per month—although this may vary depending upon individual circumstances. This is necessary to monitor the progress of treatment and to watch out for any adverse reactions that may occur. HBV DNA and/or HBeAg will need to be regularly monitored to ascertain whether eradication of the virus has been achieved.

DETERMINING A RESPONSE TO THERAPY

During therapy, the specialist monitors the patient's symptoms and blood tests frequently. This is done both to determine whether the person has responded to therapy and to monitor for any side effects of therapy. Prior to the eradication of HBV from the body, people characteristically have a "flare" of the disease. This flare is noted by an increase of transaminase activity, which is sometimes as high as ten to twenty times the upper limit of normal, and also by the return or worsening of symptoms. While this course of events typically causes the person experiencing them some alarm, this "flare" is actually indicative of a favorable outcome, namely HBV clearance from the body. One way that antivirals work is by assisting the immune system in attacking the virus. Picture a war going on inside the liver between the enemy (HBV) and the soldiers (antiviral medication). Just before the enemy is kicked out of the body, there is a great deal of upheaval ("flare"). The hope is that this battle will conclude with the antiviral medication having conquered HBV.

When a person responds to therapy, she will no longer have a detectable level of HBV DNA, will become HBeAg negative and HBeAb positive, and will normalize transaminase levels (ALT and AST). However, HBcAb will be positive lifelong. (See Table 9.1 on page 101 for further clarification.) Symptoms associated with hepatitis B, such as fatigue, weakness, and loss of appetite, will be diminished, or even totally gone. Symptoms associated with some of the extrahepatic manifestations of chronic hepatitis B, such as fever, rash, and/or joint pain, may also improve. Liver scarring and inflammation have also been demonstrated to improve significantly in many people who have responded to therapy. Indicators of successful treatment include the following:

• HBV DNA will become non-detectable.

• HBeAg will become negative.

• HBeAb will become positive.

• HBcAb will remain positive lifelong.

• Transaminase levels will become normal.

• Symptoms will improve.

ALFA INTERFERON THERAPY FOR CHRONIC HEPATITIS B

People with chronic hepatitis have a defective immune response to the interferon that their bodies produce naturally. So, as early as the 1970s, researchers began investigating interferon therapy for people with chronic hepatitis B. However, it wasn't until 1992 that the FDA approved interferon therapy for the treatment of chronic hepatitis—at a dose of 5 million units of interferon alfa-2b (Intron A) daily, or 10 million units three times per week. Therapy may last a minimum of three months, but usually lasts for four to six months. Approximately one-third to one-half of infected people will eradicate the virus with interferon treatment. This compares to a mere 5- to 10-percent chance each year of virus eradication without treatment by spontaneous remission.

HBV eradication is manifested by the disappearance of HBV DNA, followed by the disappearance of HBeAg. The normalization of elevated transaminase levels should occur soon thereafter. Approximately 10 to 15 percent of these people will lose the carrier state, meaning they will no longer be carriers (as manifested by the loss of HBsAg), within one year of commencing therapy, and over time, this percentage increases. In fact, one group of researchers found that approximately 65 percent of people with chronic hepatitis B eventually lost the carrier state as a result of being treated with interferon. When this occurs, congratulations are in order, as these people no longer have chronic hepatitis B, are no longer infectious to others, and will experience minimal, if any, further damage to their livers.

If transaminase levels remain elevated, the possibility of the emergence of a mutant strain of HBV (chronic hepatitis B, negative for HBeAg but positive for HBV DNA) should be considered. It is important for the patient's doctor to evaluate why transaminases remain persistently elevated after apparent virus eradication.

Those Most Likely to Respond to Interferon Therapy

Although it is impossible to predict which people with chronic hepatitis B will respond to therapy, some indicators can identify the people who will be most likely to respond. The characteristics of these people include the following:

- Elevated levels of transaminases (ALT and AST) greater than 100 IU/ml.

- Low level of HBV DNA, less than 200 pg/dl (picograms per deciliter).

- Liver biopsy findings of moderate to severe inflammation.

- Short duration of disease.

- No evidence of decompensated cirrhosis (for example, no bleeding esophageal varices, ascites, etc.).

- Female gender.

- Acquisition of infection as an adult.

- No evidence of hepatitis delta virus (HDV).

- Non-immunocompromised (for example, HIV negative; not an organ transplant recipient).

- HBeAg positive (non-mutant form of HBV).

- Non-Asian origins.

Factors That May Adversely Influence Response to Interferon Therapy

Unlike the above factors, which are beyond a person's control, there are some variables that a person does have control over that can influence her response to therapy. Alcohol use is one such variable. Alcohol is a potent liver toxin and can induce HBV to replicate. Therefore, minimal consumption of alcohol, if not total abstinence, is recommended for people with chronic hepatitis B, especially those undergoing interferon therapy.

People with chronic hepatitis B who become infected with the hepatitis A virus (HAV) have been found to suffer from a particularly severe, and sometimes fatal, course of infection. Therefore, everyone with chronic hepatitis B should receive the vaccination against HAV if they have not already been exposed to this virus. Vaccination should preferably take place prior to the start of interferon therapy. (See Chapter 24 for more information on vaccinations.)

It has been shown that marijuana use may decrease the effectiveness of interferon therapy and may inhibit the body's own natural production of interferon. Therefore, it is advisable for people with chronic hepatitis B to avoid marijuana, especially while on interferon treatment.

Immunosuppressed conditions, such as treatment with corticosteroids (for example, prednisone), may cause activation of HBV. Therefore, unless absolutely required, people with chronic hepatitis B should avoid these types of medications when other treatment options exist.

Relapse After Interferon Therapy

Rarely will a person revert into the infectious state once the virus has been eradicated. In fact, over a ten-year period following virus eradication, only between 5 to 10 percent of people will experience a relapse of disease. Any relapse is usually temporary, and most of these people revert to a noninfectious stage.

OTHER TREATMENT OPTIONS FOR CHRONIC HEPATITIS B

Interferon works well for many people with chronic hepatitis B. However, interferon is not without side effects. At times, the side effects may be so severe that discontinuation of the drug becomes necessary. (For the management of these side effects, see Chapter 11.)

Alternatively, some people do not respond to treatment with interferon. Asian people who acquired hepatitis B at birth—especially those with normal transaminases; people with mutant strains of HBV (those that are HBeAg negative but positive for HBV DNA); and liver transplant recipients are among those who tend *not* to respond to interferon. In addition, some people are at risk of serious complications if treated with interferon. For instance, people with decompensated liver disease may develop liver failure if treated with interferon. It should be noted, as well, that interferon must be given by injection, a route that is somewhat unpleasant to most people.

For all of the above-mentioned reasons, a number of alternative antiviral and immune-system modifying medications are being investigated for treatment of people with chronic hepatitis B. The following pages describe briefly some of the most promising medications for use in the treatment of chronic hepatitis B. Of these therapies, lamivudine (Epivir-HBV) is the only drug currently FDA-approved for the treatment of chronic hepatitis B.

Nucleoside and Nucleotide Agents

Nucleoside and nucleotide analogues are oral antiviral agents. A *nucleoside* is a compound that forms the building blocks of deoxyribonucleic acid (DNA) and ribonucleic acid (RNA)—the compounds in which genetic information is stored. A *nucleotide* is like a nucleoside except that it has a phosphorus molecule attached to it. An *analogue* is a compound that resembles another compound in structure and function. Some of these drugs appear to be quite effective in suppressing HBV replication and disease activity. However, these medications often do not lead to long-term remissions. Moreover, the development of mutant strains of HBV, which are resistant to therapy, commonly occurs during treatment or, with even greater frequency, after treatment has been discontinued. Whether continuous long-term therapy with these drugs will be necessary, and what, if any, side effects can occur with long-term therapy are under investigation.

The following pages discuss nucleoside and nucleotide agents that have been, or are in the process of being, investigated for the treatment of chronic hepatitis B.

Lamivudine (Epivir-HBV) Therapy for Chronic Hepatitis B

Lamivudine is a nucleoside analogue, manufactured by GlaxoWellcome, Inc. Lamivudine was initially evaluated in 1991 as a treatment for people with AIDS. It was found to be a potent inhibitor of human immunodeficiency virus (HIV) replication. As approximately 10 percent of HIV-infected people are also infected with chronic hepatitis B, it was also observed that lamivudine was capable of inhibiting the replication of HBV as well. Lamivudine, marketed as Epivir-HBV, was FDA approved for treating people with chronic hepatitis B in December 1998. In fact, it is now recommended by most experts as the first line of therapy for treatment of people with chronic hepatitis B.

It appears that in contrast to interferon, lamivudine may work well on most people regardless of their individual characteristics. Therefore, people who notoriously respond poorly to interferon—those with normal liver enzymes, Asians, those with HBV mutations, those who are immunosuppressed, and those who acquired infection at birth—appear to respond well to lamivudine. Also, compared with interferon therapy, in which approximately one-third of the individuals will eradicate HBV DNA, almost everyone treated with lamivudine will become HBV DNA-negative, and at a more rapid rate than the typical person who responds to interferon. Plus, it has been shown that almost 40 percent of people treated with lamivudine for up to eighteen months eradicated HBeAg as well. Most important, it has been demonstrated that people treated with lamivudine experience decreased inflammation and are less likely to progress to scarring (as per liver biopsy samples) than similar people treated with interferon. Furthermore, lamivudine may provide some benefit in circumstances in which interferon use is inadvisable (such as in people with decompensated cirrhosis) or ineffective (such as in treating HBV infection occurring after liver transplant or treating people with normal liver enzymes who acquired infection at birth). In fact, a recent study showed that people who lack HBeAg but who have active viral replication (due to mutant strains), not only respond well to lamivudine with evidence of HBV DNA loss, but have a low incidence of viral resistance. Thus, lamivudine should be the treatment of choice for people with mutant strains of HBV.

Because it is administered orally, lamivudine is very easy to take. It is also very well tolerated. Since it has only been studied since 1991, long-term side effects are not completely known. So far, it has been associated with very few side effects. The most commonly occurring ones include headache, diarrhea, fatigue, nausea, abdominal pain, muscle aches, coughing, and skin rashes. These occur infrequently, however. In fact, in one study, these side effects occurred with the same frequency in people who were not treated with lamivudine.

Unfortunately, lamivudine does have some drawbacks and does not appear to be the answer for everyone with chronic hepatitis B. Upon discontinuation of lamivudine, approximately 80 percent of those treated will relapse, as noted by a return of HBV DNA and a flare of transaminases. Therapy with lamivudine should be promptly restarted in this circumstance.

It appears that mutations of HBV occur frequently while a person is on lamivudine therapy. These mutated strains of HBV are generally felt to be weaker and capable of causing less liver damage than non-mutated strains of HBV. Therefore, it is thought that continued treatment with lamivudine for prolonged intervals or possibly lifelong is justified in order to reap the benefits of treatment. Further study will need to be conducted to confirm this hypothesis.

The recommended dose of lamivudine is 100 milligrams, taken orally once a day. Treatment may be as short as three months but is recommended to continue until HBV DNA is repeatedly non-detectable, HBeAg is negative, and preferably until HBeAb is positive. Since there is such a high HBV relapse and mutation rate, studies are evaluating long-term treatment for a year to eighteen months or even longer. Possibly the combination of lamivudine plus interferon, or more likely lamivudine plus one or even two additional nucleoside analogues will delay or prevent emergence of viral resistance. Studies are being conducted to confirm this. So far, it does not appear that interferon-lamivudine combination therapy is yielding superior results to lamivudine therapy alone.

Famciclovir

Famciclovir is another nucleoside analogue. In a study evaluating the effectiveness of this drug in eleven patients with chronic hepatitis B, more than half of the subjects showed a marked decrease in HBV DNA levels after only ten days of treatment. Another study demonstrated that most people responding to famciclovir had only a partial response to therapy. Famciclovir has also been shown to be effective for liver transplant recipients who become reinfected with HBV after the transplant. So far, famciclovir does not appear to have any serious side effects. Efficacy of the combination of famciclovir with lamivudine appears to be limited. Further study needs to be conducted on this drug before it can be recommended.

Lobucavir

Lobucavir is a nucleoside analogue. In preliminary studies, more than two-thirds of people with chronic hepatitis B who were treated with lobucavir successfully eradicated HBV DNA from their blood within three months of treatment. However, after discontinuation of therapy, rebound of HBV DNA levels was common. Lobucavir has not been associated with any severe side effects. However, in animal studies, an increase in tumor growth was noted in the rodents given lobucavir. While this side effect has never been demonstrated in humans, further study on lobucavir has been suspended.

Adefovir

Adefovir is a nucleotide analogue. Preliminary studies have shown that this drug has significant antiviral activity in people regardless of whether their ALT levels are normal or elevated. Further study needs to be conducted to determine the drug's effectiveness for both types of people with chronic hepatitis B.

Other Nucleoside Analogues

Some other nucleoside analogues, such as ganciclovir, have been tried, but have been found to be only temporarily effective, or—in the case of fialuridine (FIAU), for example—limited in use due to severe side effects. Nucleoside analogues, including 5'-thiafluorocytosine (FTC) and the carbocyclic analogue of 2'-deoxyguaosine, are also undergoing investigation for use in people with chronic hepatitis B—both those with and those without HBeAg.

Thymosin

Thymosin is a *polypeptide* (a group of amino acids linked together) hormone that is produced by a gland located in the neck, known as the thymus gland. Studies have shown that thymosin can stimulate the immune system—thus, it has immunomodulatory properties. Studies suggest that thymosin can eradicate active hepatitis B viral infection from the body. In one study, thymosin alfa-1 treatment (Zadaxin; manufactured by SciClone Pharmaceuticals, Inc.) for twenty-six or fifty-two weeks (1.6 mg subcutaneously, twice a week) resulted in loss of HBV DNA and HBeAg from the blood in approximately 40 percent of people one year after completion of treatment. Furthermore, among the 40 percent of the people who responded, liver inflammation was significantly reduced. Thymosin alfa-1 also appears to be safe with few side effects. Further study needs to be conducted to confirm these results and to determine the effectiveness of combination therapy using thymosin alfa-1.

HBV Vaccine as Therapy

The immune system of most adults is strong enough to eradicate HBV from the body when exposure occurs. The failure of some adults to clear the virus is due to many factors, one of which is a poorly functioning or defective immune system. Researchers have sought to counter this circumstance by administering the hepatitis B vaccination to people with chronic hepatitis B in an attempt to stimulate an immune response against the virus. This strategy has been tried on a small group of people, and the results look promising. However, further research in this area is needed before it is offered as a therapy.

Interleukin-12

Interleukin-12 (IL-12) is a natural protein made in the body. This protein acts to regulate the intensity and duration of the body's immune response. Furthermore, IL-12 has been shown to induce interferon production in the body. Therefore, this agent can potentially assist the immune system in eradicating HBV from the body. Further study on this protein is needed before it can possibly be offered as an effective treatment for individuals with chronic hepatitis B.

Combination Therapy

From the medical knowledge gained from treating people with HIV, doctors have learned that a combination of medications may work better than one medication alone. The superior efficacy of combination therapy has become evident in the treatment of chronic hepatitis C, which is discussed in Chapter 13. As more medications become available to treat people infected with chronic hepatitis B, treatment with one drug may eventually become a thing of the past, at least for those people who are classically poor responders to individual-drug therapy (monotherapy). Furthermore, combination therapy may eliminate the problem of drug-resistant, mutant forms of HBV, which commonly emerge in people treated with nucleoside analogues. Further research needs to be conducted to evaluate the effectiveness of various combinations of drugs, such as a nucleoside analogue and interferon, or more likely, two or even three nucleoside analogues together.

ALTERING THE COURSE OF CHRONIC HEPATITIS B WITH TREATMENT

For people with chronic hepatitis B, treatment with interferon has been shown to decrease the incidence of long-term complications such as liver failure and the subsequent need for liver transplantation. The result is a prolonged life expectancy.

Lamivudine has been shown to reduce the risk of liver cancer, although to date this benefit has only been demonstrated in experimental studies involving woodchucks.

In some people, treatment totally eliminates HBV, and in others, treatment slows down the progression of the disease although not eliminating it totally. Therefore, it makes sense for everyone with chronic hepatitis B to seek treatment. People probably have a decreased risk of liver cancer if HBsAg is eradicated prior to the development of cirrhosis. However, since liver cancer may still occur in people with chronic hepatitis B who do not progress to cirrhosis, further study is needed to confirm this relationship. Similarly, a person who eradicates HBsAg prior to the development of cirrhosis may still be at risk for the development of complications, but the risk of complications is probably significantly reduced. Therefore, even those people who have had a successful response to therapy should be monitored lifelong by their doctors.

IS ANTIVIRAL THERAPY FOR EVERYONE WITH CHRONIC HEPATITIS B?

Everybody with chronic hepatitis B should begin antiviral therapy if they are actively infectious—as indicated by the presence of HBV DNA and HbeAg and elevated transaminase levels (AST and ALT)—and they do not have decompensated cirrhosis (complications arising from cirrhosis, such as bleeding esophageal varices). However, not everyone with chronic hepatitis B falls into these categories. People with chronic hepatitis B without the above criteria for treatment may have a low likelihood of response to antiviral medication or may actually worsen by starting therapy. These people may nevertheless opt to try therapy, but they will need very close observation. The following is a discussion of specific instances in which antiviral therapy may not be indicated or may, in fact, be harmful.

Those With Normal Transaminases

People with chronic hepatitis B should not be treated with interferon if their transaminases are normal. These people have only a minimal chance of eradicating the virus from their bodies. In fact, these people may actually experience a worsening of the disease when interferon treatment is stopped. Some liver experts have suggested initial treatment with a short course of steroids, such as prednisone, to stimulate viral replication, followed by treatment with interferon. However, in many cases, this dual treatment regimen has caused a worsening of the disease, and, as such, it cannot be recommended.

Treatment with a nucleoside analogue (for example, lamivudine and famciclovir) has a better chance of suppressing HBV replication. However, the use of nucleoside analogues may cause HBV to form mutant strains, which leads to resistance to further therapy. Studies treating this category of people with a combination of interferon and a nucleoside analogue are underway.

Those With Decompensated Cirrhosis

People with chronic hepatitis B who have decompensated cirrhosis (see Chapter 6) should refrain from treatment, especially treatment with interferon. People with decompensated cirrhosis who are treated with interferon are likely to experience severe complications such as liver failure, infection, and hemorrhage. If a person with decompensated cirrhosis opts to be treated with interferon, reduced dosages should be used. In addition, it is recommended that these people be placed on a list for and prepared for liver transplantation (see Chapter 22).

Those With Mutant Strains of HBV

People with mutant strains of HBV (HBeAg-negative, but HBV DNA-positive) are notoriously difficult to treat with success, especially with interferon. Loss of the carrier state (eradication of HbsAg from the body) is uncommon and relapses are frequent. However, since HBV replication can be suppressed in many of these people, an attempt to treat them is recommended. While relapses are frequent when using conventional treatment with interferon, studies have shown that lamivudine may be effective for those with mutant strains of HBV (see page 103) and is thus the treatment of choice.

TREATMENT OF CHRONIC HEPATITIS D

Hepatitis delta virus (HDV) is a virus that can live only in a person who is infected with HBV. Approximately 70,000 people in the United States are infected with HDV. Hepatitis D tends to be a particularly severe infection, with significant long-term consequences causing greater than 1,000 deaths each year. Compared with people who have chronic hepatitis B alone, those with chronic infections of both HBV and HDV have a more aggressive disease course, and they develop cirrhosis faster and at an earlier age. In fact, approximately 15 percent of people with chronic hepatitis D develop cirrhosis within two years of initially becoming infected with this virus. Therefore, treatment of people with chronic hepatitis D is crucial.

Unfortunately, HDV appears to be a particularly stubborn virus, as the virus does not respond particularly well to interferon treatment over sustained periods of time. When treatment with interferon alfa-2a is undertaken at 9 million units, three times a week for forty-eight weeks, about half of those being treated will show signs of response—normalization of transaminases, eradication of hepatitis delta virus from the blood, and improvement of inflammation on liver biopsy samples. Unfortunately, this response is short-lived, as most people will relapse when therapy is discontinued.

Since this is such an aggressive virus, everyone with chronic hepatitis D should attempt to be treated with interferon. Further studies entailing longer treatment with interferon as well as maintenance dosing are under investigation. Other therapies, such as special nucleotide agents known as antisense oligonucleotides and agents that could block the life cycle of HDV are also being researched. Of course, the only way to cure hepatitis D is to prevent it in the first place. Prevention of hepatitis D is possible by preventing hepatitis B with the hepatitis B vaccination, which will be discussed in Chapter 24.

MONITORING THOSE WHO ARE NOT TREATED

People with chronic hepatitis D and/or chronic hepatitis B who are not treated should have periodic follow-up visits with their liver specialists. It is recommended that these visits occur from two to four times per year. During a typical visit, a physical exam will be conducted and blood work will be obtained. Once a year, a sonogram of the liver will need to be obtained, or possibly more often, depending upon the person's individual characteristics. The purpose of these visits is to assess the patient's status and to determine if she is stable or is progressing to cirrhosis, liver failure, and/or liver cancer. The specialist will seek to assess whether the patient has silently converted into an active stage of the disease, wherein she is highly infectious to others and consequently an appropriate candidate for treatment. A repeat liver biopsy is sometimes performed approximately every five years in order to assess disease progression—although intervals may vary at the discretion of the doctor.

CONCLUSION

Treatment options for chronic hepatitis B and chronic hepatitis D are increasing and are very promising. However, one stumbling block to treatment is the emergence of drug-resistant mutant strains of HBV. One possible solution is combination therapy, using two or more drugs, each with different modes of attack against HBV. This treatment strategy has been used successfully in people infected with HIV and in those with chronic hepatitis C. The best treatment, of course is prevention. This is discussed in Chapter 24.

The next chapter discusses treatment of another chronic virus, the hepatitis C virus (HCV), which has several effective treatments presently available and some promising new ones on the horizon.

13

Treating Hepatitis C

There are approximately 250 million chronic carriers of the hepatitis C virus (HCV) worldwide. In the United States, where about 2 percent of the population is infected with HCV, hepatitis C is the most common reason for adults with chronic liver disease to require a liver transplant. In fact, approximately 730 liver transplants per year are due to chronic hepatitis C. It is estimated that approximately 8,000 to 10,000 Americans die each year from chronic hepatitis C. The National Institutes of Health (NIH) estimates that without effective treatment, this number may triple within the next few decades. However, chronic hepatitis C should not be viewed as inevitably leading to death. It is important to keep in mind that some effective treatments are available and that some new and improved treatments are being developed. So, it is unlikely if people with chronic hepatitis C seek appropriate medical care that this estimated future death toll will be a reality. In fact, many people with chronic hepatitis C may live a long and healthy life and may not require therapy at all.

The goals of therapy are to suppress viral activity and replication, to decrease inflammation in the liver, to prevent future inflammation and liver damage, to decrease a person's chances of progressing to cirrhosis and liver cancer, and to diminish any symptoms that are present. These goals are capable of being achieved only through antiviral therapy.

This chapter discusses the treatment of chronic hepatitis C. It analyzes who will benefit the most from treatment and the circumstances under which people do and do not require treatment. Alfa-interferon (Intron A) was the first effective treatment for chronic hepatitis C. It was approved by the FDA in 1991. People tend to vary greatly in their response to alfa-interferon. And, in fact, most people fail to have a long-term response to this treatment. The different types of interferon and the different interferon treatment regimens are discussed in detail in this chapter. Also discussed in this chapter is a major advancement in the treatment of chronic hepatitis C—combination therapy of interferon and ribavirin (Rebetron), which became the standard therapy after its FDA approval in 1998. Finally some promising experimental treatment options are discussed.

TREATMENT OF ACUTE HEPATITIS C

This incidence of acute hepatitis has dropped dramatically in the past few years. In the 1980s, approximately 200,000 new infections occurred each year. Recent statistics, however, show that only approximately 30,000 new infections are occurring each year. Since the symptoms associated with acute HCV are either nonspecific or nonexistent, only a small percentage of these people will be diagnosed during the acute stage of the disease. Yet, in view of the extraordinarily high incidence of progression to chronic disease (approximately 85 percent), it is important to identify and treat these people in an attempt to eradicate the virus at the acute stage. In fact, studies have shown that a short course of interferon therapy—one to three months—provided to people with acute hepatitis C significantly reduced the likelihood of progression to chronic liver disease. In one study, eradication of HCV RNA was seen in 41 percent of people treated with interferon versus only 4 percent of those who were not treated. Therefore, treatment with interferon is recommended for people diagnosed with acute hepatitis C.

THE REASONS TO TREAT CHRONIC HEPATITIS C

Chronic hepatitis C will not go away on its own. In most people, it is a slowly progressive disease. Not only does HCV do its damage slowly, but it usually does its damage silently. This explains why many people with chronic hepatitis C (especially those who have no symptoms), when advised by their doctors to start treatment with an injectable medication that has potential side effects, react with confusion.

"Why should I be treated? I feel fine!" is a comment that liver specialists commonly hear. The answer to this question is that people with chronic hepatitis C are at risk for developing cirrhosis, liver failure, and liver cancer. Once cirrhosis has developed, the likelihood of responding to treatment is greatly reduced. And once a person develops liver failure and/or liver cancer, conventional medical therapies are unlikely to help and may actually worsen the patient's condition. Therefore, it is of utmost importance to attempt to eradicate HCV from the body in order to stop or slow down progression of disease before the development of any liver-related complications. And the earlier a person seeks treatment, the more likely she is to reap its benefits—benefits that include long-term eradication of HCV from the body and a reduced incidence of progression to cirrhosis, liver failure, and liver cancer. Furthermore, people who are treated in the early stages of disease are less likely to experience the adverse side effects sometimes associated with antiviral therapy.

THOSE WHO SHOULD OR SHOULDN'T START ANTIVIRAL THERAPY

Whether or not to start treatment for chronic hepatitis C is an important decision that should be made jointly by the doctor and the patient. Many variables must be taken into consideration when making this decision, as not everyone with chronic hepatitis C needs to be treated with antiviral medication. All individuals with elevated transaminase levels, elevated hepatitis C viral loads (HCV RNA), and either scarring and/or inflammation on liver biopsy specimens are advised to consider treatment, unless specific reasons to avoid treatment exist. The following is a discussion of whether or not people with persistently normal ALT levels should start antiviral therapy and of some specific instances in which antiviral therapy may not be indicated or may even be harmful.

Those With Normal ALT Levels

Approximately one-third of all people with chronic hepatitis C have persistently normal ALT levels, despite having elevated viral loads (HCV RNA). The exact significance of this finding is not known and may, in fact, vary from person to person. Some experts believe that these people may never have serious liver disease, and thus, have been referred to as "healthy chronic carriers" of HCV. Other experts believe that some people with chronic hepatitis C who have normal ALT levels may eventually develop liver inflammation and scarring and that some will even progress to cirrhosis. To complicate matters further, the degree of elevation of HCV RNA does not correlate with the severity of inflammation or damage found on liver biopsy samples. This leaves the doctor without any simple parameters with which to judge severity or worsening of disease.

Accordingly, many studies have recommended treatment with interferon for people with chronic hepatitis C who have normal ALT levels, regardless of the HCV RNA level. Initially, it was thought that this group of people might respond better to therapy than people with elevated ALT levels. However, the results from the majority of these trials failed to show any significant benefit from treatment with interferon. Most of the time, HCV RNA did not decrease at all, and even increased in some people. Some people (approximately two-thirds) even experienced a temporary elevation of their ALT levels both during and after completion of the study. This suggests that either interferon itself caused liver toxicity, thereby resulting in a temporary elevation in the ALT level, or that interferon actually instigated a flare-up of disease, as evidenced by a corresponding elevation of the HCV viral load (HCV RNA) among some of these people.

So, should people with persistently normal ALT levels be treated? Well, the National Institutes of Health (NIH) consensus statement in 1997 regarding the management of hepatitis C recommended that people with persistently normal ALT levels refrain from treatment. However, since it appears that some people with normal ALT levels do progress to serious liver disease, an alternative option—to undergo a liver biopsy—should be considered. In this manner, the doctor will be able to evaluate the amount of inflammation and scarring present in the liver. If little or no inflammation or damage is present, the person should refrain from treatment. If significant damage has occurred, especially if cirrhosis appears imminent, individuals should be given the option of antiviral treatment (interferon or Rebetron) or the opportunity to participate in an ongoing trial of antiviral medication for people with chronic hepatitis C and normal transaminases. The effectiveness of antiviral medications other than interferon, as well as Rebetron (Intron A plus ribavirin), is currently being evaluated for this group of people.

One point that is crucial to remember is that transaminase levels in people with chronic hepatitis C typically fluctuate. So it is to be expected that people whose transaminases are elevated most of the time will occasionally have normal transaminase levels. These people must be distinguished from those with persistently normal transaminases. The temporary normalization of transaminase levels should not be equated with improvement of disease or used as a justification not to seek treatment.

Those for Whom Antiviral Therapy Isn't Advisable

Among certain people, the risks of treatment with interferon outweigh the potential benefits. The following discusses some instances in which interferon treatment may not be advisable.

Those With Psychiatric Disorders

Interferon, whether administered alone or in combination with ribavirin, may cause significant depression, anxiety, and altered thought processes. Therefore, people who suffer from a significant underlying psychiatric disorder should refrain from treatment with interferon, as interferon may cause psychiatric problems to worsen or perhaps even to become life-threatening in nature. Those that suffer from a temporary psychiatric problem should postpone interferon therapy until the disorder is under control for a significant amount of time or has totally resolved. If a person has a stable chronic psychiatric disorder, but is motivated to begin treatment for chronic hepatitis C, treatment can often successfully be accomplished by having the person closely and carefully comanaged by a psychiatrist and a liver specialist.

Those With Decompensated Cirrhosis

People who have decompensated cirrhosis—those who have experienced complications due to cirrhosis, such as bleeding esophageal varices or ascites—are not considered appropriate candidates for interferon therapy. These people usually have low platelet counts (thrombocytopenia), which may get even lower when treated with interferon, thereby putting these people at risk for life-threatening bleeding. People with decompensated cirrhosis should be referred to a liver transplant center for evaluation (see Chapter 22).

Those Who Have Undergone Kidney Transplantation

Approximately 20 to 30 percent of all individuals on hemodialysis for kidney failure are infected with chronic hepatitis C. These people are often awaiting kidney transplantation. Treating individuals with chronic hepatitis C with interferon after kidney transplantation is risky, as it may cause rejection of the newly transplanted kidney. Therefore, it is strongly recommended that people with chronic hepatitis C, who are also undergoing dialysis for the treatment of kidney failure, should be treated for hepatitis C prior to undergoing a kidney transplant. Studies have demonstrated that these people respond to interferon treatment for chronic hepatitis C similarly to people who have normally functioning kidneys.

Those With Autoimmune Disorders

Interferon may worsen an underlying autoimmune disorder, particularly autoimmune hepatitis (AIH), which is discussed in Chapter 14. People who have both AIH and chronic hepatitis C should be treated for AIH first. Of course, prior to making treatment decisions, a liver biopsy must be performed first to confirm that AIH is the predominant liver disease. After AIH is successfully treated, an attempt may be made to treat chronic hepatitis C, but the risk of a severe relapse of AIH exists.

Other autoimmune disorders, such as thyroid disease, may also worsen on interferon treatment. People with thyroid disorders may undergo interferon therapy; however, dosages of thyroid medication need to be closely monitored and often need to be altered.

DETERMINING A RESPONSE TO THERAPY

Response to therapy is determined by the normalization of alanine transaminase (ALT) and eradication of HCV from the blood. Eradication, if achieved, is manifested as non-detectable levels of HCV RNA on blood tests. Therefore, a *nonresponder* is a person who does not normalize her transaminases, and who continues to have detectable levels of HCV RNA in her blood while on therapy. These individuals are also known as being *refractory to therapy.*

A *responder* is a person who normalizes transaminases and eradicates HCV RNA while on therapy. Responders fall into one of two categories. Some lucky people have a *sustained response,* meaning that the virus has remained undetectable for more than six months beyond the date therapy was discontinued. People who have a sustained response to therapy are unlikely to have a relapse of disease in the future. This has been demonstrated to hold true for at least ten years beyond the discontinuation of therapy. However, studies ranging from thirty to forty years still need to be conducted in order to assess the actual stability of this long-term response. The other category of responders is known as *relapsers,* meaning that when they are taken off therapy, HCV RNA again becomes detectable in their blood and their transaminase levels again become elevated. Although a relapse may happen at any time, it is most common within the first six months after therapy is discontinued, and usually can be noted as early as one month after discontinuation of therapy. As noted above, once a person has eradicated HCV RNA from her blood for more than six months beyond the discontinuation of therapy, it is very unlikely that the virus will return.

MONITORING PATIENTS BEFORE AND DURING THERAPY

Before starting therapy, a person should have a full series of blood tests. These should include transaminases, HCV RNA, bilirubin, prothrombin time, and complete blood count with differential and platelets (CBC), thyroid tests, antinuclear antibody (ANA; see Chapter 14), glucose (blood sugar) level, alpha-feto-protein (AFP), and human immunodeficiency virus (HIV). (See Chapter 3 for an explanation of some of these tests.) A liver biopsy is not required but is highly recommended prior to beginning therapy for a variety of reasons (see Chapter 5). It is not necessary to repeat a liver biopsy at the end of therapy—unless as part of a clinical study protocol. A complete physical exam—including an eye exam if a person has high blood pressure or diabetes—should be obtained.

The patient should expect to see her doctor and undergo blood tests monthly during therapy—although intervals may vary at the discretion of the doctor. On these occasions, the patient should discuss with her doctor any side effects of therapy she is experiencing and should feel free to ask the doctor any questions that pertain to the therapy. Typically, three months after starting therapy, the doctor will run blood tests to determine whether the person is responding to therapy. This is indicated by a normal ALT and non-detectable HCV RNA in the blood. If the person is responding to therapy, repeat HCV RNA blood tests typically are performed at the end of therapy—for example, twelve months from the commencement of treatment—to document end-of-treatment response. Other blood tests and additional viral loads may be drawn at the discretion of the doctor.

ALFA INTERFERON THERAPY ALONE FOR CHRONIC HEPATITIS C (MONOTHERAPY)

Three years before the hepatitis C virus was discovered, researchers already had established that alfa interferon was effective therapy for some people with chronic hepatitis C—which was known prior to 1989 as non-A non-B hepatitis. Currently, three brands of alfa interferon—Intron A (interferon alfa-2b), Roferon (interferon alfa-2a), and Infergen (interferon alfacon-1 or consensus interferon)—are FDA-approved to treat people with chronic hepatitis C. Each of these brands have been approved for use in the treatment of people who have never been treated before *(treatment naive)* or who have been treated with interferon and either relapsed after therapy was discontinued (relapsers) or who did not respond to interferon therapy at all (nonresponders or refractory to response). The three FDA-approved interferons—as well as some other not-as-yet-approved interferons, such as interferon alfa-n1, interferon beta, interferon alfa-n3—appear to be roughly equally effective in *treatment-naive* people.

Certain characteristics are common among people who are most likely to have a long-term response to monotherapy (treatment with only one therapy—in this case, interferon). This includes the following individuals:

• People with a recent infection with HCV.

.• People with a low viral load (HCV RNA less than one million copies/ml).

• People without cirrhosis.

• People without genotype 1b (see Chapter 10).

• People with no or little quasispecies variation (see Chapter 10).

• People without excessive iron on liver biopsy specimens.

• Females.

• People who are less than forty-five years old.

However, it should be kept in mind that people to whom these characteristics do not apply may still respond to therapy. As such, lack of these characteristics should not, in and of itself, dissuade a person from starting interferon therapy. Response to alfa interferon can usually be determined after three months of starting therapy—although some experts believe that as little as one month is enough time to judge whether or not a person will respond. People who fail to normalize ALT and fail to eradicate HCV RNA from their blood after three months of monotherapy are unlikely to respond if given more of the same therapy. These people should change to a different treatment regimen, discussed on page 170.

Everyone with chronic hepatitis C who is a candidate for therapy should attempt to be treated. People who respond to therapy have been shown to have decreased inflammation and scarring on liver biopsy specimens. It appears that even people who do not respond to therapy still receive a benefit from treatment with interferon. Thus, even in cases where interferon does not totally eradicate HCV from the body, it may still decrease inflammation of the liver, thus potentially slowing progression of disease and decreasing the chances of developing cirrhosis and liver cancer.

Six Months of Alfa Interferon Therapy

Alfa interferon (Intron A) was initially FDA-approved for three times a week for only six months. With this treatment regimen, approximately one-half of patients will initially respond to therapy—they will have a normal ALT level and a nondetectable viral load (HCV RNA) in their blood. However, within six months of discontinuing alfa interferon therapy, one-half to as many as three-quarters of these people relapse—both ALT becomes elevated and HCV RNA becomes detectable in the blood once again. Thus, long-term response rates after an initial course of six months of alfa interferon given three times a week to people with chronic hepatitis C ranges between only approximately 12 to 25 percent.

While alfa interferon on its own (monotherapy) works well for some people, as noted above, long-term response is uncommon for most people. Therefore, other regimens of treatment have been studied, such as a longer duration of therapy; higher dosages of alfa interferon; daily dosing of interferon usually at a higher than normal dose during the initial period of therapy of one to three months (induction therapy); combination of alfa interferon with other medications (particularly ribavirin—Rebetron); and combination of interferon with other forms of therapy such as phlebotomy (the removal of blood through a vein). These regimens, in addition to other drugs that have been studied for use in people with chronic hepatitis C, are discussed below.

Longer Alfa Interferon Treatment Regimens

Since long-term eradication of HCV occurs in only a small percentage of people treated for six months, studies were conducted to evaluate a longer duration of treatment and also treatment with higher dosages of interferon. While higher doses of interferon do not appear to significantly increase response rates, longer treatment regimens lasting one year have proven to be beneficial. Studies have found that when treatment with alfa interferon is given three times a week for one year, long-term response increases to between 20 to 30 percent. Thus, in 1997, the FDA approved the extended treatment interval of alfa interferon to one year.

After three months of interferon therapy, people with both a normal ALT and a nondetectable HCV RNA are likely to have a sustained long-term response. It is recommended that these people continue interferon therapy for a total of twelve months. Studies are underway to evaluate the efficacy of even longer treatment regimens (eighteen to twenty-four months). As noted above, interferon may have some benefit even among people who do not experience complete viral eradication. Therefore, people who do not have normalized ALT levels and in whom the viral load (HCV RNA) has remained elevated (non-responders) should continue some form of antiviral therapy. This is especially important for people with severe inflammation and scarring on liver biopsy specimens. Since these people are on their way to cirrhosis, an all out effort should be made to slow or stop progression of disease. It is recommended that these non-responders begin combination therapy with Rebetron (Intron A and ribavirin; see below). Other treatment options include daily dosing with interferon for a few months (induction therapy), other forms of interferon (for example, Infergen), lifelong interferon therapy, or enrolling in a research trial of a promising new treatment.

INTERFERON (INTRON A) COMBINED WITH RIBAVIRIN— (REBETRON) THERAPY

From knowledge gained by the medical profession in the treatment of people with HIV, it has become clear that combining two or more antiviral drugs together can be a particularly effective form of therapy to fight viruses. This method of combining medications together has been referred to as *cocktail therapy* (not to be confused with an alcoholic mixed drink).

The addition of ribavirin to interferon is a major advance in the treatment of chronic hepatitis C. Ribavirin is an orally administered synthetic antiviral agent.

It is known medically as a guanosine nucleoside analogue—a component of DNA and RNA, the genetic building blocks of life. When used alone, it is ineffective against HCV—it may temporarily normalize ALT levels, but has no effect on HCV RNA. However, when used in combination with alfa interferon, the so-called "cocktail therapy," it has been found to be quite effective against HCV. The recommended dose depends on the person's weight, and is usually about five to six tablets a day (each tablet is 200 mg) taken in two divided doses. A typical daily regimen might be, for example, two or three tablets in the morning and three tablets in the evening, for a total dosage of approximately 1,000 mg to 1,200 mg per day.

The exact way that ribavirin fights against viruses is not known. Also, it is not known why ribavirin works against HCV only when combined with interferon. However, it has been demonstrated that ribavirin works in union with (synergistically with) interferon, boosting interferon's antiviral and immune activity against HCV.

WHO MAY BENEFIT FROM INTERFERON AND RIBAVIRIN COMBINED

The addition of ribavirin to interferon (Intron A), packaged together as Rebetron (marketed by Schering-Plough) has been shown to be a more effective treatment than interferon alone. This applies to people who have never been treated with interferon before (the treatment naive); people who have relapsed after initially responding to interferon (relapsers); and people who did not respond to interferon at all (nonresponders).

The Treatment-Naïve

Studies have shown that Rebetron, used for forty-eight weeks by people who had never been treated with interferon before, achieved a long-term sustained response in 38 to 47 percent of the subjects—as compared with 6 to 20 percent of the subjects treated with interferon alone. Rebetron, when used for twenty-four weeks, achieved a 31- to 35-percent long-term sustained response rate—versus 6 to 8 percent for people treated with interferon alone. And people treated with Rebetron have demonstrated greater improvements on liver biopsy specimens as compared with those treated with interferon alone.

Relapsers

Among people who relapsed after initially responding to interferon therapy (relapsers), the use of Rebetron for only six months resulted in a sustained long-term response in approximately half of these people. Thus, after relapsing, treatment of people with Rebetron proves to be more effective than treatment for one year with interferon alone. As with the treatment-naive, inflammation on liver biopsy is also reduced.

Non-Responders

Studies have shown that approximately 6 to 26 percent of the patients who did not respond to interferon alone (non-responders), achieve a sustained response of viral eradication with Rebetron therapy. As such, combination therapy appears to be beneficial even to some people within this group of difficult-to-treat patients.

PREDICTORS OF RESPONSE TO REBETRON

The characteristics of a person that may predict a good response to Rebetron therapy appear to be somewhat similar to those that apply to interferon alone. However, one of the great benefits of Rebetron is that some people with characteristics of a poor response to interferon therapy—such as those with cirrhosis, high viral loads, or genotype 1—may in fact respond to Rebetron, particularly if treated for a full forty-eight weeks.

As noted above, people who achieve a sustained long-term response when treated with interferon alone usually eradicate HCV RNA from their blood within three months from the start of therapy. In contrast, at least half the people who achieve a sustained response from combination therapy take longer than three months and up to six months (and possibly longer) to eradicate the virus. Therefore, it is important for everyone using Rebetron to continue therapy for at least six months before calling it quits.

SIDE EFFECTS OF RIBAVIRIN

From the standpoint of mathematical probability, it is clear that the more drugs a person takes, the greater the likelihood that she will experience adverse side effects—hence, the downside of combination drug therapy. Therefore, it is not unexpected that the incidence of discontinuation of therapy is greater among people taking Rebetron (approximately 6 percent) than among those taking interferon alone (approximately 3 percent). But not everyone experiences adverse side effects, and some have no side effects at all. (See Chapter 11 for a discussion of the side effects associated with interferon alone.)

Following is a discussion of the side effects associated with ribavirin. Meanwhile, an important point to remember is that there is not a tremendous difference in the long-term response rates for treatment-naive individuals treated for only twenty-four weeks versus forty-eight weeks—approximately 31 to 35 percent for the former versus 38 to 47 percent for the latter. Therefore, people who are experiencing severe side effects from combination therapy should be given the option of discontinuing at week twenty-four.

One advantageous side effect of ribavirin is that it often causes an increase in the platelet count. Therefore, people who have low platelet counts, as is often seen in those with cirrhosis, may obtain this additional benefit from being treated with combination therapy. Furthermore, this ribavirin-induced platelet count elevation can offset platelet count reduction that interferon commonly causes.

Ribavirin-Induced Anemia

Ribavirin can accumulate in red blood cells (RBCs), destroying them. The destruction of red blood cells is known as *hemolysis*. Hemolysis results in a low red blood cell count known as *hemolytic anemia*. This is detected on blood tests as a low hemoglobin (less than 10 grams/dl). *Hemoglobin* is an iron-containing protein that is part of a red blood cell. This is perhaps the most serious side effect related to ribavirin, occurring in approximately 10 percent of people taking this drug. Symptoms associated with anemia include fatigue and shortness of breath. In cases where anemia occurs as a result of ribavirin therapy, it will typically occur during the first few weeks of therapy. Therefore, it is important to be diligent with follow-up visits to the doctor's office especially during the initial period of time after beginning Rebetron.

Ribavirin-induced anemia is both dose-dependent and reversible, meaning that if the ribavirin dose is lowered or discontinued, the anemia will resolve. People who are already anemic may not be suitable candidates for Rebetron, as it will most likely worsen their anemia. Ribavirin-induced anemia is particularly dangerous for people with an underlying cardiac condition. Anyone with a prior history of heart disease should be evaluated by a cardiologist to determine if she is a suitable candidate for therapy. All men over the age of forty and all women over fifty should obtain an electrocardiogram (EKG) prior to beginning therapy.

Erythropoietin is a protein made by the body that can stimulate the formation of new red blood cells. Preliminary studies have shown that when erythropoietin is administered (10,000 to 40,000 units subcutaneously per week) to some people on Rebetron, hemoglobin levels return to normal. This therapy may prove to be an effective way to combat ribavirin-induced hemolytic anemia.

Birth Defects

Ribavirin is *teratogenic*—capable of causing birth defects. Therefore, people who are pregnant, or who are contemplating pregnancy, are not candidates for Rebetron therapy. Furthermore, everyone should use contraception while on therapy and for six months following the discontinuation of therapy.

Gastrointestinal Symptoms

Some people become nauseous and develop abdominal discomfort from ribavirin. This is easily remedied by taking ribavirin with food. If these symptoms continue, a dose reduction of ribavirin by one or two pills per day may become necessary.

Other Symptoms

Some other side effects include fatigue, pruritus, cough, insomnia, depression, and rash. When these side effects do occur in connection with ribavirin therapy, they are usually not very severe, and typically dissipate upon discontinuation of therapy.

OTHER TREATMENT OPTIONS FOR CHRONIC HEPATITIS C

Response rates to therapy have been higher than ever; however, many people for various reasons are in need of a different treatment regimen. The following is a discussion of other treatment options available to those who have not responded to standard treatment regimens.

Infergen

Infergen (consensus interferon or interferon alfacon-1; manufactured by Amgen) is a genetically bioengineered synthetic form of alfa interferon. Compared to other type-1 alfa interferons, it has been shown to have significantly greater antiviral activity. It has been found to be an effective treatment for some people who had either relapsed or who did not respond to an initial course of treatment with alfa-interferon. In fact, 58 percent of the individuals who experienced a relapse after initially responding to treatment with alfa-interferon had a sustained long-term response when retreated with 15 micrograms of Infergen three times a week for forty-eight weeks. And an additional 13 percent of the individuals who did not respond to an initial course of alfa-interferon responded to 15 micrograms of Infergen three times a week for forty-eight weeks. Thus, Infergen appears to be a particularly effective alternative treatment option particularly for some people who relapsed after an initial course of interferon therapy.

Studies are underway to confirm the effectiveness of Infergen for people who relapsed or who did not respond to Rebetron combination therapy.

Induction Therapy

Researchers have shown that administering interferon three times a week may not be adequate to sustain long-term viral eradication in many people. Some preliminary studies have shown that at least during the first four to twelve weeks of therapy, people require higher doses—for example, 5 to 10 million units (MU) of Intron A—administered *daily* in order to achieve an optimal response. This is then followed by the traditional dose of 3 MU of Intron A three times a week. This is known as *induction therapy*. It has been noted that blood levels of HCV RNA decrease the fastest when interferon is initially administered daily at a higher-than-normal dose. Furthermore, daily attack on the virus with interferon does not give HCV a two-day reprieve. During the two-day "vacation period" that HCV has under the current three-times-a-week regimen, the virus has ample time in which to regain strength and replicate. This may explain why so many people do not respond at all or else relapse after initially responding to therapy.

Studies are underway to confirm the effectiveness of administering interferon or Rebetron in daily doses. Initial results appear promising. Thus, daily dosing, at least during the initial treatment period, is likely to become a preferred treatment regimen, particularly for people with genotype 1 and/or with viral loads of greater than 2 million viral particles.

Pegylated Interferon

Anyone would prefer to take a drug just once a week, rather than three times a week or worse, daily. Well, two pharmaceutical companies, Roche and Schering-Plough, are studying this concept for interferon therapy in people with chronic hepatitis C. Their drugs are known as PEGASYS (pegylated interferon alfa 2a) and PEG-Rebetron (pegylated Rebetron), respectively.

Polyethylene glycol (PEG) is a substance that can attach to a protein, resulting in longer-acting, sustained activity of the protein. If the activity of a protein, such as interferon, is prolonged by the attachment to PEG, the frequency of interferon's administration each week would be decreased. Under this reasoning, a once-a-week dosing of pegylated interferon would hopefully be as effective as interferon administered three times a week. If results turn out as hoped, pegylated interferon stands to be a more convenient way to administer interferon. This, in turn, would result in improved patient compliance, as one injection per week is easier to handle than three. In fact, preliminary data has shown that approximately 36 percent of the individuals had a sustained nondetectable hepatitis C viral load (HCV RNA) after one year of treatment with pegylated interferon alfa-2a (PEGASYS), with similar side effects as those occurring in people taking interferon three times a week. Further evaluation is needed before definitive conclusions can be drawn.

Initial results with pegylated Rebetron are pending. If response rates prove to be as expected, this therapy may, in fact, become the standard of care for people with chronic hepatitis C.

Iron Reduction Therapy

Phlebotomy—a form of iron reduction therapy—involves taking blood out of the body via a catheter that is temporarily placed in a vein in the arm. This blood is then discarded. It cannot be used for blood donation or for any other purpose. Phlebotomy is the primary form of treatment for people with an iron overload disease, such as hemochromatosis (see Chapter 18). People with chronic hepatitis C often have a high iron content, in both their blood and livers. It is believed that such people may have a low response rate to alfa-interferon alone. Some studies have shown that among this group of people, phlebotomy may improve the overall response to interferon therapy.

Chelation therapy—another form of iron reduction therapy—involves the infusion of deferoxamine (Desferal) either into a vein or beneath the skin (subcutaneously). Deferoxamine works by binding to iron and promoting its elimination from the body. Its effectiveness as an adjunct to interferon therapy is being evaluated. So far, no definitive conclusions have been made concerning the long-term benefits of iron-reduction therapy for people with chronic hepatitis C.

Long-Term or Lifelong Suppressive Interferon Therapy

Long-term suppressive therapy of viruses is not a new concept. Certainly, this form of continuous therapy, possibly lasting lifelong, has proven successful in treating people infected with HIV. The primary goal of suppressive therapy in people with chronic hepatitis C is to impede the progression of liver disease. Thus, even if HCV is not eradicated from the body, suppressive therapy may prevent cirrhosis, liver failure, and liver cancer.

It has been shown that there are substantial benefits to interferon therapy, even in people who do not eradicate HCV, as liver damage and inflammation have been shown to be reduced as a result of treatment. Furthermore, it is believed that treatment with interferon may decrease the likelihood of developing liver cancer. And, in non-cirrhotic individuals who had a sustained response to interferon, the chance of progression to cirrhosis and liver cancer is probably negligible. As such, people who have not eradicated HCV using traditional regimens of interferon treatment may still benefit from long-term, or possibly even lifelong, therapy. Studies are now in progress to assess the effectiveness of long-term suppressive therapy. Certainly, pegylated interferon would appear to be the drug of choice for lifelong therapy.

Amantadine

Amantadine (Symmetrel; manufactured by Endolaboratories) is an oral antiviral medication used to treat people with influenza A (the flu), as well as people with Parkinson's disease—a neurological disorder. Thus far, only one study has shown amantadine to be an effective treatment for people with chronic hepatitis C. Minimal side effects were encountered in this study. Unfortunately, this finding has not been duplicated in other studies. Combination therapy with amantadine and interferon has been attempted for people with chronic hepatitis C. However, the results have been somewhat disappointing. Therefore, the initial enthusiasm for treating people with chronic hepatitis C with amantadine has greatly diminished. Further study is ongoing.

Ursodeoxycholic Acid

Ursodeoxycholic acid (UDCA) is a bile salt that has been shown to be beneficial in the treatment of some liver diseases. In people with primary biliary cirrhosis (see Chapter 15), UDCA can normalize transaminase levels and delay progression of disease. Studies have monitored the effect of UDCA, both alone and in combination with interferon, in people with chronic hepatitis C. When used as the sole agent for people with chronic hepatitis C, UDCA appears to temporarily normalize transaminase levels. When used in combination with interferon, UDCA results in a higher incidence of transaminase normalization compared with the incidence of transaminase normalization in people treated with interferon alone. However, it does not appear that UDCA has any significant effect on reducing the hepatitis C viral load or in improving inflammation or scarring in the liver. Therefore, the long-term benefits of UDCA appear limited.

Thymosin alfa-I (Zadaxin)

Thymosin alfa-1 (TA1) is a group of linked amino acids that is produced by the thymus gland, a gland located in the neck. Studies have shown that synthetic TA1 (Zadaxin; manufactured by SciClone Pharmaceuticals) can stimulate the immune system. Thus, thymosin has immunomodulatory properties. TA1 used alone to treat people with chronic hepatitis C produces no significant improvements. However, preliminary studies suggest that TA1 used in combination with interferon may lower viral levels and improve inflammation and damage in the liver. So far, the side effects of Zadaxin have proved negligible. Further study on the drug combination of interferon and Zadaxin is expected.

Other Approaches

A major advance for potential future treatment strategies for hepatitis C was the discovery of the actual structure of two of the crucial enzymes involved in HCV replication by researchers from Vertex Pharmaceuticals. These enzymes are known as the NS3 protease and the NS3 helicase. The next step that Vertex is evaluating is the development of a drug that will inhibit these specific enzymes—an HCV-protease and a HCV-helicase inhibitor. The development of a drug that would inhibit these key enzymes in the HCV life cycle would be a powerful weapon in the treatment of hepatitis C.

Specific clinical trials are ongoing evaluating the drug VX-497 manufactured by Vertex Pharmaceuticals. VX-497 is an inhibitor of the enzyme *inosine monophosphate dehydrogenase* (IMPDH). This enzyme is essential for the production of a nucleotide—a compound that forms the building blocks of DNA and RNA. Therefore, blocking the production of IMPDH may also block viral replication. In experimental trials, VX-497 has been demonstrated to be a potent antiviral, much more potent than ribavirin. And, in combination with interferon, VX-497's antiviral activity appears to be even greater. Research in this key area of investigation is continuing.

Interleukin-12 (IL-12) is a natural protein made in the body that can regulate the intensity and duration of the immune response. IL-12 has been shown to induce the natural production of interferon in the body. Therefore, this agent can potentially assist the immune system in eradicating HCV from the body. However, further study is needed on this protein.

Heptazyme, manufactured by Ribozyme Pharmaceuticals, Inc., is a type of ribozyme—a kind of RNA molecule with the unique ability to cut targeted genetic material. In the case of heptazyme, the targeted genetic material is contained within HCV. Thus heptazyme incapacitates HCV so that replication is no longer possible. When this key genetic material is severed, HCV dies and, therefore, no further viruses can be produced. Further study on this promising therapy is ongoing and results are eagerly being awaited.

CAN CHRONIC HEPATITIS C BE CURED?

So, the ultimate question is—can chronic hepatitis C actually be cured? Well, people who have a negative (less than 100 copies/ml) HCV RNA six months after the discontinuation of interferon are unlikely to experience a relapse of disease—indicated by a reappearance of HCV RNA in the blood. In fact, studies done on people who responded to treatment over ten years ago have shown a good long-term response, with persistently normal transaminase levels and HCV RNA levels. Only about 5 percent of the individuals who were HCV RNA-negative six months after treatment experienced a relapse years later. Even some liver biopsy samples revealed the disappearance of scarring (fibrosis, not cirrhosis) that had been there ten years earlier. This data suggests that in some people, chronic hepatitis C can be cured with interferon therapy. Longer follow-up studies will hopefully confirm these promising results.

Studies have also demonstrated that people whose ALT levels significantly decreased or normalized after interferon treatment had a decreased likelihood of liver cancer than people who were never treated with interferon. Studies have also demonstrated that people with cirrhosis who responded to interferon have a reduced incidence of liver cancer. However, it is important to remember that since cirrhosis is irreversible, these people must still be monitored lifelong for potential complications. Finally, it has been shown that people who either normalized their liver enzymes or who eradicated HCV due to interferon therapy had a greatly improved quality of life in relation to their physical health and emotional well-being.

Even if it does not cure chronic hepatitis C, treatment with interferon or Rebetron may slow disease progression to such an extent that the long-term complications of liver disease, such as cirrhosis, liver failure, and liver cancer, may be prevented for the lifetime of some people.

MONITORING THOSE WHO ARE NOT BEING TREATED

People with chronic hepatitis C who are not treated for whatever reason should be monitored by a doctor at least twice a year. However, the frequency of these visits may need to be increased depending upon specific circumstances. For example, people with decompensated cirrhosis may need more frequent visits in order to manage complications, such as ascites. Visits consist of a history of new symptoms that have occurred, a physical exam, and some blood tests. If cirrhosis is present, an alpha-feto-protein blood test and a sonogram will be necessary once or twice a year. It is important to remember that blood work, symptoms, physical exams, and imaging studies are often inadequate to predict the progression of chronic hepatitis C. To best determine progression of disease—the actual amount of new inflammation and scarring that has occurred—a liver biopsy, performed approximately every five years, is necessary.

CONCLUSION

In this chapter, you learned about some of the remarkable advances that have been made in the treatment of hepatitis C since the virus was first identified. As research on medications to treat people infected with chronic hepatitis C advances, it is becoming evident that treatment with one drug alone may eventually become a thing of the past. This applies especially to those people who are classically poor responders to therapy. Certainly, we have learned that two drugs, each having a different mechanism of action against HCV, work better than one drug alone. Will the future of therapy for people who fail to respond to two medications be the addition of yet another agent? Will interferon always be included in the regimen? Only time will tell.

In the meantime, investigational trials of new drugs and new drug combinations are growing. It is to be expected that from this extensive research, some promising new treatment regimens will emerge. Since most people with chronic hepatitis C have a slowly progressive disease, many individuals will die *with* HCV rather than *from* HCV. Yet, it is not possible to predict with 100-percent accuracy which people will have a benign course of liver disease and which people will have an aggressive course of disease. Thus, treatment should be seriously considered by everyone with chronic hepatitis C.

The first chapter of Part Three discusses autoimmune hepatitis, a type of liver disease caused by an attack on the liver by a person's own immune system. The remaining chapters of Part Three cover other liver disorders and their treatments.

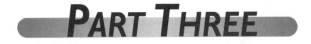
PART THREE

Understanding and Treating Other Liver Diseases

14

Autoimmune Hepatitis

Beth, a usually energetic twenty-two-year-old nurse, had been feeling relentlessly fatigued during the last few months. When her usually regular menstrual cycle stopped for three months, she became very concerned. The results of an at-home pregnancy test came up negative. So what was the problem? Maybe it was the extra shift she'd recently added to her already busy work schedule at the hospital. Or maybe the thyroid medication she just started taking to treat her recent diagnosis of hypothyroidism was to blame.

One day at work, a fellow nurse approached Beth and said in a concerned manner, "Beth, you look jaundiced—you should see a doctor right away." Beth looked in the mirror and was surprised to see that her eyes and skin were in fact yellow.

Beth consulted with her family doctor who referred her to a liver specialist. The specialist took a lengthy history from Beth, which included questions about exposure to viral hepatitis, medication history, and family history of liver disease. A physical exam was performed. In addition to jaundice, the doctor detected that Beth had an enlarged liver and spleen. A battery of blood tests was taken, which revealed that her bilirubin level and liver enzymes was more than ten times the normal values. The test for viral hepatitis was negative, but some of Beth's autoimmune markers were positive. A liver biopsy was performed and confirmed the suspected diagnosis of autoimmune hepatitis. The specialist placed Beth on two medications, and within three weeks, she was back to her normal, healthy self.

Gloria, a fifty-nine-year-old postmenopausal school teacher, went to her doctor for her yearly check-up. With the exception of some minor aches and pains, which she attributed to her history of osteoporosis, Gloria was feeling well. After performing a physical exam and drawing some blood for routine tests, the doctor told Gloria that, as usual, she passed her yearly exam with flying colors. He told her he would telephone her the following week with the results of her blood tests.

"Some of your LFTs were mildly elevated," the doctor told her a week later. "You need to return to the office for additional blood work." Although the doctor tried to alleviate Gloria's fears by telling her there was probably nothing to worry about, she was still concerned. A week after the additional blood tests were done, Gloria went back to the doctor to discuss the results. "You have a mild case of a liver disease known as autoimmune hepatitis," the doctor told her. "You'll need to see a liver specialist to discuss a liver biopsy and treatment options."

Gloria went to the specialist for the biopsy, which revealed mild inflammation without any scarring. The liver specialist confirmed the diagnosis of autoimmune hepatitis. But because Gloria was feeling fine and her liver was only mildly inflamed, the doctor advised her not to start any medical treatment at the present time, as the medication for this disorder can worsen osteoporosis in postmenopausal women.

A utoimmune hepatitis (AIH) is the subject of this chapter. Since this is a liver disease marked by a defect of the immune system, this chapter discusses the immune system as it relates to AIH. Although there is no single test that can accurately diagnose AIH, this chapter also discusses the factors that typically lead to a diagnosis of this disease, as well as the symptoms that are commonly associated with it. AIH responds remarkably well to treatment in certain people. Conventional treatments, which are generally quite effective, are reviewed, as are their potential side effects. A discussion of long-term prognosis for people with AIH, options when medical therapy fails, and some promising new therapies conclude this chapter.

WHAT IS AUTOIMMUNE HEPATITIS?

Autoimmune hepatitis (AIH) is an uncommon liver disease that has the potential to lead to cirrhosis. It is characterized by inflammation of the liver and/or liver damage caused by an attack on the liver by a person's own immune system. This disease was first recognized in 1950, when it was noted that there was an association among young women who stopped menstruating (a condition known as *amenorrhea*); who suffered from arthritis; who had a severe form of chronic hepatitis that rapidly progressed to cirrhosis; and who had an elevated protein (gamma globulin) found on their blood tests.

Some similarities between AIH and systemic lupus erythematosus (SLE)—another autoimmune disease—led to AIH being named "lupoid hepatitis" in 1956.

Today, however, much more is known about this disease. For starters, it has been clearly confirmed that AIH and SLE are two totally separate disorders. Thus, the name "lupoid hepatitis" is obsolete. Furthermore, it has been established that despite a greater occurrence rate among young women, AIH may also occur in men, and it may occur in either gender at any age. Finally, case studies have established that AIH has varying manifestations. It is not always a severe, rapidly progressive disease, as originally believed. In fact, it may have a mild, asymptomatic (without symptoms) natural history.

While this disease may occur at any age, there are two age intervals within which the disease most commonly manifests itself. More often, AIH is discovered in people between fifteen and thirty years old, and less often in people over the age of fifty. Both groups are predominantly women. In fact, women account for approximately 70 to 80 percent of cases of AIH. When AIH occurs in men, it is usually in the older age group.

THE IMMUNE SYSTEM AND AIH

The main function of the immune system is to protect the body against harmful substances. Many times each day, the immune system is called upon to distinguish between substances that belong to the body, such as blood and internal organs, and substances that are foreign to the body, such as drugs, fumes, or viruses. In addition, it must distinguish between foreign substances that are potentially harmful and those that are safe. The immune system is hard at work protecting the body twenty-four hours a day.

Unfortunately, there are occasions when this vital and intricate system malfunctions. When the immune system fails to perform its duties properly, one of two scenarios may arise. Either the body receives diminished protection, as occurs in immune deficiency diseases, such as AIDS. Or the immune system may fail to correctly distinguish between what belongs to the body and what is a foreign substance. The term *autoimmune* is used to describe what happens when a person's body produces an immune response against its own tissues or organs. In other words, the body incorrectly identifies one of its organs (the liver, for example) as foreign, as not belonging to the body, or as "the enemy." When this occurs, the immune system produces protective antibodies that actually attack the "enemy" organ. These antibodies are known as *autoantibodies*. (See Chapter 7 for a brief discussion of the immune system as it relates to antibodies and antigens.)

Examples of common autoimmune diseases include Grave's disease, in which the thyroid is under attack; insulin-dependent diabetes mellitus, in which the pancreas is under attack; rheumatoid arthritis, in which the joints are under attack; and ulcerative colitis, in which the colon is under attack. Sometimes the body even attacks more than one organ, and a person can actually have more than one autoimmune disorder at a time. In the case of autoimmune hepatitis, the organ under siege is the liver. AIH is considered a type of chronic hepatitis because this autoimmune process can continue indefinitely, or at least until cirrhosis and/or liver failure occur.

THE DIFFERENT TYPES OF AIH

There are two established categories of AIH: type I and type II. Some researchers believe that there is also a type III. While there is currently insufficient evidence to actually confirm the existence of type III (which may actually be a variant of type I), for the purpose of this book, AIH will be considered to fall into three separate categories—the final one being type III AIH. The categories of AIH are classified by the type of autoantibody present in the blood.

- Type I AIH, also known as classic AIH, was identified in the 1950s. It is characterized by the presence of the two autoantibodies: *antinuclear antibody* (ANA) and *smooth muscle antibody* (SMA). This is the most common form of AIH in the United States.

- Type II AIH was identified in the 1980s. It is characterized by the presence of another autoantibody known as the *liver kidney microsomal antibody* (LKM Ab). This autoantibody is present primarily in young women and children with AIH. In these people, other autoantibodies, such as ANA and SMA, are characteristically absent. Untreated people with type II AIH appear to have a rapidly progressive course of disease leading to cirrhosis. This type of AIH accounts for only about 4 percent of AIH cases in the United States.

- Type III AIH is also known as *autoantibody-negative AIH*. These people lack all autoantibody markers, yet have all of the other features of AIH. People with type III AIH respond to treatment in a manner similar to those people with autoantibodies.

THE POSSIBLE CAUSES OF AIH

The exact cause of AIH is not known. However, it is believed that this disease arises when some factor occurs in a genetically predisposed person that triggers the body to initiate an autoimmune attack against the liver. Such "triggering" factors are not clearly established but may possibly include the following: viruses, such as hepatitis A, B, and C, the measles virus, and the Epstein Barr virus (EBV); bacteria, such as salmonella and *Escherichia coli* (E. coli); medications, such as halothane (a type of anesthesia); or possibly even certain herbs, such as Dai-saiko-to.

Genetic factors have also been implicated, as it is believed that some people with AIH have a genetic defect on chromosome 6. (A chromosome contains most or all of the DNA or RNA that make up the genes of an individual.) This genetic defect is thought to predispose some people to manifest the signs and symptoms of AIH, which are discussed on page 183. Thus, it is thought that the disease itself is not inherited, but that the predisposition (susceptibility) to have the disease is. In fact, AIH is rarely found in more than one member of the same family.

THE SYMPTOMS AND SIGNS OF AIH

There are a variety of ways in which a doctor may discover that a person has AIH. In its most clandestine form, AIH may be detected by accident—upon the discovery of abnormal LFTs (see Chapter 3) in a person who is asymptomatic (without symptoms). At the opposite extreme, AIH may be discovered during an acute attack, usually characterized by grossly elevated LFTs, jaundice, severe itching, and fatigue. This occurs in up to 25 percent of the cases. Most of the people in these cases do not actually have "acute" AIH, but turn out to be having "acute flare-ups" of a previously undiagnosed asymptomatic chronic AIH. Other people fall somewhere in between, having vague symptoms, such as a general sense of lethargy, muscle and joint aches, or mild abdominal discomfort.

In more advanced cases, symptoms and signs of decompensated cirrhosis, such as ascites, encephalopathy, or bleeding esophageal varices, may be the initial features of AIH. (See Chapter 6 for a discussion of cirrhosis.) Other people may have symptoms due to other autoimmune disorders associated with AIH, such as a thyroid disorder, diabetes, or others discussed on page 185. Menstrual irregularities are common in women with AIH; some stop menstruating altogether (a condition known as *amenorrhea*).

On a physical exam, the doctor may detect jaundice (yellowing of the skin and eyes) and spider angiomatas (enlarged blood vessels), which are usually located on the upper body or face. The liver and spleen are often enlarged. Other signs include *hirsutism* (excessive hair growth) and acne.

People with AIH typically have a chronic fluctuating course. AIH is characterized by exacerbations (worsening) and remissions (abatement) of disease, which occur at varying intervals.

DIAGNOSING AIH

There is no single test that will accurately diagnose AIH. However, many factors taken together can provide the basis for an accurate diagnosis. Most important, in order to have an accurate diagnosis of AIH, it is necessary to first eliminate all other causes of chronic hepatitis, such as viral hepatitis, hemochromatosis, and excessive alcohol consumption.

In contrast to other liver diseases, such as chronic hepatitis C or hemochromatosis, AIH is a liver disease in which the degree of LFT elevation and the severity of symptoms often (although not always) correlate with the degree of liver damage and inflammation. Many times, the dramatic improvement of symptoms and normalization of LFTs with treatment will virtually prove or confirm the diagnosis of AIH. However, LFTs, autoimmune blood tests, genetic markers, and liver biopsy findings, when evaluated together, more typically are used to confirm the diagnosis. These tests are discussed on the following pages.

Liver Function Tests (LFTs)

In severe cases of AIH, the LFTs are very elevated. Liver enzymes may be as much as ten to twenty times normal values. For example, AST and ALT may be around 400 to 800 IU/L, and the bilirubin level may be around 10 mg/dl. In milder cases, the LFTs are only slightly elevated, around 60 to 200 IU/L, and the bilirubin level is normal. In any scenario, when LFTs are elevated, other more specific blood tests for AIH should be run. (See Chapter 3 for an explanation of the liver function tests.)

Specific Autoimmune Blood Tests

Specific autoimmune blood tests include a check for elevated immunoglobulin levels, specifically an elevated IgG level, and for the presence of antinuclear antibody (ANA) and/or smooth muscle antibody (SMA). As mentioned previously, ANA and SMA are both known as *autoantibodies*. Many autoantibodies are typically produced by the body in AIH, but ANA and SMA are the most common. These autoantibodies—which do not cause AIH—are considered markers of AIH. However, they are not specific for AIH. This means they may also occur in liver diseases other than AIH, as well as in diseases of other organs. Approximately 64 percent of people with AIH have both ANA and SMA present in their blood. Other people have one, but not both, of these autoantibodies. The presence of both autoantibodies is not necessary for the diagnosis to be made. In fact, it is possible for people to lack all autoantibodies and still have AIH. These people are known as autoantibody-negative AIH (type III AIH). (See page 182.)

When ANA and SMA are present in liver diseases other than AIH, their values tend to be very low and are thought to be of little significance. These autoantibodies are reported to doctors on blood work by *dilution titers* (the dilution of blood containing a specific antibody). A titer of 1:160 (one to one hundred sixty) or greater is highly suggestive of AIH. Titers of less than 1:80 (one to eighty)—which are not necessarily indicative of AIH—are often found in other liver disorders and may be of no clinical significance. Note that autoantibody titers can fluctuate from one blood test to the next, and during therapy for AIH, they may disappear altogether. Moreover, the levels of these autoantibodies do not correlate with the severity of disease.

Genetic Markers

It is believed that there is a genetic predisposition or susceptibility to the development of AIH. Research has focused primarily on chromosome 6. *Human leukocyte antigens* (HLAs) are special antigens located on chromosomes that are believed to be factors in the hereditary predisposition of people to different diseases.

There are certain HLAs found to be located on chromosome 6 that are associated with AIH. These are known as HLA DR3 and HLA DR4. These HLAs can be detected by special blood tests, although these blood tests are not readily available in all laboratories. People with AIH who have HLA DR3 tend to be relatively young and have a very aggressive disease that is poorly responsive to medical therapy. People who have HLA DR4 tend to be relatively old and have a less aggressive disease that responds quite well to medical treatment.

Liver Biopsy

Liver biopsy, which was discussed at length in Chapter 5, is the only test that will accurately determine the extent of damage done to the liver by AIH. Moreover, there are findings on a liver biopsy that are highly suggestive of AIH that assist the specialist in making a diagnosis of AIH. Thus, a liver biopsy is an important tool for confirming the diagnosis of AIH and for determining its severity. Treatment decisions are usually based on the results of a liver biopsy.

OTHER AUTOIMMUNE DISORDERS ASSOCIATED WITH AIH

Other autoimmune diseases may also occur in people with AIH. In fact, about one-third of people with AIH also have another autoimmune disease. The diseases most commonly associated with AIH include thyroid abnormalities, rheumatoid arthritis, and ulcerative colitis. These and other autoimmune disorders associated with AIH are listed below.

- Thyroid disorders—hyperthyroidism (overactive thyroid) and (hypothyroidism) underactive thyroid.

- Diabetes mellitus and insipidus—glucose (sugar) abnormalities.

- Ulcerative colitis—intestinal disorder characterized by inflammation of the large intestine (colon) and bloody diarrhea.

- Blood disorders, including hemolytic anemia, a low blood count due to breakdown of red blood cells (hemoglobin and hematocrit); and thrombocytopenia (low platelet count).

- Celiac sprue—gluten (wheat) intolerance.

- Myasthenia gravis—a neuromuscular disorder characterized by extreme muscle weakness.

- Sjögren's syndrome—a chronic disease characterized by dry eyes and dry mouth.

- Glomerulonephritis—a kidney disorder.

- Rheumatoid arthritis—chronic disease characterized by pain and swelling of the joints.

- Vitiligo—a skin disorder characterized by patches of discoloration.

- Synovitis—inflammation of the lining of joints, characterized by joint swelling and pain.

THE OVERLAP SYNDROMES

Sometimes people will have features of AIH as well as the features of another liver disease. These are known as overlap syndromes. The following is a discussion of these overlap syndromes.

AIH and Primary Biliary Cirrhosis

AIH overlaps with primary biliary cirrhosis (PBC) about 8 percent of the time. These people have the clinical features of AIH, but have the presence of the autoantibody *antimitochondrial antibody* (AMA) in their blood, which is diagnostic of PBC. These people typically respond well to conventional treatment for AIH. See Chapter 15 for more information about PBC.

AIH and Primary Sclerosing Cholangitis

AIH may also overlap with a disease known as primary sclerosing cholangitis (PSC). This occurs about 6 percent of the time. PSC is an uncommon liver disease characterized by inflammation and damage to both the intrahepatic and extrahepatic bile ducts. PSC can lead to cirrhosis. PSC occurs most frequently in men and is commonly associated with ulcerative colitis. Therefore, people with AIH (especially men) who also have ulcerative colitis should undergo testing for PSC. People with both AIH and PSC typically have a poor response to steroid treatment. This type of overlap syndrome occurs most frequently in children. See Chapter 15 for more information about PSC.

AIH and Autoimmune Cholangitis

Autoimmune cholangitis is an autoimmune liver disease characterized by inflammation of the liver and positive autoimmune markers (ANA and/or SMA), in addition to injury to the bile ducts. This disease has also been referred to as *mitochondrial antibody-negative PBC*. Treatment with steroids has different responses in different people. See Chapter 15 for more information about autoimmune cholangitis.

AIH and Hepatitis C

AIH and the hepatitis C virus (HCV) antibody may occur together in three separate situations. First, antibodies to hepatitis C can be falsely present in about 5 percent of people with AIH. This usually represents a nonspecific autoimmune reaction. These people do not actually have the hepatitis C virus, despite the fact that their blood test results are positive for the antibody to hepatitis C. For these people, once AIH is in remission, the hepatitis C antibody usually disappears.

Second, when people with hepatitis C are treated with the drug interferon—a medication used to treat viral hepatitis—AIH may be triggered. People who suffer from both hepatitis C and AIH usually have a worsening course of disease when treated with interferon.

Finally, a person may have hepatitis C in addition to AIH—most commonly type II AIH, manifested by the presence of the liver kidney microsomal autoantibody (LKM Ab). These people are sometimes classified as having autoimmune hepatitis type IIb. For these people, treatment decisions become somewhat problematic, as the use of interferon to treat hepatitis C will worsen the course of AIH. Similarly, prednisone, used to treat AIH, can cause the hepatitis C virus to replicate. This is manifested by an elevated hepatitis C viral load (HCV RNA) on blood tests.

Treatment methods for people with both AIH and hepatitis C are discussed in this chapter on page 194. See Chapters 10 and 13 for more information about hepatitis C.

TREATMENT FOR AIH

The goal of treatment of AIH is to ameliorate symptoms, to decrease the inflammation of the liver, to induce a long-term remission of the disease, and to prevent progression to cirrhosis. When treatment is successful, people have a normal life expectancy. This section discusses the medications used for AIH and includes information about the successes, relapses, and failures of treatment. The potential side effects of treatment and who is most likely to benefit from treatment are also covered.

Medications for the Treatment of AIH

People with AIH are typically treated with a combination of two medications: prednisone and azathioprine (Imuran). Both drugs have anti-inflammatory properties, meaning that they are capable of diminishing inflammation. Although prednisone alone (in high doses) is an option, the combination of drugs is usually preferred. This combination is usually associated with a lower incidence of drug-related side effects. A discussion of the side effects of prednisone begins on page 189 and a discussion of the side effects of azathioprine begins on page 191.

The initial dose of prednisone is anywhere from 10 to 30 milligrams (mg). This is usually combined with azathioprine, which is given in a dosage between 50 and 100 milligrams. Azathioprine is considered a steroid-sparing drug. This means that its anti-inflammatory properties allow for smaller doses of prednisone to be used. Therapy may last months or years or may even be lifelong. Generally, once remission is achieved—as judged by the resolution of symptoms and normalization or near normalization of LFTs—dosages of medications are slowly decreased, and eventually medication is discontinued. If a person should relapse after the medication is discontinued, lifelong therapy is advisable using low doses of prednisone and azathioprine. Studies have shown that some of these people will remain in remission despite discontinuing prednisone, provided they continue the use of azathioprine.

Successes of Treatment

Early and aggressive treatment can slow progression of AIH, and some researchers feel that it may even reverse the course in some people with early stages of liver scarring. AIH generally responds very well to the combination regimen mentioned above, and remission is usually achieved in approximately 65 to 80 percent of the cases. It takes about a year-and-a-half to two years for most people to go into remission. Some people respond much faster—perhaps within six months—while others take years. Approximately 14 to 50 percent of these people remain in long-term remission after medications are discontinued. People who remain in remission usually have a normal life expectancy.

Successful response to treatment may be assessed from a combination of factors. For example, results of blood work will demonstrate a decrease of LFTs and immunoglobulin (IgG) levels. Liver biopsy specimens show a decrease of inflammation and in some cases even scarring (fibrosis, not cirrhosis) is improved. Also, symptoms usually resolve when treatment is successful. In fact, many people feel better after only one to two weeks on therapy.

Relapse After Treatment

Relapse of the disease may occur between six months to three years after treatment is stopped. People who relapse benefit from long-term maintenance therapy with low doses of prednisone (for example, 10 milligrams) and azathioprine (for example, 50 milligrams). Compared with multiple rounds of treatment and withdrawal of medication, long-term maintenance therapy is actually associated with a lower incidence of side effects. Some people on long-term treatment with prednisone and azathioprine may eventually be tapered off the prednisone altogether and kept solely on azathioprine.

If a person has remained in remission more than six months after cessation of therapy, the probability of relapse at some future point during his lifetime is only 8 percent. Some researchers believe that people who have cirrhosis on initial liver biopsy specimens rarely remain in remission once treatment is discontinued. Resolution of symptoms and normalization of LFTs may occur before a decrease of liver inflammation. Therefore, some doctors choose to repeat a liver biopsy before discontinuing therapy to assess the actual degree of liver inflammation remaining. By proceeding in this manner, the rate of relapse will be diminished, as premature discontinuation of medication will not occur.

No Response to Treatment

Up to 20 percent of people with AIH do not respond to conventional treatment. The reason for this is unclear and is subject to differing opinions among researchers. Some researchers believe that the types of people who are less likely to respond to treatment are those with cirrhosis and those who developed the disease at an early age. However, others believe that the presence of cirrhosis does not affect a person's response to therapy and that the presence of cirrhosis should not affect treatment decisions.

Some researchers believe that a genetic susceptibility among some people accounts for their rapid disease progression and lack of response to treatment. Studies have shown that people who tested positive for HLA DR3 fail to respond to treatment more frequently and more commonly require liver transplantation than those people who tested positive for HLA DR4. Therefore, higher doses of conventional therapy or the use of other drugs may be advantageous for HLA DR3-positive people.

Potential Side Effects of Treatment With Prednisone and/or Azathioprine

Approximately one-third of people undergoing treatment for AIH develop some side effects. Generally, side effects can be diminished by using lower doses of medications. However, approximately 10 percent of people on medications for AIH develop side effects that are so debilitating that they must discontinue therapy. These people may want to consider entering a clinical trial of an experimental medication. See Promising New Therapies for AIH on page 193.

Side effects of both prednisone and azathioprine are dependent upon the dosage and duration of use. The higher the dose and the longer the duration of use, the greater the likelihood that side effects will be experienced. Note that people with cirrhosis appear to have more side effects from drug therapy than those without cirrhosis.

Prednisone and Its Side Effects

Prednisone, known by the brand name Deltasone, is a synthetic hormone. It is similar to the hormones known as corticosteroids or steroids that the body produces naturally. The major action of all steroids is to decrease or suppress inflammation. Steroids belong to a category of medications known as immunosuppressants or anti-inflammatories. Prednisone works remarkably well for people with AIH and is also effective for people suffering from other types of autoimmune disorders.

Some drugs, such as antacids, can interfere with the actions of prednisone and decrease its effectiveness. Medications such as diuretics can interact with prednisone to cause a low blood-potassium level. This underscores the importance of a person keeping his doctor informed of all medications (even herbs or over-the-counter drugs) that he is taking.

As with all potent medications, prednisone use may potentially cause adverse side effects, which are more common when high dosages are administered for a long period. The side effects usually take about a year to manifest—even at high doses. When recognized early, they can generally be managed by decreasing the dose of prednisone. The use of azathioprine, a steroid-sparing drug, in combination with prednisone, allows the dosage of prednisone to be lowered. Low doses (for example, 10 milligrams) rarely result in side effects.

No matter what side effects occur, prednisone should never be discontinued abruptly. Severe side effects may occur unless the dosage is reduced gradually. Thus, as with other powerful medications, it is essential that a person using prednisone remain under the close supervision of a doctor. Since prednisone may actually worsen many medical conditions, including diabetes, high blood pressure, and osteoporosis, the person taking the drug should always make sure that his doctor is aware of his entire medical history—not merely as it relates to the liver. Since prednisone may worsen the severity and increase the spread of serious fungal infections, such as candidiasis, its use should be avoided in the presence of such infections. Furthermore, prednisone may hide symptoms—such as fever and pain—that commonly signify the presence of an infection, and thereby decreases the likelihood that an infection will be detected and treated. Moreover, prednisone may increase fatty deposits in the liver, causing a person to develop a fatty liver. (See Chapter 16 for a discussion of this condition.) See Table 14.1 on page 191 for potential side effects associated with prednisone use and how they are typically managed.

Azathioprine and Its Side Effects

Azathioprine, also known by its brand name Imuran, has been used since 1968 as a steroid-sparing agent. Azathioprine possesses immunosuppressive properties. Its major action, that of decreasing inflammation, makes it useful in the treatment of many autoimmune disorders. Because of its steroid-sparing aspect, it allows a person to be treated with lowered dosages of prednisone. Exactly how azathioprine suppresses the immune system isn't exactly known, but its actions probably exemplify its ability to inhibit the replication of cells.

Each tablet of azathioprine contains a dosage of 50 milligrams. It will normally take approximately three months for azathioprine to start producing its desired effects. Therefore, it is advisable to start taking this medication as soon as possible in conjunction with prednisone. This will enable the dosage of prednisone to be decreased significantly around three months from the time treatment with azathioprine is started.

The likelihood of side effects from taking azathioprine depends upon the dosage and the duration of usage. Most side effects can be reduced, and often eliminated, by lowering the dosage. As azathioprine can irritate the stomach lining, it is preferable to take it with meals. Occasionally, azathioprine will need to be discontinued temporarily—especially in cases when a severe fungal infection occurs or when blood counts have decreased dramatically. Therefore, it is essential that anyone who is taking azathioprine be monitored by an experienced doctor.

The most common side effect of azathioprine is bone marrow depression. When this occurs, a person's platelets and white and red blood cells can decrease to dangerously low levels. People with reduced platelet levels are at increased risk of unexpected bruising and bleeding. When the levels of white blood cells drop, a per-

Table 14.1. Potential Side Effects of Prednisone and Management Possibilities

Potential Side Effects	Management Possibilities
Psychiatric symptoms, such as mood swings, personality changes, depression, and irritability	Decrease dosage; consult with a therapist; reduce additional stress
Insomnia	Decrease dosage; take melatonin before bed
Fluid retention; high blood pressure; Congestive heart failure	Low-sodium diet; blood pressure medication
Osteoporosis and other bone disorders	Calcium and vitamin D supplements; alendronate [Fosamax] or etidronate [Didronal]; calcitonin nasal spray; sensible exercise program; hormone replacement therapy (HRT)
Gastrointestinal ulcers and inflammation	H2 blocker, such as famotidine (Pepcid); pump inhibitor, such as lansoprazole (Prevacid), or omeprazole (Prilosec)
Impaired wound healing	Decrease dose prior to surgery
Muscle loss	Weight-training program
Headache	Low-sodium diet; acetaminophen in moderation
Diabetes	Insulin or oral hypoglycemic (sugar-lowering) medications
Glaucoma/cataracts	Frequent eye check-ups
Weight gain due to increased appetite	Low-fat, low-sodium diet; exercise
Menstrual irregularities	Oral contraceptives
Acne	Acne medication

son is at increased risk for infection. These people may experience frequent episodes of fevers, sore throat, or mouth sores. When the levels of red blood cells decrease, a person may feel fatigued and weak. It is important for anyone taking azathioprine to have his blood work regularly monitored by a doctor. And people who have low blood counts for other reasons should probably avoid the use of azathioprine altogether.

It's important to note that women who are pregnant, or who are planning to become pregnant in the near future, should not use azathioprine, as this drug has been shown to cause birth defects. Also, people with cancer of any organ are advised to avoid azathioprine.

Drug interactions are also a common concern for people taking azathioprine, as they have been shown to increase side effects. While taking azathioprine, the following drugs should be avoided:

- Allopurinol—gout medication.

- Dilantin and Phenobarbitol—seizure medication.

- Rifampin—tuberculosis medication.

- Vasotec/Monopril/Zestril/Capoten—angiotensin-converting enzyme inhibitor medications used to control high blood pressure.

- Coumadin—blood thinner.

The biggest concern for people on azathioprine is an increased risk of cancer. This risk, while typically very small, increases in likelihood in situations of long-term use at high dosages. Skin cancer, lymphoma, and leukemia are the cancers most attributable to azathioprine use, although these cancers occur as a side effect only in rare circumstances.

Oddly enough, azathioprine can also be toxic to the liver. In the unlikely event that this occurs, it will be manifested by elevations of LFTs. This side effect is very infrequent, occurring in less than 1 percent of people using the drug. Despite its potential side effects, the benefits of azathioprine, especially its steroid-sparing property, usually outweigh its potential risks. See Table 14.2 on page 193 for potential side effects associated with azathioprine use and some possible ways they are managed. As with the side effects of prednisone or any other drug, a person should always inform the doctor of any side effects he may be experiencing for optimal management.

Who Benefits and Who Doesn't From Treatment

The benefits of treatment must always be weighed against the potential side effects and risks associated with treatment. People who will typically benefit from treatment include those with severe symptoms, those with severe damage on liver biopsy specimens, and those with severely elevated liver enzyme abnormalities of about five- to tenfold above the upper limits of normal. In all other cases, the decision to begin therapy should be made on a case-by-case basis.

There are some people who are not likely to benefit from treatment. For example, the initiation of treatment is usually unnecessary in people with mild hepatitis, as determined from results of a liver biopsy, and liver enzyme abnormalities about less than three fold above the upper limits of normal. In these people, the decision to initiate therapy is determined by the degree of symptoms. If symptoms are significant, then a trial of low dose treatment should be attempted. If the person is asymptomatic, no therapy should be started. People without symptoms still need close monitoring and should have repeat liver biopsies performed approximately every five years to assess progression of disease.

Table 14.2. Potential Side Effects of Azathioprine and Management Possibilites

Potential Side Effects	Management Possibilities
Nausea; vomiting; loss of appetite	Eat multiple small meals; take azathioprine with, or immediately after meals; take azathioprine in divided doses
Diarrhea	Avoid dairy products; add white rice to diet
Rash and itching	Stay out of the sun; use over-the-counter anti-itching medication, such as the antihistamine Benadryl
Bone marrow depression	Have periodic blood work done; reduce dosage; temporarily withdraw azathioprine
Infection	Avoid people who are ill; wash hands carefully and frequently; reduce dosage
Cancer	Self breast and/or testicular exam; avoid excess sun exposure; use high-potency sunscreen; avoid smoking and drinking alcohol
Mouth sores	Attentively care for and clean mouth
Birth defects	Use birth control; discontinue if pregnant; avoid breast-feeding

Treatment is also not indicated for people who have cirrhosis without liver inflammation. People with decompensated cirrhosis should not be treated with medications, but should consider liver transplantation. Women who are postmenopausal are at increased risk for the development of osteoporosis while on prednisone. Therefore, some studies maintain that the benefits are outweighed by the risks in this group. However, other investigators have found a similar occurrence of side effects from prednisone in postmenopausal women and premenopausal women. As always, the risks versus the benefits of treatment must be assessed on a patient-by-patient basis.

PROMISING NEW THERAPIES FOR AIH

When conventional therapy has failed or when the side effects of conventional medicine limit its utility, other medications should be tried. There are some medications that are in use for the treatment for AIH but are still considered "investigational." Clinical trials are being performed to assess their effectiveness in the treatment of AIH.

Cyclosporine and tacrolimus (FK-506) are two medications commonly used to prevent liver transplant rejection. These *antirejection drugs,* which are discussed in Chapter 22, possess potent anti-inflammatory properties. Limited studies involving their use in people with AIH have revealed reductions of LFTs when taken for a period of one year. Further studies need to be conducted to clearly define the incidence of relapse and to determine whether the benefits of these medications outweigh their potential risks.

Budesonide is a steroid that is associated with fewer side effects than prednisone. Preliminary studies show great promise for the use of budesonide as a treatment for people with AIH.

Ursodeoxycholic acid (Actigall; URSO) is a natural bile acid that is found in small quantities in humans, but is found in large quantities in bears. It may be a useful additional medication to prednisone and azathioprine in treating people with AIH.

6-Mercaptopurine (6-MP) has been shown to be a potential substitute drug for azathioprine for those people who are unable to tolerate or who are unresponsive to azathioprine. Thus, 6-MP may be of benefit for use in place of azathioprine as an additional therapy to prednisone.

Other medications, including *cytoprotective agents* (substances that can protect cells), such as polyunsaturated phosphatidylcholine and arginine thiazolidinecarboxylate, *immunosuppressive drugs* (medications that stifle the actions of the immune system), such as brequinar and rapamycin, and thymic hormone extracts have all shown some anecdotal benefits; however, further study is required before any definite conclusions can be made.

TREATMENT OF AIH AND HEPATITIS C

Treatment of people with both AIH and hepatitis C is particularly difficult. In general, treatment decisions should be aimed at the predominant disease. Thus, when autoantibody titers are greater than 1:160 and liver biopsy results are consistent with AIH, treatment with steroids should be initiated. If autoantibody titers are low (less than 1:160) and the liver biopsy results are consistent with hepatitis C, the hepatitis C infection may be cautiously treated with interferon. However, when the diagnosis is in doubt, an initial trial of prednisone is generally a better and safer route to take.

On one hand, prednisone may increase the replication of the hepatitis C virus (HCV). On the other hand, administering interferon to a person with AIH may have severe consequences, perhaps even precipitating an episode of encephalopathy (mental confusion). All things considered, the danger of administering interferon to a person with AIH exceeds the danger of administering steroids to a person with hepatitis C.

LIVER TRANSPLANTATION—WHEN ALL ELSE HAS FAILED

When all medical therapies have failed or if complications from cirrhosis have developed, liver transplantation must be considered. The success rate of transplantation in people with AIH is excellent. There is approximately a 92-percent survival rate of at least five years after liver transplantation. Autoantibodies generally disappear within two years from the time of transplantation. The disease may recur after transplantation, but it can usually be managed successfully by adjustment of immunosuppressive drug dosages. Although dosages may be decreased after transplantation, total discontinuation of immunosuppressive drugs is not recommended.

THE LONG-TERM PROGNOSIS FOR THOSE WITH AIH

People who are appropriately and aggressively treated generally have a prolonged survival time. Treatment may reduce the chances of developing cirrhosis or at least slow its progression. Some researchers have shown that in certain people, treatment can actually reverse liver scarring. Studies have also shown that people successfully treated have a life expectancy similar to that of the general population, even if cirrhosis was present at the time AIH was initially diagnosed. During the first three years of therapy, people with AIH have about an 11-percent probability each year of progressing to cirrhosis. After the initial three-year period, they have a 1-percent per year chance of developing cirrhosis. People with severe AIH who do not receive treatment have only about a 30-percent chance of surviving another five years. It has been shown that many of these people will develop cirrhosis within two years of their diagnosis.

Any liver disease that leads to cirrhosis may potentially also lead to liver cancer. People with AIH and cirrhosis are at increased risk for the development of liver cancer. Fortunately, the incidence of liver cancer among people with AIH is much lower than it is among people with liver disorders such as hemochromatosis or chronic viral hepatitis. People with AIH in whom the development of cirrhosis is prevented by successful therapy will not be at risk for liver cancer.

CONCLUSION

As discussed in this chapter, autoimmune hepatitis is a liver disease that has a wide spectrum of severity. While some people are quite ill, others have a course so mild that no therapy is required. As there is no single test that definitively identifies people with AIH, multiple indicators are usually necessary to confirm the diagnosis. Determining who is a good candidate for treatment is crucial, as the medications used for treatment of AIH may have significant side effects. When people are treated promptly and aggressively, most have a relatively long-term survival rate. The next chapter discusses another liver disease—primary biliary cirrhosis (PBC). As noted in this chapter, PBC may occur in conjunction with AIH. While PBC is suspected to also be an autoimmune disease, the features and treatment of PBC differ drastically from those of AIH.

15

Primary Biliary Cirrhosis

Edith, a fifty-three-year-old homemaker, had been feeling somewhat fatigued for the past year. She had always been an energetic woman—involved in two local benefit organizations, while running a household, doing all the chores and errands, and taking care of four children. She blamed her uncharacteristic rundown feeling on her advancing age. But when Edith started feeling itchy all the time, she couldn't blame that on her age. So she changed her brand of laundry detergent thinking it could be an allergy and tried several over-the-counter topical creams that her pharmacist had recommended. But nothing worked. Finally, when her constant scratching started keeping her husband awake at night, he insisted that she see a dermatologist.

The dermatologist worked with Edith for two months, but none of the various medications and therapies he prescribed brought her relief. Another dermatologist told Edith that her condition was caused by her nerves and advised her to see a psychiatrist. Feeling frustrated and depressed by this point, Edith thought that might be a good idea. The psychiatrist concluded that Edith was suffering from depression and wanted to start her on an antidepression medication; however, he required that she first get a check-up from her doctor. Edith's doctor conducted a thorough physical exam and drew blood for a comprehensive battery of blood tests. The tests revealed that Edith's liver enzymes were elevated, and she was referred to a liver specialist. The specialist ran additional blood tests and had Edith obtain a sonogram of her liver. After reviewing the test results, the liver specialist told Edith that she had a rare liver disease known as primary biliary cirrhosis. "This is most likely what has been causing your fatigue, itching, and depres-

sion," he told her. The results of a liver biopsy confirmed the specialist's diagnosis, and Edith began treatment.

Georgia, a seventy-two-year-old retired bookkeeper, paid a visit to her rheumatologist. Her arthritis, which she had suffered from for years, was bothering her more than usual. Not only did Georgia's joints hurt, but she was experiencing numbness and tingling in her fingers as well. She told her rheumatologist that when she spent time outdoors in cold weather, the tips of her fingers actually turned blue. Even wearing thick gloves did not help. The rheumatologist's examination of Georgia revealed that, with the exception of arthritis and a slow thyroid, Georgia was in good health. The doctor drew some blood from Georgia and also gave her a prescription for a new arthritis medication.

When Georgia called a week later for the results of her blood tests, her rheumatologist informed her that some of her liver enzymes were abnormal and she would need additional testing. Georgia was referred to a liver specialist who ran additional blood tests on her and conducted a physical exam. The specialist diagnosed Georgia as having primary biliary cirrhosis—a rare liver disease. She subsequently learned from the specialist that arthritis, thyroid disorders, and Raynaud's phenomenon (the cause of her blue fingertips) are diseases commonly associated with primary biliary cirrhosis. A liver biopsy confirmed the specialist's diagnosis, and Georgia began treatment.

Primary biliary cirrhosis (PBC)—a relatively rare liver disease that occurs primarily in middle-aged women—is the topic of this chapter. You'll learn about the characteristics and possible causes of PBC. Also covered in this chapter is how PBC is diagnosed and what its associated symptoms are. In addition, the many other disorders frequently associated with PBC are detailed. The current medications that are used to treat PBC are discussed, and some promising new treatment strategies are reviewed. Finally, the natural history and prognosis of people with PBC, while somewhat unpredictable, concludes this chapter.

WHAT IS PRIMARY BILIARY CIRRHOSIS (PBC)?

PBC is a chronic liver disease characterized by the slow destruction of the intrahepatic bile ducts. As discussed in earlier chapters, *chronic* connotes a duration of greater than six months. In fact, PBC may be accurately characterized as a lifelong illness. Like autoimmune hepatitis, which was discussed in Chapter 14, PBC is also believed to be an autoimmune disorder. An autoimmune disorder is a condition in which the immune system malfunctions and produces an immune response (an attack) against its own organs. In PBC, as with autoimmune hepatitis (AIH), the organ under attack is the liver. However, unlike AIH, in which the immune system attacks liver cells, in PBC the immune system attacks the cells lining the bile ducts within the liver.

As discussed in Chapter 1, bile ducts carry bile—a substance that aids in the digestion of fats and in the neutralization of poisons. When the bile ducts become inflamed and eventually destroyed, the surrounding liver tissue subsequently becomes damaged. This leads to scarring and cirrhosis. This explains the derivation of the name primary "biliary cirrhosis." This name can be a bit misleading since most people with PBC do not yet have cirrhosis at the time of initial diagnosis, and some may never even progress to cirrhosis in their lifetimes. Because this is a disease wherein the bile ducts become inflamed (a condition known as cholangitis) by a process that is not due to an infection, the alternative name, *chronic nonsuppurative* (not pus producing) *cholangitis,* has been suggested to be a more accurate description of this disease. However, this alternative name is not widely accepted and is therefore not in use.

PBC is known as one of the cholestatic liver diseases. Cholestatic liver diseases are characterized by cholestasis—failure of bile flow. In PBC there is an eventual failure of bile flow within the liver, which is known as intrahepatic cholestasis. Cholestatic liver diseases are also characterized by a certain pattern of blood-test abnormalities (elevated levels of AP, GGTP, and bilirubin; see Chapter 3). In addition, PBC is a liver disease that is commonly associated with many other disorders. A discussion of these disorders begins on page 203.

THE RISING REPORTS OF PBC

PBC was first described in 1851, but prior to the 1950s, very few cases of PBC were reported. Today, it is estimated that approximately 4 to 15 people per million population each year have PBC, and that there are approximately 20 to 150 people per million population with PBC. The most likely explanation of why PBC is more commonly reported now involves the increased awareness of this disease among the medical profession and the improved methods of detection through routine blood work.

THOSE WHO ARE AT RISK FOR PBC

PBC occurs in all countries and among all races, although people from Northern Europe appear to have a particularly high rate of occurrence. First degree family members—parents, siblings, and children—of a person with PBC appear to be approximately 1,000 times more likely to develop PBC compared with the general population. Therefore, family members should be checked for PBC. Women are more likely to have PBC than men. In fact, approximately 90 to 95 percent of people with PBC are women. The reason for this disproportionate predisposition among women is unknown. PBC most often afflicts people between the ages of forty and sixty; however, people have been diagnosed with PBC while still in their twenties and even as late as their nineties.

THE CAUSES OF PBC

The exact cause of PBC is unknown. However, PBC is believed to be a disease of autoimmune origin occurring in people with a genetic susceptibility to the disease. The autoimmune nature of PBC is supported by its frequent association with other autoimmune disorders, such as rheumatoid arthritis. The laboratory findings of a special autoantibody known as the *antimitochondrial antibody* and an elevated immunoglobulin M (IgM) level lend additional support to this autoimmune characterization. As mentioned previously, the disease's autoimmune attack is targeted specifically against the cells lining the bile ducts within the liver.

Many factors have been cited as potentially triggering the autoimmune response that leads to the development of PBC. Such factors include tainted well water; certain types of infections, such as the Epstein-Barr virus; and some medications, such as interferon and chlorpramazine—an antipsychotic medication. A consequence of the autoimmune attack is that the bile ducts become damaged. Once the bile ducts have become damaged, the bile acids within the ducts spill out, causing inflammation, damage, and eventually, scarring of liver tissue.

THE SYMPTOMS AND SIGNS OF PBC

There is a wide spectrum of symptoms associated with PBC. At one end of the spectrum, a person with PBC can be asymptomatic (have no symptoms), even though he has elevated AP and GGTP levels (see Chapter 3). In fact, some asymptomatic people with PBC even have normal levels of liver enzymes. In these instances, a positive antimitochondrial antibody (AMA) is the sole indication that the disease is present. Up to 60 percent of people discovered to have PBC have no symptoms. Diagnosis in such people has become more common due to routine blood tests, which are performed during the course of a regular check-up. Note, however, that most people who are initially asymptomatic eventually do develop symptoms. This occurs in about three to four years from the time of initial diagnosis. However, symptoms can take as long as ten years to manifest. Interestingly, even in advanced stages of PBC, some people will still have no symptoms. At the other end of the spectrum, a person with PBC may have severe symptoms of liver failure, such as upper gastrointestinal bleeding from esophageal varices (enlarged varicose veins in the esophagus) or encephalopathy (altered mental status). People who fall somewhere between these two extremes may experience relentless fatigue and pruritus (itching). In fact, this is the most typical presentation of PBC.

The cause of fatigue in people with PBC is not known, but it is the most common symptom, occurring in approximately 78 percent of people with PBC. The degree of fatigue does not correlate with the severity of the disease and may be just as debilitating for a person in an early stage of PBC as it is for a person in a later stage of PBC. Pruritus is the second most common symptom, occurring in approximately 65 percent of people with PBC. Generally, the itching becomes worse at night. Although the cause of pruritus is not known, it can be successfully treated using *cholestyramine*—an orally taken bile-acid binder.

Other symptoms associated with PBC may include unexplained weight loss, abdominal discomfort, and depression. Often, people with PBC will have the symptoms of an associated autoimmune disorder, such as joint pains from rheumatoid arthritis or dry eyes and mouth from Sjögren's syndrome. The treatment of these specific symptoms will be discussed in Chapter 20.

On a physical exam, the doctor may find an enlarged liver and spleen. Sometimes the liver is somewhat tender. A person's skin tone may be darker than usual due to excess deposits in the skin of a pigment known as *melanin*. This is a sign of advancing disease. Ironically, these people are often asked where they got their healthy tans. Dark skin tone may sometimes be a sign of jaundice (a yellowing of the skin or eyes), which is indicative of the final stage of PBC. Another sign of PBC is a condition known as *finger clubbing*—the tips of the fingers become enlarged and rounded like clubs.

There are two distinctive physical findings that occur frequently in people with PBC that immediately alert doctors to arrive at a diagnosis, and thus, are considered hallmarks of the disease. The first physical finding is actually of two conditions—*xanthalasmas* and *xanthomas*. These are irregular fatty yellow nodules or patches on the skin due to disturbances in cholesterol metabolism. (They also occur in some people who have markedly elevated cholesterol levels from causes other than PBC.) Xanthalasmas occur in approximately 20 percent of PBC cases and are found around the eyes. Xanthomas commonly occur in the creases of the hands, arms, and legs, or on the elbows and knees. The second distinctive physical trait found in people with PBC is excoriations (severe scratch marks associated with breaks in the skin that often bleed) on the body due to intense scratching to relieve pruritus. These excoriations are commonly found in areas of the body that are easily accessible, such as the upper back, chest, and arms. Interestingly, in the later stages of the disease, both of these physical hallmarks of PBC occasionally improve.

DIAGNOSING PBC

PBC may be diagnosed by a combination of the symptoms that a person is experiencing, the physical findings detected on an exam, the results of blood work, the findings of a liver biopsy, and the results from imaging studies. These various diagnostic techniques are discussed below.

Blood Tests

PBC is most often diagnosed when abnormalities are found on blood tests. Usually, an isolated elevated alkaline phosphatase (AP) level is initially discovered. This typically leads to additional blood work testing for a specific autoantibody, antimitochondrial antibody (AMA), associated with PBC. Additionally, cholesterol levels are usually elevated in people with PBC. The following is a discussion of these blood tests.

Liver Function Tests

In people with PBC, the AP and GGTP levels are elevated out of proportion to the transaminases (AST and ALT). Thus, a typical person with PBC may have an AP and GGTP level around ten times the upper limit of normal, while their transaminase levels may be normal or only around one-and-one-half to four times the upper limit of normal. This pattern of blood test abnormalities is referred to as cholestasis—specifically intrahepatic cholestasis. The bilirubin level is usually normal in the early stages of the disease (a condition known as anicteric cholestasis). However, the bilirubin level typically becomes elevated as the disease progresses. For more information concerning these blood tests, see Chapter 3.

Autoantibodies

In 1965, it was discovered that people with PBC have an autoantibody known as the *antimitochondrial antibody* (AMA) present in their blood. This finding greatly advanced the diagnostic accuracy of this disease and allowed doctors to recognize the disease in its earliest and most treatable stages. In 1987, this diagnostic accuracy was further enhanced by the identification and cloning of specific antigens against AMA. The major antigen against AMA was discovered to be a component of pyruvate dehydrogenase—an enzyme involved in carbohydrate metabolism.

Approximately 95 percent of people with PBC have evidence of AMA. The finding of AMA in a person almost always confirms the presence of PBC. The level of AMA is reported in titers, such as a titer of 1:160 or 1:640. However, the level of the titer does not correlate with the severity of the disease nor is it significant in regard to prognosis. Immunoglobulin M (IgM) is also commonly elevated in people with PBC. Other autoantibodies, such as SMA and ANA, may also be present, although their presence is not necessarily significant. See Chapter 11 for more information concerning autoantibodies.

Cholesterol Levels

With PBC, cholesterol levels may become markedly elevated, especially in the later stages of the disease. In fact, levels of cholesterol may reach over 1,000 milligrams per deciliter, but there's no need to panic. As it turns out, people with PBC do not have an increased risk of heart disease due to this high cholesterol level. Furthermore, a person cannot reduce this elevated cholesterol level by adhering to a low-cholesterol diet.

Liver Biopsy

In cases of PBC, a liver biopsy (discussed in detail in Chapter 5) is necessary in order to determine the extent of damage present and the exact stage of the disease. Furthermore, a liver biopsy confirms the diagnosis, gives an estimate of how long the disease has been present, and provides important information that will assist the doctor in determining appropriate treatment options. As opposed to other liver disorders, PBC has been neatly classified into four distinct stages that can only be determined by a liver biopsy. *Stage 1* is characterized by the finding of damaged bile ducts. *Granulomas*—nodules filled with a variety of inflammatory cells—are often detected in this stage. *Stage 2* is characterized by the finding of a proliferation of small bile ducts known as bile ductules. *Stage 3* is characterized by fibrosis, and *stage 4* is characterized by cirrhosis. Occasionally, a single specimen from a liver biopsy may show evidence of more than one stage of the disease. In such cases, the most advanced stage present should be considered the correct stage. People may progress through the different stages at varied, and largely unpredictable, rates. For example, a person may stay in stage 1 for many years, and then rapidly progress from stage 2 to stage 3. Or a person may rapidly progress through stage 1 and then stay in stage 2 for many years.

Imaging Studies

Imaging studies generally do not add significant additional information concerning the status of a person diagnosed with PBC. However, these imaging studies are important in cases when the diagnosis is in question or when a person is experiencing abdominal pain. A situation in which a sonogram may be ordered to help determine a diagnosis is one in which there is an extrahepatic cause for LFT abnormalities, such as gallstones. Since people with PBC are at increased risk for the development of gallstones, sonograms are useful in cases of abdominal pain. See Chapter 3 for more information on imaging studies.

DISORDERS ASSOCIATED WITH PBC

PBC is frequently associated with autoimmune disorders of other organs. As a result, it is often a rheumatologist, dermatologist, or endocrinologist, rather than a liver specialist, who actually discovers that a person has a liver disorder. As many as 84 percent of people with PBC have been found to have an associated autoimmune disorder. The following is a discussion of these autoimmune disorders of organs other than the liver.

Thyroid Disorders

Up to 20 percent of people with PBC have some type of thyroid dysfunction. While the thyroid of a person suffering from PBC may sometimes be overactive (a condition known as hyperthyroidism), an underactive, slow-functioning thyroid (a condition known as hypothyroidism) is more common. Fatigue is a common symptom of hypothyroidism, which may be a contributing factor to the relentless fatigue experienced by many people with PBC. Therefore, it is important for the doctor to search for a thyroid disorder in people with PBC, especially in those who are experiencing fatigue. Treatment with thyroid medication often improves this type of fatigue.

Rheumatologic Disorders

Since many rheumatologic disorders have an autoimmune origin, it is not surprising that there is a high degree of association between rheumatologic disorders and PBC. Rheumatoid arthritis, which is characterized by joint aches and joint deformities, is often seen in people with PBC. People with PBC also commonly have Sjögren's syndrome, which is characterized by *xerophthalmia* (dry eyes) and *xerostomia* (dry mouth). *Dysphagia* (trouble swallowing) occurs in approximately half of the people who have xerostomia, partly due to a lack of sufficient saliva. People with xerostomia are also at an increased risk for the development of dental cavities. In particularly severe cases, some people may even have difficulty speaking. *Scleroderma,* also common in people with PBC, is a disease characterized by thickening and hardening of the skin and even some internal organs, due to excessive collagen deposits. When this disease affects the esophagus, it may cause dysphagia.

Raynaud's phenomenon is another rheumatologic disorder that commonly occurs in people with PBC. Raynaud's phenomenon typically causes the fingertips to turn blue and to become numb when exposed to cold weather or when the person is exposed to emotional stress. Sometimes this phenomenon is seen in conjunction with the following: excessive calcium deposits in parts of the body, known as *calcinosis;* abnormal movements of the esophagus, known as *esophageal dysmotility;* scleroderma of the fingers and toes, known as *sclerodactyly;* and small, thin, red spots on the skin or mucous membranes, known as *telangiectasia.* This group of disorders is collectively known as the CREST syndrome (Calcinosis, Raynaud's, Esophageal dysmotility, Sclerodactyly, Telangiectasia).

Finally, systemic lupus erythematosus (SLE), a disease affecting multiple organs and characterized by fever, skin rash, and arthritis, may also occur in people with PBC.

Dermatological Disorders

Many skin disorders are associated with PBC. As previously discussed, pruritus is the second most common manifestation of PBC. Xanthomas are also commonly seen in people with PBC. Vitiligo, a condition manifested by smooth nonpigmented patches on various parts of the body, is believed to be an autoimmune phenomenon and is common in people with PBC.

Kidney Disorders

Recurrent urinary tract infections (UTIs) occur in approximately 20 percent of women with PBC. These UTIs are often asymptomatic and do not require antibiotic therapy. Other kidney disorders have been noted to occur in people with PBC, but are uncommon.

Lung Disorders

Sarcoidosis is a disease characterized by the formation of granulomas (nodules filled with a variety of inflammatory cells) in the lungs, skin, liver, lymph nodes, and bones. This disease resembles primary biliary cirrhosis (PBC) in that both diseases are characterized by the formation of granulomas. PBC and sarcoidosis occasionally coexist together.

Gastrointestinal Disorders

Many gastrointestinal disorders, including gallstones and diarrhea, occur in people with PBC. Right upper quadrant abdominal pain (pain over the area of the liver) has been noted in approximately 17 percent of PBC cases. The degree of pain typically does not correlate with the severity of PBC. Also, the cause of the pain is usually not discovered. In fact, in many cases, the pain resolves without any treatment at all.

Gallstones

Up to 40 percent of people with PBC have gallstones. They are usually discovered by chance when a sonogram is obtained as part of an initial evaluation. Thus, while gallstones are the cause of right upper quadrant pain in some people with PBC, in others, they do not cause any symptoms at all.

Diarrhea

Diarrhea may have many causes in people with PBC—three of which are to be discussed. First, diarrhea may be a side effect of some medications used in the treatment of PBC, such as URSO and colchicine, or of cholestyramine, a medication used to control itching. (These medications are discussed in more detail further on in this chapter.)

Second, people in advanced stages of PBC who are cholestatic are unable to absorb fats efficiently—a condition known as fat malabsorption. This is caused by a failure to secrete bile salts necessary to absorb fats due to bile duct destruction that occurs within the livers of people with PBC. The fats that these people are unable to absorb are eliminated from their bodies in their stools, which tend to be light in color, loose in consistency, and frothy in texture. These stools are characterized by their ability to float on top of water, and it commonly takes as many as five attempts to flush them down the toilet. This type of stool is known as *steatorrhea*. Other symptoms of fat malabsorption and how to treat it are discussed in Chapter 23.

Third, an autoimmune disease known as *celiac sprue* can be the cause of diarrhea in people with PBC. Celiac sprue is a disease characterized by an inability to absorb *gluten* (a protein found in wheat, rye, oats, and barley). This is known as a gluten-intolerance. Celiac sprue is approximately ten times more likely to occur in people with PBC than among members of the general population. The association of PBC with celiac sprue is important to recognize since people suffering from these diseases jointly can obtain relief from diarrhea and its associated weight loss by adhering to a gluten-free diet.

Bone Disorders

People with PBC often suffer from severe bone problems, including bone loss, bone pain, and bone fractures. These bone disorders are often a source of great suffering and can severely disable a person. In fact, severe bone disease coupled with recurrent bone fractures in people with PBC may be an indication that liver transplantation is warranted.

Osteoporosis (a decrease in bone quantity) is the most common bone abnormality occurring in people with PBC. Some people with PBC may also have a genetic susceptibility for the development of osteoporosis. In others, the degree of osteoporosis correlates with the severity and duration of jaundice possible due to malabsorption of vitamin D, a fat-soluble vitamin. The hip and spine are the areas of the body most commonly affected by osteoporosis. Thus, people with osteoporosis are susceptible to hip fractures and often suffer from bad backs. It has been demonstrated that, after liver transplantation, osteoporosis often improves in people with PBC. The medical treatment of osteoporosis is discussed in Chapter 20.

Osteomalacia—a softening of the bones similar to rickets—can also occur in people with PBC, but it is not as common as osteoporosis. This condition is caused by a deficiency of vitamin D. Since people in advanced stages of PBC often have difficulty absorbing vitamin D, they are at risk for osteomalacia.

Since vitamin-D deficiency results in calcium malabsorption, supplementation with vitamin D and calcium is typically recommended for people with either of these two bone conditions. Note, however, that these supplements have not been shown to significantly prevent bone disease in people with PBC. Other potential therapies relating to bone disorders will be discussed in Chapter 20.

THE TREATMENT OF PBC

Since PBC cannot be cured, treatment is aimed at slowing the progression of disease and at controlling its symptoms. Treatment of the symptoms associated with PBC will be discussed in Chapter 20. The following is a discussion of the treatment of the disease itself. People with PBC may be treated with a single medication, a combination of medications, or will need to undergo a liver transplantation.

Single Medications

A variety of medications have been evaluated for the treatment of people with PBC, some of which have been found to be beneficial. Unfortunately, the adverse side effects of these drugs outweigh the potential benefits that they provide. Examples include *prednisone,* a steroid, which may accelerate the rate of bone loss associated with PBC; *cyclosporine,* an antirejection drug, which may cause high blood pressure and kidney dysfunction; and *chlorambucil,* a chemotherapy drug, which may be toxic to bone marrow.

Medications that have been studied but that have not been shown to provide significant benefits to people with PBC include *D-penicillamine,* a copper-binding drug; *azathioprine,* an antirejection, immunosuppressive drug; and *malotolate,* an anti-inflammatory drug.

There are other medications that appear to benefit people with PBC, but are undergoing evaluation to confirm their effects. Examples of such medications include S-adenosylmethionine (SAMe), a type of amino acid; and tacrolimus, an antirejection, immunosuppressive drug.

At present, the most effective drug treatment for PBC appears to be with one of the following three medications—ursodeoxycholic acid, methotrexate, and colchicine. The following is a discussion of these medications.

Ursodeoxycholic Acid

Ursodeoxycholic acid (also known as UDCA or ursodiol) is the drug most commonly used to treat PBC. In fact, it is the only drug that is FDA approved for the treatment of PBC. Ursodeoxycholic acid was initially found to be beneficial for people with PBC in the early 1980s and became FDA approved in 1998. It is manufactured by Axcan Schwarz under the brand name URSO. URSO is taken with food in oral pill form at a dosage of 12 to 15 milligrams per kilograms of body weight each day administered in four divided doses. Each pill is 250 milligrams.

Ursodeoxycholic acid is a naturally occurring bile acid, but unlike many other bile acids in the body, it is not toxic to the liver. It is found in humans in small quantities, but is found in large quantities in bears. Ursodeoxycholic acid was initially used to dissolve gallstones, a treatment that is no longer common. The exact mechanism by which ursodeoxycholic acid works in people with PBC is not known. However, it has been established that increasing the amount of ursodeoxycholic acid in the body will generally decrease the amount of liver-toxic bile acids in the body. This, in turn, should diminish or prevent destruction of bile duct cells. In fact, people treated with ursodeoxycholic acid have been shown to have decreased bile duct destruction.

URSO provides significant benefits to people with PBC. Levels of liver function tests, IgM, AMA, and cholesterol typically show notable improvement. People find that URSO, on occasion, relieves some of the symptoms associated with PBC, such as fatigue and itching. Most important, ursodeoxycholic acid has been found to slow the progression of PBC. Thus, people with PBC who are treated with URSO have been found to live longer, have less liver-related complications, and need liver transplants less often when compared with those who are not treated with URSO.

Side effects of URSO are minimal. Most studies have indicated that less than

3 percent of people develop adverse side effects from URSO. When side effects are experienced, they include diarrhea, decreased white-blood-cell count, elevated glucose levels, elevated creatinine levels, peptic ulcers, and skin rashes. Overall, URSO is a well-tolerated, safe, and effective medicine for the treatment of people with PBC.

The beneficial effects of ursodeoxycholic acid are experienced by approximately 80 percent of people with PBC who use this medication. These effects are most likely to occur the sooner a person is treated—for example, when the person is treated during the first or second stage of the disease. People who have PBC who do not respond to ursodeoxycholic acid should consider combination therapy involving ursodeoxycholic acid with another medication, or they should consider trying a different medication. People whose bilirubin levels continue to worsen despite treatment with ursodeoxycholic acid or any other medication should be evaluated for liver transplantation.

Methotrexate

Methotrexate is an immunosuppressive drug, meaning that it suppresses the immune system. When people with PBC are treated with an oral dose of 15 milligrams per week, liver enzyme levels have been shown to improve or decrease. In some people, fatigue and itching are relieved. Some studies have shown that methotrexate, taken alone or in combination with other drugs, may improve liver inflammation and intrahepatic bile duct injury. However, methotrexate may cause adverse side effects, and this serves to limit the drug's usefulness. In fact, in one study, approximately 14 percent of people taking methotrexate developed severe but reversible lung inflammation. Further studies are currently being conducted regarding the treatment with methotrexate.

Colchicine

Colchicine is a medication with anti-inflammatory properties. It has been purported to reduce scarring (fibrosis, *not* cirrhosis) in some people with liver disease, and as such, may be said to have *antifibrotic* properties. Liver enzymes tend to improve in people with PBC who are treated with colchicine in two daily oral dosages of 0.6 milligrams each. However, liver enzymes do not improve to the same degree as with ursodeoxycholic acid or methotrexate. Colchicine has not been shown to reduce liver inflammation or bile duct damage. Colchicine's side effects are minimal. The most common of these, diarrhea, occurs in less than 10 percent of the cases. This symptom usually resolves once the dose of colchicine is decreased to once per day. Some researchers believe that colchicine may slow the rate of progression of PBC. Although the benefits of treatment with colchicine do not appear to be as substantial as those derived from treatment with ursodeoxycholic acid, colchicine is useful as an alternative treatment in people who cannot tolerate ursodeoxycholic acid. Furthermore, colchicine may prove to be a useful additional therapy to ursodeoxycholic acid.

Medication Combinations

Many drug combinations have been tried in the treatment of people with PBC. The rationale is that the combined effect of two or more drugs, each with different mechanisms of action, might prove synergistic (complementary). Promising combinations that have been tested include ursodeoxycholic acid and methotrexate, ursodeoxycholic acid and colchicine, and ursodeoxycholic acid and prednisone. While some studies using these combinations have shown some beneficial results in people with PBC, additional comprehensive studies involving larger groups must be done before any definitive conclusions can be drawn.

Liver Transplantation

Medical therapy has been shown to slow the progression of PBC, thereby delaying the need for a liver transplant in some people with PBC. Nonetheless, these people continue to advance to cirrhosis and its complications, or continue to have symptoms associated with PBC, such as severe fatigue, osteoporosis, or uncontrollable pruritus—any of which may render a liver transplant necessary. People with PBC do very well after liver transplantation. See Chapter 22 for a complete discussion of this topic.

LIVER DISEASES THAT RESEMBLE PBC

Two other liver disease resemble PBC in some respects. They are autoimmune cholangitis and primary sclerosing cholangitis. As treatment and prognosis may differ in these diseases, it is most important to distinguish between them and PBC.

Autoimmune Cholangitis

Autoimmune cholangitis is characterized by liver enzyme abnormalities suggestive of cholestasis and biopsy results resembling those of people with PBC. However, the autoantibody AMA is not present in the blood of people with autoimmune cholangitis. Instead, other autoantibodies, namely ANA and SMA, are found in the blood. Accordingly, this disease is often referred to as AMA-negative PBC. While some studies demonstrate that people with autoimmune cholangitis benefit from treatment with prednisone, either alone or in combination with azathioprine (see Chapter 14), other studies have found a greater benefit from the use of ursodeoxycholic acid. Whether autoimmune cholangitis is a totally separate entity from PBC or simply PBC without the manifestation of a positive AMA on blood tests remains a subject of ongoing debate and research.

Primary Sclerosing Cholangitis

Primary sclerosing cholangitis (PSC) like PBC is a chronic cholestatic liver disease that results in damage to the intrahepatic bile ducts. Unlike PBC, PSC also results in damage to the extrahepatic bile ducts. Also unlike PBC, most people with PSC are male, and approximately two-thirds of people with PSC have an inflammatory disease of the colon (the large intestine) known as ulcerative colitis. Symptoms of PBC and PSC may overlap, as fatigue and itching are common to people with either disease.

There is a drastic difference in the way that the two diseases are diagnosed. Unlike the presence of AMA as a diagnostic marker in people with PBC, there are no diagnostic autoantibodies that occur in people with PSC. Instead, PSC requires a special procedure called an *endoscopic retrograde cholangiopancreatography* (ERCP) to be done in order for the disease to be accurately diagnosed. In an ERCP, a lighted tube (a special endoscope) is inserted into the patient's mouth and then is snaked through the stomach and into the small intestine. There is a tiny opening in the small intestine called the *ampulla of vater* that leads to the extrahepatic bile ducts. A thin wire is inserted into this opening and then into the extrahepatic bile ducts. This wire allows access into the extrahepatic bile ducts so that contrast dye needed to visualize the bile ducts on an x-ray can be injected. An x-ray can then be taken of the extrahepatic bile ducts to determine if they have suffered damage, thus making a diagnosis of PSC.

Complications from PBC and PSC are somewhat different. Extrahepatic bile duct blockages, due to bile duct damage and bile duct stones, occur in PSC but not in PBC, as only the intrahepatic bile ducts are damaged in PBC.

Medical treatment of people with PSC has been somewhat disappointing. Drugs that have been used with success in treating PBC patients have not shown an ability to slow the progression of PSC or to prevent its complications. Nor have these drugs exhibited much success at prolonging the survival of people with PSC. Liver transplantation is the best option for people with advanced PSC. For these people, results have been good with approximately 80 percent of transplant recipients surviving at least five years.

THE NATURAL HISTORY AND PROGNOSIS FOR THOSE WITH PBC

PBC is a slowly progressive disease with a very long natural history. The average time span from initial diagnosis to death from complications of the disease is approximately twenty years. However, the rate of disease progression is quite variable, and therefore the natural history of PBC is typically unpredictable. Furthermore, the natural history of the disease may be altered by therapy. As noted above, ursodeoxycholic acid can slow down the progression of PBC, and, therefore, can prolong a person's life.

Untreated asymptomatic people live approximately five years longer as compared to untreated symptomatic people—approximately 10 to 17 years versus approximately 7 to 12 years, respectively. Some researchers have shown that asymptomatic people with associated autoimmune disorders have a worse prognosis than asymptomatic people without associated autoimmune disorders.

Once a person's bilirubin level becomes elevated, a poor prognosis is universal—regardless of whether the person is symptomatic or not. Some studies have found that most people with PBC live less than two years once their bilirubin levels begin to progressively rise. These people should be promptly referred for liver transplantation. Liver transplantation is the only treatment that significantly alters the natural history of PBC. See Chapter 22 for more information on liver transplantation.

PBC AND CANCER RISK

It is estimated that about 1 to 2 percent of deaths due to cirrhosis in the United States occur in people with PBC. Liver cancer can develop in anyone with cirrhosis, regardless of the cause. However, the chance that a person in the final stage of PBC (stage 4; cirrhosis) will develop liver cancer is rather low. In fact, a person in the final stage of PBC is much less likely to develop liver cancer than a person with chronic hepatitis B, chronic hepatitis C, or hemochromatosis. It has been estimated that only approximately 2 to 6 percent of people with PBC will develop liver cancer. Note, however, that the incidence of liver cancer among people with PBC appears to be significantly higher in men than in women. Furthermore, liver cancer has been shown to be a common cause of death in men with PBC, yet an uncommon cause of death in women with PBC. Thus, people in the final stage of PBC should undergo yearly screening for liver cancer. See Chapter 19 for more information on liver cancer.

Some studies, although not all, have found an increased incidence of other cancers in people with PBC, especially breast cancer. However, since the likelihood that a person with PBC will develop a cancer outside of the liver is quite low, routine cancer surveillance—more diligent than that recommended for the general population—is not mandatory.

CONCLUSION

In this chapter, you learned that PBC is a type of chronic cholestatic liver disease characterized by numerous associations with other autoimmune disorders that may affect virtually every organ in the body. PBC can have a varied presentation and unpredictable natural history. Unlike damaged liver cells, damaged bile ducts cannot regenerate. Consequently, there are no medical treatments that can cure PBC. However, progress in the treatment of PBC has been made, as some medications, in particular URSO, have been shown to slow the progression of the disease and to prolong survival. Unfortunately, some people do not respond to certain medications even though others with similar characteristics do. Future research is aimed at resolving this paradox and at finding better medical treatments.

The next chapter discusses fatty liver, a disease that is commonly, but not always, associated with overweight people. It also discusses nonalcoholic steatohepatitis (NASH), a liver disease with similarities to fatty liver, but with the potential to lead to a serious outcome.

16

Fatty Liver and Nonalcoholic Steatohepatitis

Muriel, a fifty-year-old paralegal, decided to join a gym to help her lose the thirty pounds she had gained since last year. When she joined, she received a free nutritional consultation and cholesterol check. Muriel was shocked to learn that her cholesterol level was greater than 300 mg/dl (normal levels being less than 200 mg/dl). Having just joined an HMO, she decided to make an appointment for an initial consultation. The doctor who examined Muriel found her liver to be somewhat enlarged. He drew some additional blood tests and gave her a low-cholesterol diet to follow after seeing the cholesterol level report that Muriel had obtained from the gym.

Muriel was feeling upbeat until she received a phone call a week later from the doctor, who informed her that her sugar levels were very high and the blood work related to her liver (LFTs) was abnormal. The doctor told Muriel that she probably had diabetes and that she would need to begin taking medication as part of her treatment if additional testing confirmed this diagnosis. In addition, he advised her not to drink any more alcohol and to have her liver function tests (LFTs) repeated in approximately one week. (Apparently, the doctor suspected that Muriel had alcoholic liver disease.) Muriel was somewhat puzzled. The last alcoholic drink she had was over three months ago at her nephew's Bar Mitzvah.

Muriel returned to the doctor's office the following week to be retested and stressed to him that she rarely consumed alcohol. However, the tests were abnormal again. More in-depth conversations with Muriel and her husband confirmed that she drank alcohol only on rare occasions. A sonogram of Muriel's liver revealed that she had a fatty liver. She was placed on a weight-reduction diet that was also low in choles-

terol and was advised to continue her exercise program at the gym. Over the course of the next few months, Muriel lost twenty pounds. The LFTs were repeated, and this time, they were normal. In addition, Muriel's diabetes improved so much that she no longer required medication for its treatment. The doctor concluded that that Muriel's elevated LFTs had been due to fatty liver.

Jerry, a thirty-nine-year-old used-car salesman, applied for a life insurance policy. He was stunned when his application was rejected due to the finding of "abnormal liver enzymes" that appeared on his blood tests results. "How can this be? I don't drink alcohol, and I feel fine," Jerry thought to himself.

    Jerry met with his family doctor hoping to find out what was wrong with his liver. The doctor asked Jerry if he used illicit drugs, if he drank a lot of alcohol, or if he was taking any medications. She also asked Jerry if there was any history of liver disease in his family. Jerry responded no to each of these questions. Jerry's physical exam revealed that he was in fine physical shape and the comprehensive blood tests that were performed didn't reveal any hereditary liver diseases, autoimmune diseases, or exposure to a viral hepatitis. Jerry was referred to a liver specialist, who performed a liver biopsy. The results of the liver biopsy revealed a greatly inflamed liver, loaded with deposits of fat. In addition, it showed early signs of scarring. From these findings, the liver specialist was able to determine that Jerry had nonalcoholic steatohepatitis (NASH).

Two liver conditions—*fatty liver* and *nonalcoholic steatohepatitis* (NASH)—are discussed in this chapter. Also covered is the difference between fatty liver, which is a benign (harmless) condition, and NASH, which can be a serious condition since it has the potential to lead to liver damage and even cirrhosis. The possible causes of both fatty liver and NASH, as well as their rates of occurrence, are discussed. The type of person who is at risk for development of these conditions is identified and associated symptoms, physical findings, and diagnosis are described. The natural history and prognosis of a person with either of these conditions is also addressed. Finally, treatment options are reviewed.

WHAT ARE FATTY LIVER AND NONALCOHOLIC STEATOHEPATITIS (NASH)?

Just as fat can accumulate everywhere else on the body when a person gains weight, fat can also accumulate in the liver. Thus, as the name suggests, a person will develop a "fatty" liver that looks something like a rasher of raw bacon! In its worst case scenario—in a morbidly obese person—almost the entire liver may become comprised of fat. This is in contrast to a person of normal weight whose liver is usually made up of less than 5-percent fat. Being overweight is just one of many causes of fatty liver and nonalcoholic steatohepatitis (NASH). In fact, fatty liver, which is characterized by the deposit of fat particles in the cells of the liver, is a condition that can be caused by a variety of factors, which are discussed below.

The medical term for fatty liver is *steatosis*. This is a reversible condition without the potential to lead to cirrhosis. When this condition is accompanied by inflammation (*steatohepatitis*) and scarring (*steatonecrosis*) of the liver, it is known as nonalcoholic steatohepatitis (NASH). The association between fat accumulation in the liver and cirrhosis has been recognized for centuries. However, it was not until 1980 that the term *nonalcoholic steatohepatitis* was coined to describe a condition characterized by liver inflammation and damage occurring in nonalcoholic people with fatty liver.

Unlike a fatty liver, NASH is not considered a relatively harmless condition, but rather a liver disease with the potential to cause cirrhosis and liver failure. The disease is prefaced by the word "nonalcoholic" because the results of liver biopsies from people with NASH are frequently identical to those from people with alcoholic liver disease. Yet people with NASH do not have a history of excessive alcohol use. Excessive use is commonly defined as greater than 80 grams per day for men and greater than 20 grams per day for women. (See Chapter 17 for more information about alcohol and the liver.)

THE PREVALENCE OF FATTY LIVER AND NASH

The prevalence of fatty liver and NASH is difficult to ascertain. This is primarily due to three facts: First, liver biopsies are not routinely performed on everyone with liver abnormalities. (NASH has been found in up to 9 percent of liver biopsies.) Second, the exact incidence of liver abnormalities among obese people is unknown. And third, fatty changes in the liver may occur in the absence of associated liver-related abnormalities. Thus, the actual prevalence of fatty liver and NASH is probably higher than the published statistics would lead us to believe. In fact, if it were estimated that approximately one-third of Americans are obese, and that at least 50 percent of these people have excessive fat in their livers, then fatty liver would be the most common cause of liver disease in the United States. Some studies even approximate that almost 75 percent of obese people have a fatty liver, and this statistic probably approaches 100 percent in morbidly obese people. Furthermore, 12 percent of cirrhosis cases are related to obesity. In addition, fatty liver occurs in 30 to 70 percent of diabetic people, and approximately 5 to 20 percent of people with diabetes have cirrhosis due to NASH.

CAUSATIVE FACTORS OF FATTY LIVER AND NASH

The liver is intricately involved in the metabolism of fat. This process can be disrupted by a variety of factors occurring singly or in combination. These factors include certain types of diseases, dietary indiscretions, the use of some medications, and exposure to certain types of toxins. When the liver's fat metabolism process is disrupted, fat can accumulate in the liver in excessive amounts. When this occurs, the result is fatty liver. Excess fat is stored in the liver mostly in the form of *triglycerides*. When triglycerides accumulate in the liver in the absence of liver inflammation and scarring, the condition is relatively harmless and can usually be reversed with the loss of weight. However, in some people, the excess accumulation of triglycerides triggers a progression from fatty liver to NASH, characterized by liver inflammation, damage, and eventually cirrhosis.

Fatty liver is most commonly found in people who consume excessive amounts of alcohol, obese people, and diabetics. Fatty liver due to obesity is most frequently associated with people who have excessive fat around their midsections, known as *central* or *truncal obesity*. In the case of diabetes, fatty liver is most commonly associated with non-insulin-dependent diabetes mellitus (also known as type 2 diabetes). Fatty livers are infrequently found in people with insulin-dependent-diabetes mellitus (also known as type 1 diabetes) whose glucose levels are well-controlled. NASH has been reported to occur in people who have undergone weight reduction surgery, such as gastroplasty or jejunal bypass surgery. In fact, about a year to a year and six months after surgery, approximately 6 percent of these people were discovered to have liver failure attributable to NASH.

By now it should be obvious that there are many different potential risk or causative factors for the development of fatty liver and NASH. Several of these factors are as follows:

- Obesity.

- Diabetes.

- Hyperlipidemia (elevated levels of lipids, or fats, in the blood).

- Rapid weight loss.

- Starvation.

- Total parenteral nutrition (TPN) (intravenous feeding).

- Use of steroids.

- Use of estrogen.

- Use of amiodarone (a heart medication).

- Use of tamoxifen (medication used for breast cancer).

- Use of methotrexate (a type of chemotherapy).

- Weight-reduction surgery, such as gastroplasty or jejunal bypass surgery.

- Small-bowel resection (surgical removal of the small intestine).

- Excessive alcohol use (note that, by definition, people with NASH do not have a history of consuming excessive amounts of alcohol).

When NASH was initially described in 1980, the typical person diagnosed with this liver disease was a middle-aged, obese woman, with non-insulin-dependent diabetes and hyperlipidemia—high blood levels of triglycerides and cholesterol. However, it is now recognized that NASH is not gender-specific, it may occur at any age, and it often occurs in people who are not overweight, not diabetic, and not hyperlipidemic. In fact, there have even been some studies showing that NASH occurs more commonly in men than women.

THE SYMPTOMS AND SIGNS OF FATTY LIVER AND NASH

Most people who have either fatty liver or NASH are asymptomatic (without symptoms). When symptoms do occur, they are usually nonspecific, such as fatigue and weakness. Occasionally, a person will complain of right upper quadrant discomfort (pain or discomfort over the area of the liver) or fullness. This may be due to the stretching of the liver with fat.

During a physical exam, the doctor may detect an enlarged liver. Signs of cirrhosis and its complications, such as ascites (abnormal accumulation of fluid) or splenomegaly (enlarged spleen), may be present, but only in people with NASH. These symptoms and physical findings often prompt further evaluation, including blood work, imaging studies, and possibly a liver biopsy.

DIAGNOSING FATTY LIVER AND NASH

There is no single test that can accurately diagnose either of these conditions. The elimination of other causes of liver abnormalities, especially excessive alcohol use, is crucial in order for an accurate diagnosis to be made. Normalization of liver abnormalities upon elimination of the causative factor—for example, weight reduction where obesity is the causative factor—is often sufficient to confirm a diagnosis. When the diagnosis continues to be in doubt, a liver biopsy is necessary. The following section discusses blood tests, imaging studies, and liver biopsy finding in people with fatty liver and NASH.

Blood Tests

Blood test results are often abnormal in people with fatty liver or NASH. However, there are no specific blood tests that are diagnostic for either of these conditions or that determine their severity. Transaminases (AST and ALT) are usually not higher than four times the upper limit of normal (upper limit of normal = 40 to 45 IU/L). In fact, in about one-third of people, these liver enzymes may even be normal. The degree of elevation does not correlate with the extent of fat accumulation, inflammation, or scarring found on the liver. The level of ALT elevation is usually higher than the level of AST elevation. This is the opposite of that seen in people with alcoholic liver disease (in which AST is higher than ALT), which is discussed in Chapter 17. Thus, the recognition of this pattern of transaminase elevation is one manner of distinguishing between NASH and alcoholic liver disease, which often mimics the former condition. The GGTP level is typically elevated, and the degree of elevation often correlates with the extent of fat deposits in the liver. In the absence of cirrhosis, the bilirubin level is normal. (See Chapter 3 for more information concerning these blood tests.)

Carbohydrate-deficient transferrin (CDT) is a blood test that is being evaluated as an indicator of excessive alcohol use. Transferrin is a protein that transports iron through the body. It contains about 6-percent carbohydrate. In people who drink alcohol excessively, the carbohydrate content of transferrin decreases. Assuming that its validity as an indication for excessive alcohol use becomes more well-established, it will prove helpful in distinguishing between NASH and alcoholic liver disease. CDT is not available in all laboratories as it is currently a research tool.

Imaging Studies

Most imaging studies can detect the presence of fat in the liver. In fact, the diagnosis of a fatty liver is sometimes discovered incidentally from an imaging study obtained during the evaluation of an unrelated problem. However, there are no imaging studies that can reliably distinguish between a fatty liver and NASH, or that can determine either the extent of fat deposits or the severity of disease. And since fat accumulation can also resemble cirrhosis and/or a liver tumor, the results of imaging studies are often a source of unnecessary confusion and distress. As always, when the diagnosis is in doubt, a liver biopsy is necessary.

Liver Biopsy

A liver biopsy is the only test that can reliably diagnose a fatty liver and NASH, as well as distinguish between the two. Furthermore, a liver biopsy can determine the amount of fatty deposits, the degree of inflammation, and the extent of damage to the liver. Liver biopsy findings for people with a fatty liver or NASH often mimic the findings seen in people with alcoholic liver disease. Consequently, a thorough questioning of the patient, and often the patient's family members as well, may be performed by the doctor in instances where the amount of alcohol intake is in question. Granted, this method of investigation may appear somewhat intrusive. However, since there is no single test that can accurately confirm, or eliminate, excessive alcohol consumption, this line of questioning is often necessary in order for the doctor to arrive at an accurate diagnosis and to offer appropriate treatment options. When NASH has progressed to cirrhosis, liver biopsy findings often reveal relatively little fatty deposits. This sometimes causes additional difficulty in arriving at a correct diagnosis. (See Chapter 5 for a complete discussion of liver biopsies.)

TREATMENT OF FATTY LIVER AND NASH

The treatment of a fatty liver and NASH is directly dependent upon the cause of the condition. For example, treatment is somewhat different in overweight versus normal weight people. The following section discusses the treatments for fatty liver and NASH under different circumstances. First note, however, that, as with all liver diseases, avoidance of alcohol before, during, and after treatment is essential despite the cause. This is especially true for people with NASH, as alcohol may worsen the severity of fat deposits, fatty inflammation, and fatty scarring in the liver.

Treatment of Fatty Liver and NASH in Those Who Are Overweight

Overweight or obese people with a fatty liver or NASH can usually normalize the elevations in liver enzymes, decrease some of the enlargement of their livers, and diminish the amount of fat in their livers merely through weight reduction. A weight loss of approximately 10 percent can significantly correct these abnormalities. If weight reduction is achieved early in the disease, progression to scarring and cirrhosis can possibly be prevented altogether. In fact, in one study, weight reduction actually reversed some scarring (fibrosis, *not* cirrhosis).

Three points need to be emphasized concerning weight reduction. First, weight loss must be sustained, or the disease will recur. Second, weight reduction must be achieved through reasonable methods, and it must occur at a slow pace. Excessively rapid weight reduction or starvation techniques can actually worsen or even cause fatty liver and NASH. Obviously, this is at odds with the purpose of the weight reduction. Plus, it can adversely affect a person's overall health. Finally, an exercise routine must be incorporated into any weight-reduction routine. See Chapter 23 for some guidelines regarding weight loss and exercise.

Weight reduction is also important for those overweight people with fatty liver or NASH who also have an additional liver disease—for example, hepatitis C. In these people, a 10-percent weight loss will also lower elevated LFTs, although LFTs may not revert to totally normal levels. And, it has been shown that people with chronic hepatitis C who also have excessive fat deposits probably progress to cirrhosis more quickly.

Treatment of Fatty Liver and NASH Due to Medication or Toxin

In cases where fatty liver or NASH was caused by a medication or toxin, discontinuation of the exposure will generally reverse the condition, as long as cirrhosis is not already present. Examples of medications that can lead to fatty liver or NASH include steroids (such as prednisone), the hormone estrogen, amiodarone (a heart medication), tamoxifen (a medication used for breast cancer), and methotrexate (a type of chemotherapy). A disease known as Jamaican vomiting sickness can also lead to fatty liver or NASH. It is caused by ingestion of a toxin produced by the unripe fruit of the ackee tree.

Treatment of Fatty Liver and NASH in Those With Diabetes

In people with insulin-dependent diabetes, close control of sugar levels is crucial for minimizing the amount of fat in the liver. However, for non-insulin-dependent diabetics, the group more likely to have a fatty liver and NASH, controlling sugar levels—while important for overall health—will generally not improve liver abnormalities. For non-insulin-dependent-diabetics who are overweight, weight reduction is the only effective treatment option.

Treatment of Fatty Liver and NASH in Those Who Are Not Overweight

There is no specific treatment for people with a fatty liver or NASH who are not overweight. Many medications are presently being evaluated for this group of people. The most promising one appears to be ursodeoxycholic acid (UDCA). UDCA, also known by the brand names Actigall and URSO, is a naturally occurring bile acid, that, unlike many other bile acids in the body, is not toxic to the liver. It is found in a small quantity in the human body, but in a large quantity in a bear's body. UDCA was initially used to dissolve gallstones, but is now commonly used to treat many different liver diseases, specifically primary biliary cirrhosis (see Chapter 15). Initial studies in people with NASH have shown that treatment with UDCA can lead to improvements in LFTs and to a reduction in the severity of fatty deposits in the liver.

Clofibrate, a triglyceride-lowering drug, has been tested as a treatment but has not proven to be beneficial.

Polymixin B is an antibiotic that can alter the bacterial population in the intestines. This medication may be characterized as a form of "bowel decontaminate." People on intravenous feedings (total parenteral nutrition) who received polymixin B were found to have a reduced amount of fat on their livers. This treatment option needs further study before definite conclusions can be drawn about its effectiveness in treating people with NASH.

Since people with both NASH and elevated amounts of iron in their livers appear to have an increased incidence of progression to scarring, treatment with phlebotomy (the removal of blood through a vein) for these people is a potential, yet unexplored, option.

Certain nutritional deficiencies in people with a fatty liver and NASH may provide a clue for successful treatment. Some people receiving intravenous feedings for prolonged periods of time develop fatty liver in addition to a choline deficiency. (Choline is a B vitamin.) When the choline deficiency was corrected, the fatty liver resolved. Thus, choline supplementation in people with fatty liver is an area that requires further study.

Coenzyme A is a substance that is essential to the metabolism of carbohydrates, fats, and certain amino acids. It contains pantothenic acid, a B vitamin, which is essential to growth. When people with fatty liver were supplemented with a form of coenzyme A, the extent of fat deposits in the liver decreased. More research must be done to confirm the efficacy of this type of nutritional supplementation.

One preliminary study indicated that vitamin E (alpha-tocopherol) may be a beneficial treatment for people with NASH, but more research is needed in this area.

Dietary alterations, such as correcting protein deficiencies and avoiding carbohydrate and fat excesses, may be a potentially effective treatment for people with fatty liver or NASH who are not overweight, but it is one that requires additional study to confirm its effectiveness.

Treatment of NASH in Those Who Have Developed Cirrhosis

If a person with NASH develops complications of cirrhosis, he should be evaluated for liver transplantation. NASH accounts for approximately 1 percent of transplantations in the United States, although this is thought to be an underestimate. Since people often gain weight after transplantation, all transplant recipients, but particularly those prone to NASH, must be especially diligent about maintaining a normal weight after liver transplantation. See Chapter 22 for more information concerning liver transplantation.

THE NATURAL HISTORY AND PROGNOSIS FOR THOSE WITH FATTY LIVER

Fatty liver is a relatively harmless condition that does not lead to any significant short-term or long-term consequences. Thus, people with fatty liver do not experience liver-related complications or a decreased life span due to this condition. However, there is some controversy as to whether an increased amount of fat in the liver actually does increase the liver's susceptibility to injury. In fact, it has been recognized that people who receive a fatty liver in a liver transplant have an increased complication rate as compared to people who receive a normal liver. This realization has led to the discontinuance of using fatty livers for liver transplantation. Furthermore, whether fatty liver progresses to NASH is somewhat unclear. Since this possibility probably exists, when diagnosed with a fatty liver, it is recommended to attempt to eliminate this condition when possible.

THE NATURAL HISTORY AND PROGNOSIS FOR THOSE WITH NASH

The natural history of NASH is poorly defined. It appears to be a progressive disease, but the actual risk of progression to cirrhosis is unknown. Some studies have noted that as many as 50 percent of people with NASH will likely progress to cirrhosis. Other studies have concluded that there is only a minimal risk of progression to cirrhosis. The risk of progression to cirrhosis probably lies somewhere between these two extremes. In any event, NASH appears to be a slowly progressive disease.

People with NASH whose biopsies reveal high iron deposits on their livers appear to be at increased risk for scarring, and therefore, for progression to cirrhosis. These people often carry a single gene mutation for the liver disease known as *hemochromatosis*. See Chapter 18 for more information about hemochromatosis.

In one study, 59 percent of people with NASH were alive ten years after being diagnosed. Thus, it appears that the life expectancy for people with NASH, while somewhat lower than that of the general population, is not significantly shortened.

CONCLUSION

In this chapter you learned that, while excess fat deposits in the liver is relatively harmless, there is the possibility that fat may increase the liver's susceptibility to injury. This observation leads to the belief that perhaps a fatty liver, in some cases, is simply the initial stage of NASH. The perspective on NASH has changed dramatically over the years. Initially thought to be a benign disease limited primarily to middle-aged, obese women with diabetes, it is now recognized as being a progressive disease that can affect virtually anyone. While NASH, in its early stages, may be reversible by removing the cause for fat deposits, once the disease has progressed unchecked, there is an increased risk for cirrhosis and its complications. Future research is targeted at identifying who is at risk for NASH and at developing therapies that can stop or slow the course of this disease. Researchers hope to learn more about the mechanism by which fat triggers the development of NASH.

The next chapter discusses alcoholic liver disease, a liver disease that closely resembles NASH on liver biopsy specimens, but is otherwise—as you will soon learn—very different.

17

Alcohol and the Liver and Alcoholic Liver Disease

Adele, a fifty-four-year-old administrator, noticed that for the past month she was gaining weight rapidly. In fact, the only clothes she could fit into were her maternity dresses from twenty-five years ago. She noticed that her stomach was quite distended and that her legs were swollen. She made an appointment with her family doctor to find out what was going on.

After asking her some questions, the doctor examined Adele and noticed that she had spider angiomatas on her upper chest and arms. He also noted that her palms were bright red. Even though she had gained almost thirty pounds since her last check-up two years ago, her muscles looked wasted. The exam further revealed that Adele's abdomen was distended from ascites and that her legs were swollen from edema. The doctor reviewed Adele's medical records and noted that on her patient questionnaire, she claimed to drink wine only on social occasions. When he asked Adele about this, she asserted that she only drank socially or when dining out. After giving her a prescription for diuretics (water pills) and a low-sodium diet to follow, the doctor asked Adele to return in two weeks with her husband.

Two weeks later, Adele's ascites had significantly improved, and she had lost twelve pounds due to the diuretics and low-sodium diet. In the consultation room with Adele and her husband, the doctor asked again how frequently Adele consumed alcohol. When she replied as she had two weeks earlier, Adele's husband was surprised and exclaimed, "Adele! What about the wine you drink every night with dinner and the martini you have as soon as you get home from work?" From this additional information, the doctor concluded that Adele had alcoholic cirrhosis and advised her to go into an alcoholic rehabilitation program.

Oscar, a thirty-nine-year-old computer programmer, was rushed to the hospital after his wife, Allison, discovered him unconscious on the bathroom floor. When the ambulance arrived at the hospital, Oscar was immediately taken to the intensive care unit. While a group of doctors attended to Oscar, a nurse in the ICU asked Allison what had happened. Between sobs, Allison explained that Oscar had recently lost his job, and he had started drinking again—maybe even more than before. Allison also told the nurse that Oscar's eyes had been looking somewhat yellow during the past week. Meanwhile, Oscar was placed on a respirator and the doctors had inserted two large intravenous lines into his arms and started to transfuse some blood into him. The doctors worked on Oscar throughout the night. By the morning, the doctors informed Allison that Oscar was doing better and that he was very lucky to be alive as he had a severe case of alcoholic hepatitis. Within three days, Oscar was off the respirator. He promised Allison that he would never drink again. When his condition improved, he was transferred to the alcohol rehabilitation unit of the hospital.

A lcohol and the liver and alcoholic liver disease (ALD) are the subjects of this chapter. Topics covered include how alcohol is processed by the body, specifically the liver's role in rendering alcohol harmless, and why the liver more than any other organ in the body is susceptible to harm from alcohol. Also discussed are the multitude of factors, including genetics and gender, that contribute to the development of ALD. In addition, the adverse effects on the liver of combining alcohol and other drugs, such as acetaminophen, are addressed. This chapter also explains how a diagnosis of ALD is made. It discusses the various stages of ALD and its treatment. In addition, this chapter addresses which organs, besides the liver, are adversely affected by alcohol consumption. Finally, the natural history and prognosis of people with ALD is addressed.

WHAT IS ALCOHOL AND ALCOHOLISM?

Before discussing alcohol and its effects upon the liver and alcoholic liver disease (ALD), some basic terms, which will be used throughout this chapter, must be defined. *Alcohol,* for which the chemical name is *ethanol,* is a liquid produced by a process known as *fermentation.* Alcohol is a product of the fermentation of carbohydrates (glucose) with yeast. After the process of fermentation, alcohol is purified and concentrated through the process of *distillation.* Hard liquor—beverages such as vodka, gin, rum, and scotch—results from the fermentation of carbohydrates, such as potatoes or grains. Wine results primarily from the fermentation of grapes, whereas beer results from the fermentation of barley and hops.

Proof is a term for the alcoholic strength of a beverage, which is expressed by a number that is double the percentage of alcohol present. Most types of hard liquor are approximately 40-percent alcohol (80 proof), most wines are approximately 15-percent alcohol (30 proof), and beer is generally approximately 5-percent alcohol (10 proof). The alcohol content of 1 pint of hard liquor is usually about 150 grams (5.3 ounces), the alcohol content of 1 pint of wine is usually about 45 grams (1.6 ounces), and the alcohol content of 1 pint of beer is usually 18 grams (0.6 ounces).

According to the National Council on Alcoholism and Drug Dependence and the American Society of Addiction Medicine, the definition of alcoholism is as follows: "Alcoholism is a primary, chronic disease with genetic, psychosocial and environmental factors influencing its development and manifestations. The disease is often progressive and fatal. It is characterized by impaired control over drinking, preoccupation with the drug alcohol, use of alcohol despite adverse consequences, and distortion in thinking, most notably denial. Each of these symptoms may be continuous or periodic."

THE PREVALENCE OF ALCOHOLIC LIVER DISEASE

Medical problems due to excessive alcohol intake occur in approximately 10 percent of the United States population. About 25 percent of these people develop alcoholic liver disease (ALD)—one of the most common causes of liver disease in the United States. In fact, ALD is the fourth most common cause of death among middle-aged Americans. ALD may affect people from any country, any socioeconomic background, or any religion or race. One reason why ALD is so common is that alcohol—a potentially toxic substance with significant abuse potential—may be obtained inexpensively and with ease. In fact, alcohol use is encouraged in our society, as is evident in the many advertisements, movies, and television shows that portray the consumption of alcohol as sophisticated and fun.

ALCOHOL AND THE LIVER

It is common knowledge that drinking too much alcohol can be harmful to many of the organs in the body, especially the liver. But most people do not know that it is, in fact, the liver that is primarily responsible for protecting itself and the rest of the body from the harmful effects of alcohol.

The liver provides the body with two separate ways to metabolize (break down) alcohol. By metabolizing alcohol into less toxic byproducts, the liver prevents dangerously high levels of alcohol from accumulating in the bloodstream. One way the liver renders alcohol harmless is with the assistance of *enzymes* (proteins that induce chemical changes in other substances, while remaining unchanged by the process). These particular enzymes are known as *alcohol dehydrogenase and aldehyde dehydrogenase*. They literally turn alcohol into a form of vinegar that is totally harmless to the liver and the rest of the body. Alcohol can also be broken down by an alternative method, a pathway in the liver known as the *microsomal ethanol oxidizing system* (MEOS) that contains a group of enzymes known as the *cytochrome P-450* system. The cytochrome P-450 system is a complex group of specialized enzymes within the liver that are responsible for the conversion of fat-soluble substances to water-soluble substances. Liver damage occurs when one of these mechanisms of alcohol breakdown either fails to function properly or is overwhelmed by an excessive amount of alcohol ingestion. This can happen due to a variety of other factors, in addition to drinking too much alcohol, which are discussed on page 228.

There are many misconceptions that people usually have about alcohol and the liver. The following lists some of these common misconceptions:

- Social drinking is unlikely to cause liver damage.

- If a person's liver disease was not caused by alcohol, there is no need to limit alcohol consumption.

- If a person does not drink any alcohol, they can't get liver disease.

- All alcoholics eventually get liver disease.

- If a person with ALD abstains from alcohol, he no longer has to worry about his liver.

- Alcohol provides some nutritional value.

When the liver has been damaged by alcohol and can no longer prevent dangerously high levels of this toxin from accumulating in the bloodstream, other body parts can become damaged. One reason why alcohol can so easily damage other organs is that alcohol is soluble in both water and fat. This enables it to readily enter any organ and negatively affect their vital functions. Also, alcohol-related damage to other organs can result as a consequence unrelated to the liver's inability to filter this toxin. See the inset "Alcohol and the Rest of the Body" below.

Alcohol and the Rest of the Body

While the liver is the organ most vulnerable to the toxic effects of alcohol, alcohol has the capacity to adversely affect almost any organ in the body. The following is a brief summary of the detrimental effects of excessive alcohol consumption on organs other than the liver:

- Alcohol may cause *esophagitis*—inflammation of the esophagus. Symptoms may include heartburn, chest pain, and hematemesis (vomiting of bright red blood).

- Alcohol may cause *gastritis*—inflammation of the stomach. Gastritis can cause abdominal pain, nausea, and bleeding.

- Alcohol's toxic effects on the intestines may result in the malabsorption of many nutrients, most notably resulting in deficiencies of the vitamins folate, cobalamin (vitamin B_{12}), and thiamine (vitamin B_1).

- Excessive intake of alcohol may lead to *lactose intolerance* (intolerance to dairy products), which can contribute to diarrhea.

- Alcohol may cause *pancreatitis* (inflammation of the pancreas). Symptoms of pancreatitis include severe abdominal pain, nausea, and vomiting. Pancreatitis may result in decreased production of pancreatic enzymes, which are crucial for the digestion of fat and protein. Thus, alcoholic pancreatitis may lead to malnutrition.

- Altered mental function and nervous system disorders are common among people who abuse alcohol and can be due to a variety of causes.

- Alcohol can cause damage to the heart, resulting in *alcoholic cardiomyopathy* (enlarged heart), in which the heart can no longer effectively pump blood to others organs.

- Alcoholics also commonly have high blood pressure (*hypertension*) due to the effect of alcohol on the blood vessels.

- Alcohol may cause muscles to become sore and swollen; a condition known as *myopathy*.

- Alcohol is a central nervous system depressant, typically reducing a person's inhibitions. Thus, while alcohol is thought of as a substance that enhances sexual experience, when abused over long periods of time it has the opposite effect. Alcoholic men often suffer from diminished sexual function and drive. Their testicles become smaller, their breasts become larger, and infertility is common among them. Alcoholic women also suffer from infertility, and their menses (menstrual cycles) may totally stop.

- Alcohol is directly toxic to the bone marrow. This causes a decreased platelet count, which increases an alcoholic's risk of bleeding, and a decreased white blood cell count, which increases an alcoholic's susceptibility to infection.

- Alcohol increases cancer risk. Alcohol-related cancers often occur in the head and neck, as well as in the esophagus and stomach. It has been noted that female alcoholics have an increased risk of breast cancer.

FACTORS THAT CONTRIBUTE TO THE DEVELOPMENT OF ALD

Not everyone who drinks alcohol excessively develops ALD. In fact, only about 25 percent of alcoholics develop ALD, and only 10 to 15 percent of alcoholics are found to have cirrhosis during autopsy. So why are some people more likely than others to develop ALD? There is no single answer to this question, as many variables contribute to the development of ALD. The following is a discussion of some of these variables.

Dose and Duration of Alcohol Intake

People who drink large quantities of alcohol over a long period of time are generally at greatest risk of developing ALD. But remember, the alcoholic content differs among different kinds of alcoholic beverages. Therefore, the likelihood of developing ALD is affected by the alcohol content of the beverage ingested, not by the type of alcoholic beverage consumed.

In general, consumption of about 80 grams of alcohol daily for a significant length of time is required for men to develop ALD. 80 grams of alcohol is roughly equivalent to a six-pack of beer or a liter of wine. (To convert grams to ounces multiply by 20 and divide by 567.) Women are much more susceptible to the toxicity of alcohol than are men (see Gender on page 229). It has been estimated that it takes as little as 20 grams of daily-alcohol ingestion over an extended period of time for women to develop ALD. The specific length of time it takes for ALD to develop is not known with any precision because so many different factors play a role in its development. Similarly, the amount of time that it takes for cirrhosis to develop is unknown. However, it appears that an average person must drink the above-mentioned amounts of alcohol daily for at least five years in order for cirrhosis to develop. That's right. A mere five years of excessive drinking puts a person at significant risk for developing cirrhosis! Moreover, remember that the above figures are just estimates and the results may vary depending upon many other factors.

Genetics

Genetics play an important role in the development of ALD. Most people are familiar with the stereotype of the person who "can drink anyone under the table," or of the easily inebriated person colloquially referred to as a "cheap date." Well, it has been found that people who fall into the first category are the ones most likely to develop ALD. And the "cheap dates" are the ones least likely to develop ALD. These observations have, at least in part, a genetic basis.

It has been discovered that genetic differences regarding the efficiency of the enzymes (alcohol dehydrogenase and aldehyde dehydrogenase) that establish the rate of the metabolism of alcohol exist among people. Thus, fast metabolizers of alcohol have to drink more than everyone else in order to obtain the desired effects of alcohol. As compared with people who metabolize alcohol at a normal rate, they are less intoxicated after drinking equivalent amounts of alcohol. These people are the ones most likely to develop liver damage, as they are able to consistently consume high levels of alcohol for many years. On the other hand, slow metabolizers of alcohol become rapidly intoxicated when they consume alcohol. These people develop high levels of alcohol in their bloodstreams after consuming only small amounts of liquor. Since these people require relatively minimal quantities of alcohol in order to become intoxicated, they are unlikely to consume alcohol in great enough quantities to develop ALD, and are therefore the least likely ones to develop ALD. This characteristic is common among Asian people. To some extent, this accounts for the low incidence of ALD in the Asian population compared with the United States population.

Genetic markers (specific genes) have been searched for to further explain why certain people are more susceptible to the toxic effects of alcohol on the liver than others. While many candidate genes have been suggested, to date, no specific gene has been proven to directly influence the development of alcoholic liver disease.

Gender

Gender differences play a role in a person's susceptibility to the effects of alcohol on the liver. While alcoholism is more common among men, it has been demonstrated that women are more susceptible to the adverse consequences of alcohol on the liver. In fact, women who develop ALD and cirrhosis due to alcohol do so at a younger age than men, and they have consumed a lesser total amount of alcohol. It has also been noted that women with cirrhosis due to alcohol have a shorter life expectancy than men with cirrhosis due to alcohol.

So why are women so much more susceptible to the toxicity of alcohol than men? Well, the most obvious explanation is that women generally weigh less and are smaller than men. Women on average have a smaller total body area throughout which any ingested alcohol can be distributed. But neither this fact, nor the total amount of alcohol ingested, completely accounts for why women are at a much greater risk of developing ALD. Hormonal differences have been suggested as a factor, although this theory is not yet proven. Probably the factor that most significantly differentiates the genders is that many women (not all) have less of the enzyme alcohol dehydrogenase in the lining of their stomachs than men. This enzyme is the same one that is found in the liver that breaks down alcohol into the byproducts that are less toxic to the liver (see page 225). Thus, the reduced amount of alcohol dehydrogenase enzyme in women increases the likelihood that they will absorb nonmetabolized alcohol from their stomach linings directly into their bloodstreams. Hypothetically, if a man and a woman of equal size and weight each consumes an equivalent amount of alcohol over the same span of time, the woman will have a much higher blood-alcohol level than the man. Once in their bloodstreams, high blood-alcohol levels circulate in their bodies, placing women at increased risk for the toxic effects of alcohol on their livers and other organs.

In addition, studies show that women solicit treatment for alcohol-related problems only half as often as men do. Also, by the time a woman seeks help for her problems, she tends to be sicker and at a more advanced stage of liver disease. It is believed that one reason for this is that women may hide their addictions more successfully than men, and they are not as likely to suffer the adverse social and legal problems due to drinking alcohol. Therefore, their family members, friends, and doctors are less likely to suspect them of alcohol abuse. Studies have shown that after completing treatment in an alcohol rehabilitation program, women return to drinking alcohol more often than men. Unfortunately, statistics indicate that the incidence of alcohol abuse among women is increasing in the United States.

The Presence of Other Liver Diseases

Alcohol has been shown to worsen the course of many liver diseases. Since alcohol is a potential toxin to the liver, people with any type of liver disease should refrain from drinking alcohol.

There appears to be an additive harmful effect to the liver between alcohol and some hepatitis viruses. Thus, for people with chronic viral hepatitis (see Part Two), consuming alcohol is likely to lead to a worsening of liver disease. In people with hepatitis C, alcohol has been shown to promote the replication of the hepatitis C virus (HCV), which results in elevated hepatitis C viral loads. Furthermore, it has been shown that the consumption of even minimal quantities of alcohol may accelerate the progression of liver disease to cirrhosis in people with chronic hepatitis C. In fact, HCV has been found frequently in people with ALD, especially in those people who have severe liver damage or cirrhosis, suggesting a causative relationship (that is, HCV contributed to the liver damage).

Evidence of infection with the hepatitis B virus (HBV) is more common among alcoholics than the general population. Furthermore, HBV is often found in people with cirrhosis due to ALD. People with ALD who become acutely infected with HBV typically have a much more severe course of infection than people without ALD. Therefore, as with all liver diseases, it is especially important for people with chronic hepatitis B and chronic hepatitis C to refrain from drinking alcohol.

Alcohol can increase iron absorption. Therefore, it is important for people with hemochromatosis and other diseases of iron overload (see Chapter 18) to refrain from consuming alcohol, since alcohol may worsen liver damage. It is important to remember that for any person with liver disease, excessive alcohol consumption doubles the risk of liver cancer—at the very least.

The Use of Other Drugs

As noted on page 226, the cytochrome P-450 system is one mechanism by which alcohol is broken down. This system is also responsible for the metabolism of a variety of other drugs and medications, some of which are regularly used by people who abuse alcohol. Since these drugs compete for the same pathway as alcohol to be broken down, the capacity of this pathway becomes strained. Thus, toxic levels of these drugs and/or alcohol accumulate in the body. This may lead to additional and often severe liver injury and may account for why some people develop a more rapidly progressive course of ALD than others.

The most well-established alcohol/drug toxicity is caused by the simultaneous use of alcohol with acetaminophen (Tylenol). Typically, one tablet of acetaminophen is 500 milligrams. A therapeutic dose for minor aches and pains can range anywhere from 2 to 6 grams per day (4 to 12 tablets per day). In people without ALD, dosages greater than 7 to 10 grams (typically 15 grams) over a twenty-four hour period may cause liver damage. But for people with ALD, dosages greater than 2 grams over a twenty-four hour period may cause additional and severe liver damage. Therefore, it is crucial for people with ALD to avoid taking more than 4 tablets of acetamino-phen within a twenty-four hour period. These people would be best advised to limit their intake to one to two 500-milligram tablets per twenty-four hour period.

People are often surprised to learn that acetaminophen within these limited dosages for people with liver disease is actually safer than taking aspirin (ASA) or other nonsteroidal anti-inflammatory drugs (NSAIDs), such as Motrin or Advil. Aspirin and other NSAIDs may cause bleeding disorders (particularly in the gas-trointestinal tract) and kidney disorders, in addition to liver injury. Therefore, peo-ple with ALD, especially those who already often have a bleeding disorder, should always avoid even small doses of these medications. People should also be aware that other over-the-counter medications and some prescription medicines may con-tain acetaminophen or aspirin and other NSAIDs. Therefore, it is important to care-fully read the label of any medication prior to taking it. Of course, labels should always be read carefully, and when in doubt, a person should check with his doctor or pharmacist concerning the presence of these substances in a particular medica-tion. Another drug that increases alcohol's toxic effects on the liver is *isoniazid*—a drug used to treat tuberculosis. The effect of this drug and others on the liver is dis-cussed in more detail in Chapter 24.

When alcohol is ingested in combination with other medications, it often enhances the effect and or side effects of that medication. For example, it may cause excessive sedation (sleepiness) when taken with an anti-anxiety drug, such as alpra-zolam (Xanax). Or alcohol may increase nausea, vomiting, and severe stomach cramping when taken with certain antibiotics, such as cefaclor (Ceclor). Many drugs such as H2 blockers, for example cimetidine (Tagamet) and ranitidine (Zantac), can elevate blood-alcohol levels, thereby resulting in increased alcohol toxicity. A per-son should always consult with a doctor or pharmacist prior to ingesting alcohol in combination with any other medication.

Lastly, it is important for people with ALD to refrain from using cocaine. The combined ingestion of alcohol and cocaine can accelerate liver injury, and, at high enough levels, this toxic combination has the potential to substantially injure the kidneys and muscles and can even cause death. It is unwise for anyone with any liver disease, or anyone for that matter, to use cocaine, as there is evidence that cocaine, in and of itself, may cause liver injury.

Malnutrition

Poor dietary habits may also contribute to the progression of ALD. In fact, malnutrition—defined by the lack of calories and protein consumed—is noted in almost all people with advanced ALD. Deficiencies of vitamins and minerals are also virtually universal. In people with ALD, these substances are poorly absorbed from the stomach lining as a consequence of alcohol's harmful effects on the gastrointestinal tract. The prevalence of poor dietary habits in general among people with ALD also accounts for the nutritional deficiencies that they commonly exhibit. See Chapter 23 for some helpful information on diet and nutrition.

Other Factors

Some factors for ALD come from within the body itself. These include cytokines, endotoxins, free radicals, and possible a form of autoimmune reaction. These factors are discussed below.

Cytokines

Cytokines are substances that are secreted by cells of the immune system. They are involved in regulating the intensity and duration of an immune response. Having a small amount of cytokines present is advantageous, as, at low levels, they play an important role in helping liver cells to repair damage. However, having a large amount of cytokines present is quite dangerous, since at high levels, they play a significant role in causing injury to and death of liver cells. Levels of many cytokines—specifically interleukin-1 (IL-1), interleukin-6 (IL-6), interleukin-8 (IL-8), and tumor necrosis factor (TNF)—have been found frequently in excess in people with hepatitis due to alcohol. Thus, the level of cytokines in a person's body has been implicated to play a role in the development of ALD. However, at present, there are no known specific measures that a person can take to alter the amount of cytokines present in his body. This is an area of future research.

Endotoxin

Endotoxin is a component of the cell wall of certain types of bacteria. As its name suggests, it is a poisonous substance. Increased levels of endotoxin have been found in people with ALD, and, therefore, endotoxin has been implicated as a possible cause of alcoholic liver injury. In one study, rats were fed alcohol while their endotoxin production was blocked with antibiotics. Their LFTs decreased as did their liver damage. Thus, the use of antibiotics in the treatment of ALD is presently being investigated by researchers.

Free Radicals and Oxidative Stress

Free radicals are toxic, highly reactive compounds that are naturally produced by the body. The number of free radicals increases when the body is exposed to something that it perceives as being hazardous, such as a high-fat diet, cigarette smoke, excess iron, exposure to the sun or excess radiation, and of course, alcohol. One of the more common free radicals produced in response to the ingestion of alcohol is oxygen in many deformed, toxic states, known as *oxygen free radicals*. Oxygen free radicals can tear through the liver's protective outer membranes and cause severe injury and damage. So, the liver, just like a human being, is also subjected to a lot of daily stress. Medically, this is known as *oxidative stress*. Iron can induce the formation of free radicals. And, in combination with alcohol ingestion, iron may intensify oxidative stress on the liver, leading to greater liver damage. Therefore, people with ALD should avoid taking excess iron. (See Chapter 18 for more information about iron's effects on the liver.)

As a defense against oxidative stress, the body produces a group of enzymes known as *antioxidants* that gobble up and render harmless any free radicals they can find. Commonly known antioxidants that the body does not produce include the vitamins A, C, and E. But, probably one of the hardest working antioxidants, which is produced by the liver, is called *glutathione*. In fact, it is believed that one of the ways that alcohol causes liver damage is by interfering with the body's ability to produce glutathione. Antioxidant therapy for people with ALD is currently undergoing investigation.

Immune Reactions

Some researchers believe that the damage done to the liver by alcohol may be partly attributable to an immune attack upon liver cells, as is the case with autoimmune hepatitis, which was discussed in Chapter 14. Levels of immunoglobulin A (IgA) are commonly found to be elevated in the blood of people with ALD. People with ALD also sometimes have autoantibodies (such as antinuclear antibody [ANA] and smooth muscle antibody [SMA]) in their blood at low titers. Other studies suggest that the production of antibodies against a form of acetaldehyde may be an indicator of the severity of ALD. Further research in this area is expected.

THE SYMPTOMS AND PHYSICAL SIGNS OF ALD

Symptoms of ALD are nonspecific and may be vague or even absent altogether. They may include fatigue or weakness, both of which can be associated with any type of liver disorder. Symptoms are sometimes related to the stage of disease. For example, if decompensated cirrhosis is present, a symptom may be encephalopathy (mental confusion). But, more often, symptoms do not correlate with the severity of liver damage. Diminished sexual function, diminished sexual drive (libido), and infertility may be signs of ALD. In addition, a person with ALD may experience symptoms that are unrelated to the liver, such as depression, insomnia, lack of concentration, violent behavior, and tremulousness (shakiness).

On a physical exam, the doctor may find an enlarged spleen or a tender, enlarged liver. Physical findings, such as spider angiomatas, palmar erythema, parotid enlargement, Dupuytren's contracture (these were discussed in Chapter 2), and, of course, the smell of alcohol on the breath are more common among people with ALD than with people who have other liver diseases. Men may display signs of feminization, such as gynecomastia (breast enlargement), testicular atrophy (shrunken testicles), and muscle wasting (decreased muscle mass). Many of these physical findings reflect altered estrogen (a female hormone) metabolism by the liver. While some of these signs are suggestive of ALD, none are diagnostic of this condition.

DIAGNOSING ALD

There is no specific test that can accurately diagnosis ALD. Therefore, ALD is typically diagnosed by a combination of self-recognition, doctor recognition, blood work, imaging studies, and liver biopsy. These methods of diagnosis are discussed below.

Recognition by Patient and Doctor

People with ALD often fail to realize that they have a drinking problem. In many cases, the nonrecognition of a problem may be attributable to self-denial (as with Adele at the beginning of this chapter). Therefore, it can be difficult for doctors to diagnose ALD in cases where the patient is adamantly denying excessive alcohol use. A good way for a person to determine if he has a drinking problem is by answering a few simple questions honestly. See the inset "The CAGE Questionnaire" on page 235.

The first step toward a diagnosis of ALD is a doctor's high degree of suspicion that his patient drinks alcohol excessively. Anyone a doctor suspects of alcohol abuse usually will be asked to take the CAGE screening test. Doctors may also decide to have a meeting with the person's family or to speak with his friends or coworkers—always with his patient's informed consent—in order to better assess the actual degree of alcohol abuse. While this may seem intrusive, it is important to remember that the doctor's objective is to make an accurate diagnosis, not to punish or judge, so that appropriate treatment may be given, and so that the long-term consequences of ALD may, if possible, be avoided.

Blood Tests

There is no single blood test that can accurately diagnose ALD. However, the combined results of the following blood tests may suggest a diagnosis of ALD. Although these blood tests are not as accurate as the CAGE screening test, they are very useful in identifying people in severe denial or people who are unwilling to cooperate with a doctor's questioning.

Liver Enzymes

In people with ALD, transaminases (AST and ALT) may be elevated, but are rarely higher than 300 to 400 IU/dl. The level of elevation does not correlate with disease

---

The CAGE Questionnaire

People who drink alcohol on a regular basis need to ask themselves four questions. These four questions make up the CAGE questionnaire. Its purpose is to help determine whether or not there is an alcohol-related problem. Even if only one question is answered positively, the possibility exists that the person does have such a problem. If two or more questions are answered positively, then the presence of alcoholism is very likely. The CAGE questionnaire has been found to be accurate almost 90 percent of the time.

The CAGE Screening Test for Alcoholism

- Have you ever felt the need to **C**ut down on drinking?
- Have you ever felt **A**nnoyed by criticism of your drinking?
- Have you ever had **G**uilty feelings about drinking?
- Have you ever taken a morning **E**ye opener?

---

severity. This point is underscored by the finding that some people with cirrhosis due to alcohol have transaminases that are totally normal. In people with ALD, the AST is often elevated to a level two to three times greater than the ALT. This is partly due to a vitamin B_6 (pyridoxine) deficiency, which is often found in alcoholics. If the transaminases are found to be greatly elevated (greater than 1,000 IU/dl), the most likely cause for this is that too much acetaminophen was taken during a drinking binge. This is indicative of a serious situation necessitating immediate hospitalization and emergency treatment.

In people with ALD, GGTP is almost always elevated. This liver enzyme is frequently used as a screening test for excessive alcohol intake. Unfortunately, this test is nondiagnostic for ALD since GGTP elevations may be attributable to numerous different causes. AP is also often elevated, but is likewise nonspecific for ALD. (See Chapter 3 for information on these blood tests.)

Blood Alcohol Level

Measurement of alcohol in the blood is quite accurate. However, these levels typically reflect the amount of alcohol consumed only on the previous day. So, if a person went to a party and had a few social drinks or drank alcohol for any reason the evening before the test, his blood alcohol level would be very high. This is a poor indicator of chronic alcohol abuse and ALD. One exception is the finding of a value greater than 150 mg/dl in a nonintoxicated person, as this level is extremely high.

Other Blood Tests

In people with ALD, elevated *uric acid* levels—which are typically associated with gout (painful joint inflammation)—may occur. Triglyceride levels may be elevated, whereas the minerals potassium, magnesium, and phosphorus may be low. Levels of glucose may be either high or low. Zinc levels may be low, characteristic of, but not diagnostic of, ALD. Thyroid abnormalities are often associated with ALD. The *mean corpuscular volume* (MCV) is the volume of the average red blood cell in a sample of blood. This value can appear on a routine *complete blood cell count* (CBC). In people with ALD, this value is elevated (greater than 95 fl, or micrometers cubed—μm^3) due to the toxic effect that alcohol has on the bone marrow. This condition is also referred to as *macrocytosis* (large red blood cells).

In people with ALD, immunoglobulin A (IgA) is sometimes very elevated, and occasionally there are some autoantibodies, such as ANA or SMA, present at low titers.

People with ALD often have vitamin deficiencies, which show up on blood tests when ordered by a doctor, as a result of poor nutrition and poor absorption of nutrients into their bodies. Most common are vitamin B_{12} and folate deficiencies. A deficiency of both vitamin B_{12} and folate is suggestive of ALD. Low levels of vitamin B_{12} and folate can also cause a person's MCV to be elevated. An elevated ammonia level, when present in a person with ALD, is often a sign of encephalopathy (mental confusion).

Experimental Blood Tests

Carbohydrate-deficient transferrin (CDT) is a blood test that is being evaluated as an indicator of excessive alcohol use. Transferrin is a protein that transports iron through the body. It contains about 6 percent carbohydrate. In people who drink alcohol excessively, the carbohydrate content of transferrin decreases. So far, this blood test appears to be quite accurate. However, CDT is still considered to be experimental and is not currently available except in clinical studies.

In some studies, blood tests related to collagen synthesis have been shown to correlate with the amount of alcohol consumed and with the extent of liver damage. At this time, this type of blood test is also considered to be experimental and is undergoing further investigation. If the efficacy of these blood tests is confirmed by further research, they will be quite useful in the diagnosis of ALD.

Imaging Studies

A sonogram or a CT scan may reveal a fatty liver or an enlarged liver or spleen. But these findings are not diagnostic of ALD. As with other liver diseases, imaging studies cannot accurately diagnose ALD, nor can they determine the extent of liver damage that has occurred.

Liver Biopsy

For people with ALD, symptoms, physical findings, and laboratory tests typically do not correlate with the severity of inflammation or damage found on liver biopsy samples. Furthermore, they are often not indicative of the stage of ALD. A liver biopsy is the only test that can accurately confirm the diagnosis of ALD and determine the extent of damage caused by the disease. Moreover, a liver biopsy can determine the stage of ALD. This helps predict the likelihood of reversibility and helps to determine long-term prognosis. The stages of ALD are discussed in the following section. For a complete discussion of liver biopsies, see Chapter 5.

THE STAGES OF ALD

There are three stages of alcoholic liver disease—alcoholic fatty liver, alcoholic hepatitis, and alcoholic cirrhosis. A person will not necessarily be aware of his progression from one stage into another. For example, a person may have alcoholic cirrhosis (as confirmed by a liver biopsy specimen) despite never having had an apparent episode of alcoholic hepatitis. Furthermore, all three stages may be present at the same time. Fatty liver and alcoholic hepatitis are potentially reversible, whereas alcoholic cirrhosis is always irreversible. However, a liver biopsy is the only available method for accurately determining long-term prognosis.

Alcoholic Fatty Liver

If a person drinks about 10 ounces (240 grams) of alcohol—equal to about three 6 packs of beer or 3 liters of wine—daily for about a week, he will most likely develop a fatty liver. In fact, steatosis (fatty liver) may occur after as little as three days of excessive alcohol ingestion. Many people who consider themselves social or weekend drinkers probably have had a fatty liver on several occasions. These people are usually asymptomatic (without symptoms). Their LFTs may be normal or slightly elevated. A physical exam may reveal an enlarged liver due to fatty deposits. A liver biopsy will show only fatty deposits and no other abnormalities. When inflammation is present in the liver among these people, their condition is known as steatohepatitis. The above-mentioned findings may be indistinguishable from fatty liver and nonalcoholic steatohepatitis (NASH) which were discussed in Chapter 16. Alcoholic fatty liver is generally a benign, reversible condition. If alcohol intake is discontinued at this stage, no long-term consequences will be suffered.

Alcoholic Hepatitis

Alcoholic hepatitis is inflammation of the liver due to the toxic effects of alcohol. A person may have either acute or chronic alcoholic hepatitis. About half of all alcoholics will develop at least one episode of alcoholic hepatitis in their lifetimes. The symptoms and signs of alcoholic hepatitis vary greatly. At one end of the spectrum, a person may be asymptomatic. For such a person, the discovery of alcoholic hepatitis is likely to be made when abnormal LFTs appear on a blood test done in the course of a routine exam. For these people, alcoholic hepatitis is totally reversible if the person immediately and completely stops drinking alcohol.

At the other end of the spectrum, a person with alcoholic hepatitis may be severely ill, with fever, nausea and vomiting, abdominal pain, or even signs of severe liver damage and liver failure. Between 20 and 50 percent of these people are likely to die from a bout of alcoholic hepatitis. Those who survive may take up to six months to totally recuperate. Of course, they must totally abstain from drinking alcohol for the rest of their lives.

It must be remembered that alcoholic hepatitis can occur in a person whether or not he has alcoholic cirrhosis—an irreversible condition. A finding of alcoholic hepatitis on a liver biopsy indicates that a person is at risk for developing cirrhosis. People with alcoholic hepatitis who continue to drink alcohol have at least a 50-percent chance of developing cirrhosis within ten years from the onset of alcoholic hepatitis.

Alcoholic Cirrhosis

Alcoholic cirrhosis is irreversible scarring of the liver due to alcohol. The development of alcoholic cirrhosis carries with it the risk of complications that typically pertain to cirrhosis (see Chapter 6). When an alcoholic is actively drinking, the nodules that develop in the cirrhotic liver are small. This is known as micronodular cirrhosis and is due to the fact that alcohol impairs the normal activity of liver cells. But when such a person stops drinking alcohol, there is a surge of activity in the liver, and the small cirrhotic nodules are transformed into larger cirrhotic nodules. This is known as macronodular cirrhosis.

The significance of micronodular and macronodular cirrhosis relates to the development of liver cancer. All people with cirrhosis are at risk for liver cancer. In general, people with alcoholic cirrhosis have about a 15-percent overall lifetime risk of developing liver cancer. Liver cancer more commonly occurs in a macronodular cirrhotic liver. Paradoxically, people with alcoholic cirrhosis who continue to actively drink are actually less likely to develop liver cancer than those who abstain. This should in no way be construed as an incentive for an alcoholic to continue to drink alcohol. People with alcoholic cirrhosis who abstain from alcohol have repeatedly been shown to have a healthier and longer life span compared with those who continue to ingest alcohol.

THE TREATMENT OF ALD

Many different medications and nutritional therapies have been tested for use in the treatment of ALD. Most therapies involve either inhibiting or modifying the action of one or more cytokines (see page 232). While some of these therapies have yielded beneficial results, in general, the use of these therapies for ALD remains controversial. Consistently, the most effective form of therapy and the most important step toward recovery has been abstinence from alcohol. Other crucial steps toward recovery involve seeking the assistance of a support group and entering an alcohol treatment program. No one is expected to go it alone, and there are a variety of well-respected support groups devoted to helping people with alcohol problems achieve and sustain abstinence. (See Appendix for the names and addresses of some of these support groups.)

Corticosteroids—for example prednisone, an anti-inflammatory medication discussed in Chapter 14—have, in some cases, been shown to benefit certain people with severe alcoholic hepatitis. However, due to the potential side effects of prednisone (see Chapter 14), which may worsen some of the complications of ALD, not all people are candidates for this therapy.

Colchicine (a medication with antifibrotic and anti-inflammatory properties discussed in Chapter 15) and propylthiouracil (PTU) (an antihyperthyroid or fast thyroid medication) have been the only medications that have shown in clinical studies to improve long-term survival of people with ALD. However, further study needs to be conducted before these medications can be recommended for the treatment of people with ALD.

Nutritionally, the liver actually favors alcohol as a form of fuel. Thus, alcohol typically supplants many important nutrients needed for a healthy diet. For example, when alcohol replaces fat as an energy source, the first stage of ALD results—fatty liver. This also causes triglyceride levels to rise in the body, which puts a person at additional risk of heart disease. People with ALD should attempt to increase their caloric intake with healthy nutritious foods to maintain at least between 1,500 to 2,000 calories per day. It has been shown that people with severe ALD who ingest less than 1,000 calories per day of nutritious foods have a very poor prognosis. If a person with ALD cannot tolerate a regular meal, he should attempt to utilize one of the many supplement beverages that are readily available—many of which are designed specifically for alcoholics. See Chapter 23 for more information on diet and nutrition.

THE NATURAL HISTORY AND PROGNOSIS FOR THOSE WITH ALD

If alcohol use is discontinued prior to the development of cirrhosis, any inflammation or injury that has occurred to the liver is potentially reversible. It has even been noted that people with alcoholic cirrhosis who abstain from drinking, generally have a better prognosis than people with other forms of cirrhosis. In fact, people with alcoholic cirrhosis who have not had complications of cirrhosis, such as jaundice, variceal bleeding, or ascites, typically have a 90-percent chance of living for at least five more years. Survival rates for these people are actually only slightly below that of the general population of comparable age and sex. However, once complications of cirrhosis have occurred, the chances of living for five more years decreases to 60 percent. And people with alcoholic cirrhosis have approximately a 15-percent overall lifetime risk of developing liver cancer.

For people with ALD, the key to a positive prognosis may be summed up in one word: *abstinence.* Those who do not abstain from drinking have a very poor prognosis. A persistently elevated bilirubin level and a prolonged prothrombin time (signs of decompensated cirrhosis) are the most reliable indicators of a poor prognosis. The level of certain cytokines in the blood may possibly predict prognosis in people with ALD. Some studies have suggested that cytokine levels correlate with both the bilirubin level and with mortality rates. Further investigation is needed to confirm these findings.

CONCLUSION

The most important message in this chapter is straightforward: *If a person has any type of chronic liver disease, he should not ingest alcohol. In addition, it is especially important for any person with ALD to immediately abstain from consuming alcohol.* The dosage and duration of alcohol ingestion are among the many factors that contribute to alcoholic liver damage and to the progression of ALD. This explains why some people can consume substantial amounts of alcohol without suffering adverse consequences whereas others are very susceptible to the toxicities of alcohol. Future research is likely to focus on identifying genes that make a person more susceptible to alcoholic cirrhosis and on learning more about the role of cytokines in the development of ALD. Future therapies will likely be targeted at altering or blocking the production of liver-toxic cytokines. Other therapies may focus on utilizing antibiotics against endotoxin-induced liver injury. In this chapter, you also learned that alcohol in combination with excessive iron accelerates the progression of liver disease.

The next chapter discusses hemochromatosis, an inherited disease of iron overload. It also discusses other diseases of iron overload that a person may acquire.

18

Hemochromatosis and Other Diseases of Iron Overload

Mary, a fifty-two-year-old homemaker, went to the doctor for her year-ly check-up. With the exception of the menopausal hot flashes she'd been experiencing for the past year, she felt fine. The doctor examined her and took blood for some routine tests. A week later, he telephoned Mary and told her to stop taking iron supplements because her blood test results revealed elevated iron levels. "But I don't take iron supple-ments," Mary told him. "Then you'd better come back in for addition-al blood tests," the doctor replied.

A week later, Mary returned to the office for further testing. She and the doctor discussed possible reasons for why her iron levels were ele-vated. The doctor asked Mary if anyone in her family had high iron levels or a genetic disorder known as hemochromatosis. Mary seemed to recall that an uncle from Scotland had died of a liver disorder, but no one knew what is was.

Three weeks later, the doctor contacted Mary to inform her that her elevated iron level was due to hemochromatosis. He advised Mary that she would need to have a liver biopsy and that she would have to start treatment with phlebotomies.

Patrick, a thirty-five-year-old construction worker, began to experience a lack of energy while working at his job. But what led him to make an appointment with his doctor was his diminished interest in sex. Patrick, who was well built and had a dark ruddy complexion, had a long his-tory of various muscle and joint pains, which he blamed on the physi-cal nature of his work. He also had a mild case of diabetes, which he kept under control by watching his diet. He attributed his bronze com-plexion to the long hours he spent working outdoors in the sun. Patrick's doctor performed a physical exam and drew some blood for routine blood tests. A week later, the doctor notified Patrick that his iron level was elevated as were some of his liver enzymes and he should return to the office for additional blood work. The doctor also asked him if anyone in his family had ever had liver disease. After speaking to his mother, Patrick learned that both his aunt and great grandfather—neither of whom drank much alcohol—had died from cirrhosis. After some additional tests, the doctor confirmed that Patrick had inherited hemochromatosis. He was referred to a liver specialist who performed a liver biopsy, the results of which confirmed the diagnosis. Patrick's liver was loaded with iron. He was sent for treatment with phlebotomies.

C hances are many of you have seen Popeye gulping down a can of spinach in order to get his muscle-producing supply of iron, and most of you have probably heard that iron can "pep you up" or that it's just plain good for you. Perhaps this explains why so many people take iron supplements expecting a boost of energy. For iron-deficient people, supplementing with iron may be okay. But for people with iron-rich blood, taking iron supplements may be so harmful that it can put them at risk for cirrhosis, liver cancer, impotence, and heart failure. Hemochromatosis—a genetic disease of iron overload—is the subject of this chapter. As the main repository for iron in the body, the liver is among the first organs to be affected by hemochromatosis, and often suffers the greatest adverse consequences. This chapter covers hemochromatosis, its symptoms and signs, and how it is diagnosed and treated. In addition, it reviews exciting new advances made in this area. Towards the end, this chapter provides information about iron-overload diseases other than hemochromatosis.

WHAT IS HEMOCHROMATOSIS?

Hemochromatosis is a term that is used to describe an excessive deposit of iron in the body. Excess iron deposits may occur in the liver, heart, pancreas, joints, pituitary gland, or other organs. When this happens, the affected organ ceases to function properly and becomes damaged. Hemochromatosis can either be inherited at birth or may be acquired at some point due to a variety of causes.

Hereditary Hemochromatosis

If a person has inherited hemochromatosis, it is termed hereditary (or genetic) hemochromatosis (HH). These people have inherited the gene for the disease from their parents in an *autosomal recessive* manner. This means that in order to display the manifestations of hemochromatosis and to be at risk for its long-term complications, a person must inherit one gene from each parent. People with two hemochromatosis genes are known as *homozygotes*. People who inherit the hemochromatosis gene from only one parent are known as a *heterozygotes*.

Heterozygotes will not exhibit signs of the disease, nor are they at risk for complications of the disease. They are, however, carriers of the hemochromatosis gene and can pass the gene to their children. The hemochromatosis gene is known as HFE and will be discussed below and on page 247.

Non-Inherited Iron Overload

A person can also have too much iron in the body due to non-hereditary causes, such as taking excessive amounts of iron supplements. Some medical literature refers to this as secondary or acquired hemochromatosis. However, it is more accurate to refer to this group of people as having a *secondary iron overload disease.* Therefore, the term "hemochromatosis" will be used in this book only in reference to those people who have inherited the disease. Secondary iron overload diseases and other nonhereditary liver diseases associated with elevated iron levels will be discussed beginning on page 251.

THE HISTORY OF HEMOCHROMATOSIS

Hemochromatosis was first recognized in 1871 when an association was made among excessive iron in the liver, diabetes (excessive blood sugar), and the development of cirrhosis. Believed to be a genetic disorder of the blood (*heme*), the term hemochromatosis (*chromatosis* meaning chromosome—genetic material) was coined. The hereditary nature of hemochromatosis was confirmed when it was recognized that people with the disease had inherited a gene mutation located on chromosome 6.

In 1996, a major breakthrough in hemochromatosis research occurred—the discovery of two mutations associated with the *candidate hemochromatosis gene*, which is now called HFE. These two gene mutations were given the names C282Y and H63D.

The gene mutation C282Y is present in approximately 82 to 100 percent of people with hemochromatosis and is considered to be the more specific mutation of the two associated with the disease. The H63D mutation is less clearly associated with the risk of developing hemochromatosis. The discovery of these two mutations was remarkable because it enabled scientists to develop a blood test that can diagnose this disease with substantial accuracy (see page 247). This enables diagnosis and treatment of the disease in its earliest stages.

HOW COMMON IS HEMOCHROMATOSIS?

Hemochromatosis is a very common disorder. In fact, it is the most common genetic disease in the United States and among people of European descent. Estimates from the American Liver Foundation indicate that 1 in 250 to 300 people of northern European descent has this disease (approximately 1.5 million Americans). 1 in 10 people are carriers of the disease (approximately 32 million Americans). Carriers have one copy of the mutant HFE gene. Although all ethnic groups are at risk for hemochromatosis, it has been found to be more prevalent in those of Irish, Scottish, Celtic, or British ancestry.

AN OVERVIEW OF IRON

Hemochromatosis is a disorder of iron metabolism. Therefore, to understand hemochromatosis, it is crucial to understand what iron is, how iron is absorbed and stored, and what the effects are of having too much iron in the body.

Iron (Fe) is a mineral. A *mineral* is a substance that originates in the soil and water and eventually becomes incorporated into all animal and plant life through the food chain. While iron has many important functions in the body, an excess of iron may lead to liver damage and cirrhosis. Iron is a substance that contradicts the popular saying "if a little is good, then more is better."

How Iron Damages the Liver

One way that iron damages the liver is by promoting the formation of harmful free radicals in the body. *Free radicals* are toxic, highly reactive compounds that are naturally produced by the body. The number of free radicals increases when the body is exposed to foreign substances (such as alcohol, cigarette smoke, radiation, or excessive iron) that it perceives as hazardous. Most free radicals in the body are toxic oxygen molecules. Oxygen in its toxic state can oxidize molecules in the body, corroding them—similar to the way rust forms on an iron fence, which is actually just oxidized iron.

Iron-induced oxidation of the cell walls is known as *lipid peroxidation*. The byproducts of lipid peroxidation, such as hydrogen peroxide, are believed to be toxic or harmful to the liver. Anyone with any form of liver disease should bear this in mind as iron has been shown to speed the progression and worsen the course of many liver diseases. This is especially true for alcoholic liver disease, as alcohol and excess iron have been shown to have an additive harmful effect on the liver.

How Iron Levels Are Determined

Normal iron levels routinely found on blood work range between 30 and 160 micrograms per deciliter. Iron is stored in the cells of the body as *ferritin*. The normal ferritin level found on blood tests is 15 to 200 micrograms per liter. *Transferrin* is a protein that is made by the liver and transports iron through the body. The percentage of transferrin that is saturated with iron at any given time is known as the *transferrin saturation percent*. Normal transferrin saturation values range from 15 to 50 percent. Iron, ferritin, and transferrin saturation percent together are referred to as iron studies. If a person's iron studies are above the upper limit of normal on any of these tests, he should be checked for hemochromatosis. See Diagnosing Hemochromatosis on page 246.

How Iron Is Stored and Replaced

The amount of iron lost from the body on a daily basis is approximately 1 to 2 milligrams. People must replace this daily iron loss through the foods they eat. However, the average American diet contains about 10 to 20 milligrams of iron per day, an amount that greatly exceeds the average loss. Humans do not have a major route of elimination of iron from the body. Therefore, the content of iron in the body is determined by how much iron the body actually absorbs. For example, *heme iron,* which is obtained from animal meat, is better absorbed than *nonheme iron,* which is obtained from vegetables. So, with all due respect to Popeye, a juicy steak supplies the body with far more iron than does spinach. In people who are not at risk for iron overload, approximately 10 percent (1 to 2 milligrams) of dietary iron is absorbed by the lining of the *duodenum*—the first part of the small intestine. When the body's internal sensors detect an iron deficiency, more iron is absorbed from the diet. Conversely, if there is a surplus of iron already in the body, less iron is absorbed. Any excess iron that is not absorbed or eliminated from the body is stored predominantly in the liver as ferritin. In hemochromatosis, there is a defect in the body's ability to absorb iron. Moreover, the body's ability to sense an iron overload is lost. Thus, too much iron, approximately 3 to 6 milligrams per day, gets absorbed by the duodenum. The excess iron accumulates in the liver and other organs, such as the pancreas and heart, which can result in serious damage to these organs.

THE SYMPTOMS AND SIGNS OF HEMOCHROMATOSIS

As with most liver diseases, the symptoms of hemochromatosis are usually absent until the later stages of the disease and can be vague even when present. Men tend to have more pronounced symptoms than women. This is believed to be due to the greater amount of iron overload that exists in men because premenopausal women eliminate iron on a monthly basis through menstruation. Weakness and fatigue are the most common symptoms. Some people complain of a decreased appetite and weight loss.

Since the liver is the warehouse for the storage of excess iron, it is often damaged in the early stages of the disease. This may manifest as abdominal pain or a nondescript discomfort over the right upper quadrant (over the liver). Abnormalities due to excessive iron deposits in other organs or glands of the body occur late in the disease and may include decreased body hair, reduced interest in sex, impotence in men, and a lack of menstruation in women. Glucose intolerance or overt diabetes can also develop. Occasionally—approximately 8 percent of the time—a thyroid disorder will develop. Painful joints and arthritis occur in approximately one-fourth to one-half of people with hemochromatosis, usually beginning in the hands, but can progress to the knees, back, and neck. People with hemochromatosis are also prone to osteoporosis (bone loss).

Some people notice that they have developed what appears to be a "healthy" tan. But this skin discoloration is anything but healthy. It is actually due to a combination of iron deposits in the skin and an increased production of the pigment melanin. This bronze coloration of the skin, known as *hyperpigmentation,* is most obvious in the sun-exposed areas of the body. In fact, hemochromatosis was originally called *bronze diabetes* because most people with hemochromatosis were first seen by a doctor in the later stages of the disease—after they had already developed grayish-bronze skin coloring and the symptoms of diabetes, including increased thirst and urination. Symptoms of more advanced hemochromatosis include heart failure, heart arrhythmias (an irregular heartbeat), and the manifestations of portal hypertension (discussed in Chapter 6).

On a physical exam, the doctor may detect an enlarged liver; *cardiomegaly* (an enlarged heart); bronze skin tone; testicular atrophy (shrunken testicles); swollen and tender joints; or signs of cirrhosis and/or liver failure. Any of these finding are suggestive of advanced hemochromatosis.

DIAGNOSING HEMOCHROMATOSIS

It has been shown that early detection and treatment of hemochromatosis can prevent the long-term, potentially fatal consequences of the disease. However, in the early stages of hemochromatosis, symptoms are usually absent or very vague. Symptoms in the later stages frequently mimic those of other more common diseases, such as heart disease, arthritis, and diabetes. Often, people go undiagnosed for many years. This may be because their iron studies appear normal or even low due to factors such as frequent blood donation, multiple pregnancies, menstruation, or gastrointestinal bleeding. Therefore, it is not surprising that about 90 percent of people with hemochromatosis go undiagnosed or misdiagnosed for so long.

So how would a person normally discover that he has hemochromatosis in the first place? Well, the initial step is for the person to go to the doctor for a routine check-up and blood tests, despite feeling fine. In fact, the Iron Overload Diseases Association (IODA) recommends that all Americans eighteen years and older be routinely screened for iron overload. This section will discuss the utility of blood tests, a liver biopsy, and imaging studies in the diagnosis of hemochromatosis.

Iron Studies and Liver Function Tests (LFTs)

Hemochromatosis is often detected in people when high or elevated iron studies are detected on routine blood tests. Iron studies commonly include three values—the iron level, the ferritin level (the storage form of iron), and the transferrin saturation percent (the percent of transferrin—a protein made in the liver that transplants iron through the body—that is saturated with iron at any given time). In fact, if the ferritin and transferrin saturation percent are elevated, it strongly suggests that a person has hemochromatosis—even if the iron level itself is not elevated.

Elevated LFTs are also commonly found in people with hemochromatosis. But don't be misled by normal LFTs. In the early stages of the disease, LFTs are rarely elevated.

The Hemochromatosis Candidate Gene (HFE)

As discussed on page 243, a major advance in the diagnosis of hemochromatosis has been the identification of the candidate gene for hereditary hemochromatosis known as HFE and the subsequent discovery of two specific gene mutations that are diagnostic for hemochromatosis. Approximately 82 to 100 percent of people with hemochromatosis are homozygous (have two genes) for the gene mutation C282Y. The other gene mutation, H63D, accounts for up to 20 percent of people with hemochromatosis. Two additional HFE gene mutations have been described, but their significance is unclear. The genetic DNA tests for identifying both C282Y and H63D are currently available and can be obtained simply by having some blood tests taken by the doctor. Also, there is a tissue-collection kit available that merely requires a person to swab the inside of his mouth with a cheek brush. This screening test can be performed at home. However, regardless of which screening method is used, a doctor must evaluate the results.

As discussed on page 242, hemochromatosis is an autosomal recessively inherited disease. Therefore, a person must inherit two copies of the hemochromatosis gene mutation in order to manifest the disease. If only one copy of the HFE gene is found to contain the C282Y mutation, the person is merely a carrier. Development of disease by such a person is unlikely. However, his family members may be at risk and should be tested. If both copies of the HFE gene are found to contain the C282Y mutation, the person has hemochromatosis and is at risk for the development of long-term complications. Similarly, this person's family members need to be tested too. In fact, if a family member has been diagnosed with hemochromatosis or has been found to be a carrier of the disease, it is crucial to undergo screening tests. (See the inset "Screening Family Members" on page 248.)

The H63D mutation by itself is not as clearly associated with hemochromatosis. In fact, there are many people in the United States who are homozygous for the H63D gene mutation and rarely, if ever, develop iron overload. However, if a person inherits one H63D and one C282Y mutation—a condition known as a compound heterozygote—occasionally he will develop significant iron overload. To make matters even more complicated, approximately 10 to 15 percent of people who do not carry either of these mutations still develop hemochromatosis. Obviously, there are other unknown factors or other gene mutations not yet discovered that cause hemochromatosis.

Liver Biopsy

Iron, in and of itself, can be toxic to many organs, particularly the liver. Therefore, it is important for all people diagnosed with hemochromatosis to have a liver biopsy in order to assess both the amount of iron stores in the liver and the degree of damage done to the liver by this overload of iron. A biopsy is the only reliable test for determining whether cirrhosis is present. This information is helpful for both the patient and the doctor as it will assist in determining long-term prognosis and for assessing management and treatment.

Screening Family Members for Hemochromatosis

Since the gene for hemochromatosis is so common, many generations of people may be carriers, and yet none may ever manifest the disease. Therefore, all first-degree relatives of people with hemochromatosis and especially the siblings of such people should be screened for hemochromatosis. Screening should initially include a blood test for iron studies and LFTs. If these are found to be abnormal, the test for the hemochromatosis candidate gene should be obtained.

Due to the excellent screening techniques that are available, fewer people are now being diagnosed in the later stages of the disease when liver damage may have already occurred. Once again, it is important to stress that hemochromatosis, like most liver diseases, is a silent disorder. The only way to avoid the potentially lethal consequences of this disease is to have it detected in its earliest, most treatable, stages.

There are some instances when a biopsy may not be necessary. First, if a young person—perhaps someone in his twenties—is identified as having hemochromatosis through the genetic screening of family members, it is unlikely he will already have developed significant scarring of the liver. Under these and similar conditions, a person may forego a liver biopsy. Also, in a situation where a person refuses to have a biopsy, the diagnosis itself may still be made using blood tests. The finding of an elevated transferrin saturation and ferritin level would suggest hemochromatosis, and genetic testing would confirm this diagnosis. (See Chapter 5 for detailed information about liver biopsies.)

Imaging Studies

A sonogram is usually normal, but it may reveal an enlarged liver. While it will not reveal the degree to which the liver is damaged, it is a good screening test to evaluate for the presence or absence of liver cancer. Therefore, the doctor will most likely want a sonogram at some point in the evaluation. If a person's liver biopsy reveals cirrhosis, he will need to obtain a sonogram at least once a year because such people are at a high risk for the development of liver cancer.

CT scans may reveal evidence of iron overload in cases where the overload is very extensive. However, in milder cases of iron overload, the CT will be normal. MRIs can also detect a heavy iron overload. They are occasionally used to determine the amount of iron in the liver and the extent to which the liver has been damaged. It is important to remember that MRIs do not provide as much information as a liver biopsy. They should be substituted only for a liver biopsy in cases where it has been determined that a biopsy would be medically unsafe for a particular person. See Chapter 3 for more information on imaging studies.

TREATMENT OF HEMOCHROMATOTSIS

The goal of treatment of hemochromatosis is to remove the excess iron from the body to prevent the occurrence of organ damage. This can be easily and efficiently achieved by a method known as phlebotomy. Another way to remove excess iron is through a process known as chelation therapy. Finally, certain dietary restrictions also play a role in the treatment of hemochromatosis. The following is a discussion of these treatments.

Phlebotomy

Phlebotomy involves taking blood out of the body through a catheter that is temporarily placed in the arm. The blood that is removed from the body is discarded because it cannot be used for blood donation or for any other purpose. Approximately 500 milliliters (equal to one unit) of blood should be taken out each week. This will remove approximately 250 milligrams of iron on each occasion. For example, if a person has an excess of about 25 grams of iron, he will need to have approximately 100 units of blood removed. It usually takes about two years of weekly phlebotomies to deplete about 25 grams of iron. After each phlebotomy, a person's red blood count, measured by hemoglobin or hematocrit, should be checked. Also, iron studies—iron, ferritin, and transferrin saturation—should be checked about every three months. When the transferrin saturation falls below 50 percent and the serum ferritin falls below 50 micrograms per liter, the goal has been achieved. Mild anemia may develop at this point.

If the results of a liver biopsy reveal excessive scarring, iron should be removed from the body at a quicker rate to attempt to avoid cirrhosis and its complications. These people should have blood removed at least twice a week. Removal of excess iron can stop the progression of hemochromatosis if cirrhosis is not present at the time of diagnosis. This point underscores the importance of early diagnosis and of prompt treatment as well as the need for evaluation with liver biopsy. Phlebotomy will not be able to improve cirrhosis. Yet, despite the presence of cirrhosis, phlebotomy might alleviate some symptoms associated with hemochromatosis, especially fatigue and abdominal pain. Therefore, people with cirrhosis should still undergo phlebotomy. However, these people remain at risk for liver cancer and other complications of cirrhosis.

After the initial bulk of excessive iron has been removed, the frequency of phlebotomies is decreased to the level where 500 milliliters (one unit) of blood is removed approximately every three months. The goal should be to keep the ferritin level between 50 and 100 micrograms per liter at all times.

Some symptoms totally resolve after successful phlebotomy. Fatigue improves in over 60 percent of people who have undergone phlebotomy. Hyperpigmentation (the bronze color of the skin) also resolves in most people. Abdominal pain and enlargement of the liver, attributable to distention of the liver from iron overload, usually resolves after sufficient quantities of iron have been removed. Similarly, elevated LFTs usually normalize. Heart problems caused by hemochromatosis, such as congestive heart failure (CHF) and cardiomegaly (enlarged heart) also usually improve after excessive iron is removed.

Approximately 50 percent of people with diabetes due to hemochromatosis will be more easily managed. However, there will probably be a continued need for either insulin or *oral hypoglycemics*—sugar-lowering medications taken orally. Iron-depletion therapy has no effect on the course of hemochromatosis-associated arthritis. Treatment of joint pains should be with nonsteroidal anti-inflammatories, but in moderation, as these medications may also cause liver damage. In fact, arthritis may even develop after iron is depleted. Unfortunately, hemochromatosis-related impotence usually does not resolve. Furthermore, therapy of impotence with testosterone should be avoided due the potential additional risk factor for liver cancer, although this risk is not well documented.

Chelation Therapy

Chelation therapy—involving the infusion of deferoxamine (Desferal) either into a vein or *subcutaneously* (beneath the skin)—can also remove excess iron. This iron chelator (a binding agent) works by binding to iron and promoting its elimination from the body. This treatment takes much longer than phlebotomy, as only 10 to 20 milligrams of iron is removed each time—in contrast to 250 milligrams with phlebotomy. In addition, this treatment is more expensive than phlebotomy and is associated with some side effects, such as diarrhea, fast heartbeat, and hearing and visual disturbances. Therefore, deferoxamine infusions should be limited to people who otherwise cannot tolerate phlebotomy, such as those people with severe heart disease. Iron chelators taken orally, such as deferiprone, have been associated with significant toxicity and cannot be recommended at present.

Diet

While there is some disagreement as to how stringent a person needs to be in terms of dietary restrictions, it is probably a good idea to refrain from eating foods high in iron content. Such foods include all red meats—especially liver. Vegetable iron is not as efficiently absorbed into the body as animal iron is. Therefore, total dietary restriction of green, leafy vegetables is not necessary and not healthy.

People should avoid cooking with cast-iron laden cookware and utensils, which are often a source of hidden iron. Vitamin C increases the body's ability to absorb iron from food. Therefore, no vitamin-C supplementation, including that found in multivitamins, should be taken. Some medicines contain iron, so labels should be read carefully. There are also many foods, especially cereals, that are fortified with iron (iron has been added to them). Some weight-gain and weight-loss products are loaded with iron and vitamin C. Furthermore, some herbs commonly taken to treat liver disease (milk thistle, dandelion, and licorice) may contain iron. Therefore, people with hemochromatosis should avoid these herbs. People must become informed consumers, carefully reading labels prior to purchasing foods, beverages, herbs, supplements, or any over-the-counter medicines from any supermarket, drug, or health food store. Lastly, alcohol should be avoided for two reasons. First, alcohol may increase iron absorption. Second, alcohol, in itself, is toxic to the liver. Thus, alcohol, even in moderate amounts, may worsen liver damage in people with hemochromatosis. See Chapter 23 for more information on diet.

THE LONG-TERM PROGNOSIS FOR THOSE WITH HEMOCHROMATOSIS

Hemochromatosis is a potentially fatal disease. However, if the disease is diagnosed early and is treated promptly and aggressively, a person with hemochromatosis will enjoy a normal life span. Once cirrhosis has developed, people are at increased risk for the complications of cirrhosis and for the development of liver cancer—even if iron stores have been successfully depleted through phlebotomy. In fact, people with both hemochromatosis and cirrhosis are 200 times more likely (estimated at a 30-percent chance) to develop liver cancer compared with the general population. Between 30 and 45 percent of deaths in people with hemochromatosis are due to liver cancer. See Chapter 19 for more information on liver cancer.

Another major cause of death in people with hemochromatosis and cirrhosis is heart arrhythmias and heart failure. When heart involvement is discovered, aggressive treatment with phlebotomy and possibly chelation therapy should commence.

If complications of cirrhosis occur, the person should be considered for a liver transplant. This option will be addressed in Chapter 22.

SECONDARY OR ACQUIRED IRON OVERLOAD DISEASES

Excessive oral ingestion of iron can cause elevated iron studies. Thus, when a person is discovered to have a high iron profile on routine blood tests, a thorough investigation into all of the medicines, vitamins, and supplements both prescribed and over-the-counter that he is taking should be made. Those that contain excess iron should be eliminated from the diet.

There have also been occasional reports of people becoming iron overloaded from drinking excessive quantities of beer that had been brewed in cast iron drums or from excessively consuming foods cooked in iron cookware. If high iron studies persist after the elimination of the above-mentioned factors, another cause—such as hereditary hemochromatosis or chronic hepatitis C—should be searched for.

People who have received more than fifty blood transfusions often have elevated iron levels attributable to the excessive iron contained in all those transfusions. These people are also at risk for the development of iron-related organ damage. A chelation therapy program should be considered if continued transfusions will be needed on a regular basis.

Some people have received iron injections after being diagnosed with anemia (a low red blood cell count). Yet anemia can have a multitude of causes—iron deficiency being just one of them. If the anemia is, in fact, not due to an iron deficiency, but is due to a vitamin B_{12} deficiency (for example), toxic accumulations of iron can result if iron injections or replacements were given.

EXCESSIVE IRON AND OTHER LIVER DISEASES

Iron by itself can have harmful effects on the liver. When excessive iron exists in combination with another liver disorder, there is potential for worsening and/or accelerated liver damage. There are three liver diseases that are associated with high iron levels. They include alcoholic liver disease (see Chapter 17), nonalcoholic steatohepatitis (see Chapter 16), and chronic viral hepatitis—especially chronic hepatitis C (see Chapter 10). Elevated iron studies can occur in about 40 to 50 percent of people with one of these underlying liver disorders. However, since these people do not have hereditary hemochromatosis, their intestines do not absorb an overabundance of iron. Thus, excessive iron deposition in the liver occurs only about 10 percent of the time in this particular group. Furthermore, the degree of iron deposits in the liver is mild compared to that found in people with hemochromatosis.

Why people with these three liver disorders have high iron levels remains an area of speculation and debate among medical researchers. It is thought, but not yet proven, that possibly some of these people may in fact be heterozygotes for hemochromatosis—carriers of one mutant gene. If these people are treated with phlebotomy, their LFTs may show some improvement. However, the underlying liver disease does not actually improve, and people will continue to be at risk for cirrhosis and its complications. Therefore, it would be reasonable for the doctor to obtain hemochromatosis genetic testing on people with these liver diseases if their iron levels are elevated, before recommending phlebotomy.

CONCLUSION

After reading this chapter, you know that iron—though required by the body in small amounts for proper functioning—can be harmful to some people. This includes people with hemochromatosis, other disorders of iron overload, and some chronic liver diseases. Hemochromatosis is another liver disorder where early detection is crucial to halt the progression of disease. If a person has this disorder, it is highly recommended that their family members be screened.

The next chapter discusses both benign (noncancerous) and malignant (cancerous) liver tumors, and how they are treated. It also discusses the most common type of malignant liver tumor in the United States—metastatic liver tumors.

19

Benign and Malignant Liver Tumors

Dana, a forty-eight-year-old fashion designer, went to her family doctor for an evaluation of stomach pains and a fever. These symptoms had started after she had eaten some questionable food from a salad bar. After examining Dana, the doctor told her that she most likely had food poisoning. However, he advised her to go to a radiologist for an abdominal sonogram to make sure she didn't have gallstones. Dana went for the sonogram that day, but by the next day, she was feeling fine and decided to return to work.

Dana never showed up for her follow-up visit with the doctor to discuss the results of the sonogram, and never returned the call that was left by her doctor on her answering machine. She didn't even bother responding to the cancellation letter she had received some time later from the doctor's office, which requested that she make an appointment to discuss the results of her sonogram. About a year later, Dana went to the doctor for her yearly physical. "By the way, what was the result of the sonogram that I took last year?" Dana asked, unconcerned but curious. The doctor told her the results from the sonogram suggested that she has a benign tumor on her liver known as a hemangioma.

"A tumor!?" Dana exclaimed. "Is this a serious condition?" The doctor assured Dana that there was nothing to worry about, but he would need to order an additional imaging study to confirm the diagnosis and to assess for any enlargement. The subsequent tests confirmed the initial diagnosis of a benign hemangioma.

June, a thirty-year-old receptionist, went to her doctor for evaluation of a fever, cough, and sore throat. The doctor's diagnosis was that June had bronchitis. He gave her a prescription for an antibiotic and took some blood tests. The results of the blood tests were normal with the exception of an elevated GGTP. The doctor noted that in June's medical history questionnaire, she wrote that she'd been on birth control pills since giving birth five years earlier. The doctor advised June to see a radiologist to get a sonogram done to evaluate the cause of her elevated GGTP. The sonogram revealed a large mass on her liver, and her doctor advised her to discontinue taking the birth control pills immediately and repeat the sonogram in three months. The repeat sonogram did not reveal any decrease in size of the mass. The doctor sent June for a liver biopsy, the results of which revealed that June's tumor was a hepatic adenoma. The doctor concluded that this benign tumor was caused by June's use of birth control pills. June was referred to a surgeon for the removal of the hepatic adenoma.

Pete, a sixty-year-old retired detective, noticed that he was losing weight. He was also experiencing mild discomfort and fullness on the right side of his abdomen. Pete disliked going to doctors, and, in fact, had not been to one in over ten years. However, at the insistence of his oldest son, Pete finally made an appointment. The doctor asked Pete about his past medical history—the only significant event was an appendectomy almost forty years earlier, at which time Pete seemed to recall receiving a blood transfusion. The doctor also asked Pete about his smoking and drinking habits. Pete had stopped smoking about twenty years earlier, but he admitted to drinking more alcohol than he should. In fact, since his wife died last year, Pete stated that he began to drink daily. When the doctor examined Pete, he noted that his skin was jaundiced and that he had a rock-hard, enlarged liver. Also, Pete's ankles were swollen with fluid—a condition called pedal edema. Blood tests were drawn, revealing a bilirubin level of 6 milligrams per deciliter, a positive hepatitis C antibody, and an alpha-fetoprotein of 450 nanograms per milliliter. The doctor advised Pete to go to a radiologist to obtain a sonogram. The results of the sonogram revealed a mass in his liver. The doctor suspected that Pete had a malignant liver tumor due to cirrhosis caused by chronic hepatitis C and excessive alcohol use. A biopsy of the tumor confirmed the doctor's suspicion.

For many people, one of the worst fears is that one day a doctor will inform them that they have a tumor. However, having a liver tumor is not always a fatal condition. This chapter discusses both benign (not cancerous or fatal) and malignant (cancerous and potentially fatal) liver tumors. It addresses how they are detected, what kind of symptoms they may cause, who is at risk, and what the potential treatments are.

While there are many types of liver tumors, this chapter will detail the most common ones—*hemangiomas, hepatic adenomas, focal nodular hyperplasia, metastatic tumors,* and *hepatocellular carcinoma.* It also briefly addresses some conditions, such as *focal fatty infiltration,* that may be confused with liver tumors. With the exception of hepatocellular carcinoma, all liver tumors—whether they are benign or malignant—can occur in people regardless of whether there is an underlying liver disease. There are many promising new treatments for malignant tumors. While these treatment options will be discussed briefly, an extensive discussion of them is beyond the scope of this book. People should consult with an oncologist (cancer specialist) for further details regarding these new therapies.

LIVER MASSES

Liver masses are being detected by doctors with increasing frequency. The reason for this is simple. Advances in radiological techniques have given today's doctors access to a wide variety of imaging studies. Thus, radiological studies are regularly being performed in the course of evaluation of medical problems unrelated to the liver, such as nonspecific abdominal pain. A consequence of this frequent use of imaging studies is that liver masses are being discovered by chance. Once a mass on the liver has been detected, it then becomes necessary to conduct further testing in order to determine the exact nature of the mass. Fortunately, most of these masses will be benign (noncancerous).

The liver is a common site of tumors for a variety of reasons. As discussed in Chapter 1, the liver has a rich dual blood supply—from the portal vein and from the hepatic artery. These passageways provide a direct route for malignant (cancerous) tumor cells from other organs to navigate into the liver and deposit themselves there. This is known as liver *metastasis.* As you may recall, everything we eat, drink, and breathe—whether it be foods, medicines, or fumes—ultimately pass through the liver to be processed. Therefore, when a person ingests significant amounts of potentially toxic chemicals, such as alcohol or in some cases even oral contraceptives, the liver can potentially suffer adverse consequences. One possible outcome is the formation of a tumor. Furthermore, any diseases with the potential to lead to cirrhosis—including chronic viral hepatitis B or C and hereditary hemochromatosis—leave the liver at risk for the formation of a malignant tumor. Before discussing malignant tumors, the following section addresses a variety of benign liver tumors.

THE TYPES OF BENIGN LIVER TUMORS AND THEIR TREATMENTS

There are many types of benign liver tumors. This section will discuss three types: hemangioma, hepatic adenomas, and focal nodular hyperplasia (FNH). In general, they occur more frequently in women than in men. They are usually discovered by chance during the evaluation of nonrelated symptoms. Liver function tests (LFTs) are usually normal in people with benign liver tumors. In rare circumstances, these benign tumors can become so massive that a person may go to the doctor for abdominal discomfort caused by an enlarged liver. In these uncommon circumstances, results from blood tests occasionally reveal mildly elevated AP or GGTP levels (see Chapter 3).

There are no blood tests that specifically indicate that a tumor is in fact benign. Thus, sometimes, the doctor may be uncertain of the definite benign nature of the tumor. While malignant liver tumors may *metastasize* (spread to other organs), benign liver tumors are always confined to the liver. Diagnosing the specific nature of the tumors can generally be done by a variety of radiological techniques (imaging studies) combined with the patient's medical history. When the diagnosis remains uncertain, a liver biopsy is generally performed. Since many of these tumors have an abundance of blood vessels, liver biopsy in some cases carries an increased risk of bleeding. A smaller than normal needle can be used to decrease the occurrence of this potential complication.

Treatment of benign lesions is generally conservative. Surgery is considered primarily in cases where the tumor is causing significant abdominal pain, or if there is a high risk of rupture of the tumor. Furthermore, surgery should be done if the tumor is not confidently identified as being benign, or if it is felt that the tumor has a risk of progression to a malignancy.

What Is a Hemangioma?

Hemangiomas are the most common benign tumors of the liver. They have no malignant potential and may occur in a person with or without underlying liver disease. The name *hemangioma* derives from the fact that these tumors are filled with *heme* (blood). They resemble the small bright red spots that people commonly get on the skin of their chests and abdomens with aging. These spots, referred to as *senile hemangiomas,* are also benign. Hemangiomas occur in the liver in approximately 7 percent of the population, but some studies have reported ranges of from 1 to 20 percent. About 10 percent of people will have more than one hemangioma. Hemangiomas are more common in women, but can also be found in men, and can occur at any age.

The Symptoms and Signs of a Hemangioma

People are generally not aware that their livers harbor a hemangioma, as these tumors are usually asymptomatic (without symptoms). However, if a hemangioma grows to greater than 4 centimeters in size, a person may experience abdominal discomfort. This is attributable to the enlarged liver pushing against other surrounding organs, such as the intestines or the stomach. A person with a hemangioma may experience periodic pain if the hemangioma grows. This pain is caused by the formation of blood clots within the vessels of the expanding hemangioma. An extraordinarily rare, but very serious complication, that can occur is the rupture of a hemangioma. If this occurs, there will be excruciating abdominal pain and immediate surgery will be required.

Diagnosing a Hemangioma

Hemangiomas are usually detected by chance during a sonogram performed for the evaluation of an unrelated medical condition. However, a sonogram is not diagnostic, but only suggestive of this type of tumor. Therefore, additional radiological scans are necessary in order to confirm that the tumor in question is in fact a hemangioma. If the sonogram indicates that the mass is larger than 2.5 centimeters in size, a *tagged red blood cell (RBC) scan* is ordered. Using this scan, the person's blood is labeled with a radioactive metallic element (known as a tracer), such as technetium. Images of the liver are taken at varying time intervals. Since blood flow through the hemangioma is characteristically slow, if a hemangioma is present, the tracer will accumulate in it after a prolonged amount of time (about two hours), thereby confirming the diagnosis.

If the sonogram indicates that the mass is smaller than 2.5 centimeters in size, an MRI generally can diagnose the mass as being a hemangioma. A repeat imaging study should routinely be done after six months to a year to assess the hemangioma for any change of configuration or to determine if there has been any growth.

Liver biopsies are occasionally performed to diagnose a hemangioma, but are not recommended, as they carry an increased risk of bleeding when standard size needles are used and are often nondiagnostic when smaller needles are used.

Treating a Hemangioma

Treatment of hemangiomas is not necessary, unless they are very large and are causing significant abdominal discomfort. For these people, surgical removal (resection) of the hemangioma should be considered. The only other time that surgery is suggested is if there is uncertainty that the tumor in question is, in fact, a hemangioma. Other options, such as radiation therapy and the use of steroids have not been very successful and are not recommended. There are no pills, either prescription or over-the-counter, that will cause a hemangioma to resolve.

Reducing the Chances That a Hemangioma Will Grow

Some researchers believe that excess estrogen can cause hemangiomas to grow. In fact, growth of hemangiomas has been observed in some women during pregnancy, and in others while taking birth control pills. Furthermore, the risk of rupture may be greater in these people. Although the effect of estrogen on hemangiomas is not conclusive, it is advisable for people with hemangiomas to stay off birth control pills and all other forms of estrogen replacement.

What Is a Hepatic Adenoma?

A hepatic adenoma is a rare tumor found on the liver. It is made of hepatocytes (liver cells) that have abnormally multiplied numerous times, forming a benign mass. In contrast to hemangiomas, hepatic adenomas occur infrequently. These tumors were very uncommon in the United States prior to the widespread use of oral contraceptives, which began in the 1960s and 1970s. A typical person discovered to have this tumor is a woman in her thirties who had used birth control pills at some time in her life—usually for longer than five years. However, some tumors are discovered in women who took birth control pills for as little as six months, and some tumors are found in women up to ten years after they have discontinued using birth control pills. It is thought that the estrogen in birth control pills may be the cause of hepatic adenomas. However, since most of these pills contain a lower amount of estrogen than they did in the past, hepatic adenomas are becoming more uncommon. In occasional cases, this type of tumor has been found in women who have never used birth control pills, and in men—especially in those men who have used anabolic steroids.

The Symptoms and Signs of a Hepatic Adenoma

In contrast to the asymptomatic nature of hemangiomas, about 50 percent of people with adenomas have abdominal pain or feel an abdominal mass in the right upper quadrant, and the other 50 percent have no symptoms. Approximately 20 percent of people with a hepatic adenoma have no symptoms until the adenoma ruptures, which is marked by the sudden onset of excruciating abdominal pain. This is a serious situation that can result in massive hemorrhage and must be treated with emergency surgery.

Diagnosing a Hepatic Adenoma

About 10 to 20 percent of people will be discovered to have a hepatic adenoma by chance when imaging studies of the abdomen are obtained for an unrelated problem or complaint. In other cases, an abdominal mass may be found during a routine physical exam. Still others are detected at the time of abdominal surgery for an unrelated reason. Sonograms, CT scans, and MRIs can all be utilized to detect a hepatic adenoma. However, these imaging studies are merely suggestive of the diagnosis. Therefore, a liver biopsy is necessary to confirm the presence of a hepatic adenoma.

Treating a Hepatic Adenoma

Treatment entails the discontinuation of any estrogen-containing medications, such as birth control pills. While this tumor is typically benign, there is a small, yet significant, potential for it to progress into liver cancer. Therefore, if this tumor does not regress after birth control pills are discontinued, surgical removal of the tumor is recommended. Surgery is also advisable because of the tumor's risk of rupturing. In people opting not to undergo surgery, close follow-up scanning is crucial in order to monitor and detect tumor growth.

Special Precautions to Take for Those With a Hepatic Adenoma

As hormonal imbalances during pregnancy may trigger the hepatic adenoma to grow and rupture, pregnancy is not recommended. However, once the adenoma has been surgically removed, pregnancy should be safe. People with hepatic adenomas should avoid taking birth control pills, any form of estrogen supplementation, and anabolic steroids.

Hepatic Adenomas and Glycogen Storage Type-IA Disease

More than one adenoma may occur in people who have a rare liver disease of abnormal sugar metabolism, which is known as *glycogen storage type-IA disease*. These people have a high incidence of the adenoma rupturing and of the adenoma progressing to malignancy. Thus, people with glycogen storage type-IA disease who have multiple hepatic adenomas are often referred for liver transplantation as opposed to having the hepatic adenomas removed surgically.

What Is Focal Nodular Hyperplasia (FNH)?

Focal nodular hyperplasia (FNH) is a benign liver tumor made of liver cells that have multiplied numerous times around a malformed or abnormally formed hepatic artery. It is more common among women than among men. While estrogens probably do not actually cause the development of FNH, the hormonal effects of birth control pills and pregnancy may cause an existing tumor to grow.

The Symptoms and Signs of Focal Nodular Hyperplasia

Most people have no symptoms, but in cases where the tumor is very large, some people experience abdominal pain or notice a mass that can be felt through their skin. Unlike hemangiomas and hepatic adenomas, rupture and hemorrhage are unlikely, and progression to liver cancer has never been reported.

Diagnosing Focal Nodular Hyperplasia

As with the other benign tumors, most people are found to have FNH by imaging studies during the evaluation of unrelated complaints. These tumors have a characteristic appearance that an experienced radiologist can detect on a sonogram, CT scan, or MRI. Liver biopsy is infrequently necessary, as results are usually not diagnostic. A hepatic *arteriogram*—an x-ray of an artery after the injection of dye—is often needed to make a definitive diagnosis. If the diagnosis still remains in question, surgical removal of the lesion is undertaken to make a definitive diagnosis.

Treating Focal Nodular Hyperplasia

Since this tumor has little risk of complications, surgery is not indicated unless the person is having symptoms, such as abdominal pain, or if repeat imaging studies document an increase in size. Since hormonal imbalances can cause the tumor to grow, birth control pills should be discontinued, and future pregnancies should be avoided. Occasionally, the doctor cannot definitively determine that the tumor is benign. Thus, when the diagnosis is in doubt, surgical removal of the tumor is indicated. When surgical removal is undertaken, it usually corrects the condition.

OTHER LIVER ABNORMALITIES THAT MAY BE CONFUSED WITH A LIVER TUMOR

There are two other liver abnormalities that may be detected incidentally in the course of an evaluation for unrelated symptoms. These are *focal fatty infiltration* and *pseudotumor.*

Focal fatty infiltration of the liver is a totally benign condition. It consists of fat deposits in the liver concentrated in one area. This gives the appearance of a mass. It can be due to a variety of causes, such as obesity, diabetes, or alcoholic liver disease. It usually resolves when the underlying disease is corrected, such as with weight reduction in overweight people.

A *pseudotumor* is a fake tumor. It is medically known as *macroregenerative nodules* or *adenomatous hyperplasia.* It consists of cirrhotic nodules that give the appearance of a mass. These pseudotumors, which are found in about 25 percent of people with cirrhosis, rarely become cancerous.

WHAT IS A METASTATIC LIVER TUMOR?

A *metastatic liver tumor* is a cancer that originally started in an organ other than the liver (known as the *primary organ*), which then spread to the liver. In the United States, metastatic tumors are the most common malignancies that occur in the liver. Thus, when some doctors inform their patients that they have liver cancer, most of the time the doctors are actually referring to metastatic tumors, as opposed to primary liver cancer. Cancers originating in the colon, stomach, esophagus, pancreas, gallbladder, breast, kidney, uterus, and lungs commonly metastasize (spread) to the liver. In fact, approximately one-third of all cancers have the potential to spread to the liver.

The following is a discussion of the symptoms and signs associated with metastatic liver tumors, how a person may be diagnosed with having this condition, what the prognosis is for these people, and what some of their treatment options are.

The Symptoms and Signs of Metastatic Liver Tumors

Symptoms of metastatic liver tumors are usually related to the nature of the primary tumor. For example, if the primary tumor is colon cancer, then the symptoms may consist of altered bowel habits and rectal bleeding. Generalized weakness and weight loss are symptoms that apply to nearly all metastatic diseases affecting the liver. Occasionally, a person will go to the doctor with complaints of abdominal pain and distention. These symptoms are due to the enlargement of the liver caused by tumor cells. Jaundice (a yellowing of the skin and eyes) may occur, which suggests that the tumor has invaded the bile ducts. During a physical exam, the doctor may detect an enlarged rock-hard liver and/or ascites (an abnormal accumulation of fluid).

Diagnosing Metastatic Liver Tumors

Metastatic liver tumors are diagnosed by a combination of blood tests, imaging studies, and sometimes liver biopsy. The following is a discussion of these tests.

Blood Tests

There are no diagnostic blood tests for metastatic liver tumors. However, there are some blood tests that are indicative of, but not diagnostic of, cancer. These are known as tumor markers. One such example is the tumor marker *carcinoembryonic antigen* (CEA). When levels of CEA are very high, it is suggestive of metastatic liver cancer. Other blood test abnormalities suggestive of metastatic liver tumors include an elevated lactate dehydrogenase (LDH), AP, and GGTP. Occasionally, transaminases and bilirubin may be elevated. Some of these tests were discussed in Chapter 3.

Imaging Studies and Liver Biopsy

Diagnosis usually occurs when an imaging study, such as CT scan, sonogram, or MRI, reveals multiple tumors in the liver in a person with a known primary tumor, such as colon cancer. These liver tumors are usually detected during the evaluation of the primary tumor.

Problems in diagnosis arise when there is no identified site of the primary tumor. In this case, it may be advantageous to obtain a biopsy of the liver tumor. This is best done by using a sonogram or CT scan for guidance directly into the tumor (see Chapter 5). Unfortunately, this does not always provide conclusive evidence as to where the primary tumor is located.

The Long-Term Prognosis for Those With Metastatic Liver Tumors

The long-term outlook for a person with metastatic liver cancer depends upon the site of the primary cancer and the extent of metastatic disease (how far and to how many other organs the cancer has spread). In general, outlook is poor, with the average person living about one year from the time of diagnosis. However, there is hope that new experimental treatments will ultimately increase the survival time for many metastatic cancer patients.

Treating Metastatic Liver Tumors

As with prognosis, treatment options vary, depending on the primary cancer and the extent of metastatic disease. Some tumors, such as lymphomas (a malignant tumor of lymph tissue), show a good response to chemotherapy. Some metastases may be successfully removed through surgery. Successful surgery is most frequently seen in people with colon cancer that has spread to the liver. Unfortunately, most people with metastatic liver cancer are not candidates for surgery. Therefore, treatment has been focused on alternatives to surgery. These treatment alternatives—of which a full discussion is beyond the scope of this book—include techniques such as arterial infusion chemotherapy, percutaneous ethanol injection, transcatheter chemoembolization, cryosurgery, percutaneous laser ablation, radiofrequency electrocautery, high-intensity focused ultrasound, and liver transplantation. People should seek information specific to their cancers directly from their oncologists. These cancer specialists are most qualified to explore the various treatment options that are available.

WHAT IS HEPATOCELLULAR CARCINOMA?

A *primary malignant liver tumor* is a cancer that originates in the liver. The most common primary liver cancer in the world is known as hepatocellular carcinoma, also known as HCC or hepatoma. In fact, HCC is one of the most common cancers in the world, with its greatest frequency occurring in Southeast Asia and Africa. Although its rate of occurrence has been rising over the past twenty years in the United States, it is still uncommon, accounting for only 0.5 to 2 percent of all cancers. The cause of this rise has been linked to the prevalence of chronic viral hepatitis, especially chronic hepatitis C, in the United States. The characteristics of this cancer vary with geographic location. For example, in areas of the world where HCC is prevalent, such as in Asia and Africa, people are generally afflicted at an early age and often have a sudden onset of illness. In the United States, where this type of tumor is not as common, age of onset is generally at a later age and the tumor usually progresses slowly and silently. In general, men appear to be affected more frequently than women. In fact, in parts of the world where HCC is common, men are affected as much as eight times as frequently as women.

The following is a discussion of what causes HCC, what the associated symptoms and signs are, how a person is diagnosed, what the long-term prognosis is, and what some of the treatment options are for both operable and inoperable tumors.

The Causes of HCC

There is no simple explanation for why some people develop HCC and others do not. Most likely, there are multiple factors involved. The most significant known factor is the presence of cirrhosis due to any cause. Other factors may include genetic potential, hormonal influences, advancing age, state of general health and nutrition, lifestyle habits (especially alcohol abuse), and exposure to viruses and chemicals. While some of these factors are merely speculated to attribute to the development of HCC, other associations are definitively known. These specific factors are discussed below.

Cirrhosis

It is well established that there is a correlation between the presence of cirrhosis and the development of HCC. In fact, cirrhosis is present in approximately 60 to 90 percent of people with HCC. Furthermore, autopsy studies show that up to 28 percent of people with cirrhosis at the time of death also had HCC that went unrecognized during their lifetimes. In parts of the world where HCC is not very common, such as in the United States, cirrhosis is present in the vast majority of people with HCC. In contrast, in areas such as Mozambique, Africa, where 20 out of 100,000 people each year are afflicted with HCC, the association with cirrhosis, while common, is not as extensive—probably due to the increased incidence of chronic hepatitis B in which HCC may occur without cirrhosis. Regardless of the geographic location, it does appear that repeated liver damage, independent of the cause of damage, can predispose the liver to abnormal cell growth resulting in HCC.

The risk of developing HCC in people with cirrhosis is between 1 and 6 percent per year. The risk of developing HCC differs somewhat depending upon the cause of cirrhosis. For example, people with chronic hepatitis B have a high risk of developing HCC in their lifetimes—up to 200 times the risk that the general population has. In contrast, the risk of HCC in a person with primary biliary cirrhosis, although present, is very low. For more information on cirrhosis, see Chapter 6.

Chronic Viral Hepatitis

There is a strong correlation between chronic hepatitis B and the development of HCC. In fact, in countries with a high incidence of HCC, between 60 and 90 percent of people are found to have chronic hepatitis B. As previously noted, chronic hepatitis B infection can increase a person's risk of developing HCC up to 200 times! Furthermore, HCC can occur in people with chronic hepatitis B even in the absence of cirrhosis. This may be partly due to an unidentified gene that may make a person prone to developing HCC.

People doubly infected with both the hepatitis B virus (HBV) and the hepatitis delta virus (HDV) appear to have a lower incidence of HCC. The reason for this is not entirely clear but is possibly related to the fact that the hepatitis delta virus may actually suppress the replication of the hepatitis B virus. However, people doubly infected with both the hepatitis B virus (HBV) and the hepatitis C virus (HCV) do carry an increased risk of HCC. People with chronic hepatitis B who drink excessive amounts of alcohol have been found to develop HCC, on average, more than ten years earlier than those people who do not drink alcohol excessively. Therefore, people with chronic hepatitis B should avoid all alcohol as it can hasten progression to HCC.

It takes approximately twenty to thirty years for HCC to form in a person with chronic hepatitis B. Thus, people infected with the hepatitis B virus (HBV) at birth can develop HCC as early as twenty years of age, whereas people infected with HBV in adulthood tend to develop HCC in their sixties or seventies. The annual risk of developing HCC for people with chronic hepatitis B has been estimated to be about between 0.5 and 3 percent.

A strong correlation exists between chronic hepatitis C and the development of HCC. In contrast to hepatitis B, cirrhosis is present in all cases of hepatitis C-associated HCC. People with hepatitis C who drink alcohol excessively appear to have a greater risk of developing HCC. This underscores the importance of total abstinence of alcohol in people with chronic hepatitis C. As stated above, it appears that coinfection with both HBV and HCV greatly increases a person's chance of developing HCC. Therefore, obtaining the hepatitis B vaccination is crucial for people with hepatitis C who are not already infected with hepatitis B. (See Chapter 24 for more information on vaccinations.) It usually takes more than thirty years from the time a person becomes infected with HCV for HCC to develop. It has been demonstrated that treatment with the drug interferon prior to the development of HCC actually lowers the incidence of HCC in some people with chronic hepatitis C. This underscores the importance of early recognition and treatment of chronic hepatitis C in the early stages of disease.

See Part Two for a complete discussion of viral hepatitis, which includes chapters on each of the above-mentioned hepatitis viruses.

Chronic Liver Disease

Hemochromatosis is a genetically acquired liver disease of iron overload. As you learned in Chapter 18, iron is toxic to the liver. While, by itself, hemochromatosis does not cause HCC, once it has progressed to cirrhosis, there is up to a 200-fold increase in the risk of developing HCC as compared with the general population. Phlebotomy helps prevent progression of disease. And, if started prior to the onset of cirrhosis, phlebotomy can help prevent the development of HCC in people with hemochromatosis. However, once cirrhosis has developed, the risk of developing HCC exists. This is true even if a person with cirrhosis has undergone successful phlebotomy. Once again, this demonstrates the importance of early recognition and treatment of liver disease.

Autoimmune hepatitis and primary biliary cirrhosis are two other chronic liver diseases—discussed in Chapters 14 and 15 respectively—that can lead to cirrhosis and thus to HCC. However, the incidence of HCC in these diseases is very infrequent when compared with the incidence of HCC found in other chronic liver diseases, such as chronic hepatitis B, chronic hepatitis C, and hemochromatosis.

Lifestyle Factors—Alcohol Consumption and Cigarette Smoking

It is a well-known fact that alcohol can be toxic to the liver. In fact, most people associate the word cirrhosis with alcohol. Alcohol liver disease (ALD) is perhaps the most common cause of cirrhosis in the United States, and most cases of HCC in the United States are found in people with alcoholic cirrhosis. However, most research has shown that alcohol itself is not actually a direct cause of HCC. Rather, it is when alcohol causes liver damage and cirrhosis that HCC can develop. In people with either chronic hepatitis B or chronic hepatitis C, alcohol accelerates the course of the disease, leading to cirrhosis and HCC at an earlier age compared with people who do not drink alcohol. Thus, alcohol, in effect, acts as a *cocarcinogen*—a substance that, when combined with another carcinogenic factor, hastens the progression to cancer.

It is estimated that approximately 15 percent of people with alcoholic cirrhosis will develop HCC in their lifetimes. This is true even if these people stopped drinking after they developed alcoholic cirrhosis. People with alcoholic cirrhosis who stop drinking live an average of ten years longer than people with alcoholic cirrhosis who continue to drink; therefore, it is most likely that this increased survival time provides these people with an extra ten years in which to develop HCC. The close connection between alcoholic cirrhosis and HCC was underscored by an autopsy study performed on people who had alcoholic cirrhosis. Researchers discovered HCC in 55 percent of livers examined. A final note on this subject: People with any liver disease would be wise to abstain from alcohol due to the potentially toxic impact of alcohol on the liver.

The role of cigarettes in the development of HCC is not clear. However, some studies suggest that cigarette smoking may be a risk factor leading to HCC in some people with liver disease—especially those without evidence of chronic hepatitis B. Since cigarette smoking has been proven to be detrimental to health in so many ways, anyone who has liver disease is advised to not smoke cigarettes.

Aflatoxin

Aspergillus flavus is a fungus (mold) that produces a toxic byproduct known as *aflatoxin*. Aflatoxin has been shown to be *hepatotoxic* (harmful or damaging to the liver) and to have the potential of leading to HCC. Foods stored in hot, humid conditions for prolonged periods of time are prone to mold and thus aflatoxin contamination. In certain parts of Africa, the incidence of HCC can be directly correlated with the amount of aflatoxin-contaminated food consumed. In parts of Africa and Asia, this fungus commonly poisons foods such as peanuts, soybeans, corn, and rice. Researchers have speculated that aflatoxin leads to liver cancer by causing a genetic mutation (mutation of the p53 gene). It is believed that aflatoxins may increase the toxic effects that hepatitis viruses have on liver cancer production; that is, it may act as a cocarcinogen. Aflatoxin contamination of foods is rare in the United States; therefore, aflatoxin is not considered to be a significant cause of liver cancer in the United States.

Drugs—Anabolic Steroids and Oral Contraceptives

Some people use anabolic steroids (muscle-building hormones) for medical reasons. Others use them to increase their competitive edge in sports. Men and women who take anabolic steroids for prolonged periods of time are at increased risk for the development of HCC. Therefore, unless there is a medical reason to use anabolic steroids, their use should be avoided.

Women who take oral contraceptives for a period of greater than eight years have a slightly increased risk of the development of HCC. As noted on page 258, hepatic adenoma, which is associated with oral contraceptive use, has a small risk of developing into HCC.

The Symptoms and Signs of HCC

As previously noted, geography has a great deal of relevance in regard to HCC. This relevance is not only in the rate of occurrence of HCC, but also in the array of symptoms associated with HCC. In areas with a low rate of occurrence of HCC, such as the United States, people with chronic liver disease or cirrhosis are generally aware of their conditions and are under a doctor's care. In these people, HCC usually progresses slowly and silently, and symptoms experienced, if any, are those that pertain to cirrhosis. People are usually detected to have HCC when the tumor is quite tiny. These people usually have no symptoms whatsoever at the time. This is due to the fact that in the United States—as in many other developed countries—people with cirrhosis are commonly screened and monitored on a regular basis.

Others are first detected to have HCC due to an abrupt deterioration of an otherwise stable chronic liver disease course. Symptoms of HCC in these people can include abdominal pain, weight loss, fatigue, or manifestations of decompensated cirrhosis, such as encephalopathy (mental confusion). The liver is usually enlarged, rock hard, and nodular. Jaundice is present in some people, but is usually mild. Signs suggestive of cirrhosis may be present, or there may be obvious signs of decompensated cirrhosis, such as ascites (accumulation of fluid in the abdomen).

In contrast, in less developed areas of the world, such as sub-Saharan Africa, which has a high incidence of HCC, HCC is usually an aggressive disease with a rapid downhill course. These people are usually younger than those in geographic areas of low incidence and are often not aware that they have a chronic liver disease. These people often complain of sudden abdominal distention and tenderness, and a physical exam commonly reveals a mass in the right upper abdominal region. The doctor may hear a *bruit* over the liver during an exam. A bruit is a harsh, abnormal noise that can be heard through a stethoscope when it is placed over the liver. This is suggestive of a vascular tumor (a tumor that is chock full of blood vessels, such as HCC). Often, the initial complaint in these people with a high incidence of HCC is excruciating abdominal pain. Typically, the cause of this pain is that the tumor has ruptured. This is a medical emergency requiring immediate surgery. Low-grade intermittent fevers may also be present.

Some people will have symptoms of HCC that are exhibited in other organs of the body. This is due to secretion of substances, such as hormones, by the tumor to other parts of the body through the bloodstream. This manifestation of HCC-related symptoms in other parts of the body is known as *paraneoplastic syndromes.* Paraneoplastic manifestations may occur as one of the first symptoms of HCC in about 5 percent of people, although this percentage is higher for people in areas of high incidence of HCC. There are many types of paraneoplastic manifestations of HCC, but the two most common are a low glucose level known as *hypoglycemia,* and a high cholesterol level known as *hypercholesterolemia.* Other, less common, manifestations include a high calcium level known as *hypercalcemia,* an elevated red blood cell count known as *polycythemia,* and signs of feminization in men, such as *gynecomastia* (breast enlargement).

Diagnosing HCC

A person may be diagnosed with HCC through a combination of blood work, imaging studies, and liver biopsy. The following is a discussion of each of these diagnostic methods.

Blood Tests

In its earliest, most treatable stages, HCC can be very difficult to detect. Laboratory blood tests, such as those discussed in Chapter 3, may reveal few clues beyond an elevated AP or GGTP. Other blood test abnormalities, such as elevated liver enzymes or a decreased platelet count, are not due to HCC, but are due to the underlying liver disease, such as hepatitis or cirrhosis, respectively. Most of these tests are nonspecific and will give only vague hints that something more serious is wrong. Immediate suspicion for HCC should be raised when a person with a relatively stable course of liver disease abruptly develops a significant rise of liver function tests (LFTs). As emphasized throughout this book, the liver is a master of camouflage. Thus, a large tumor can be present in the liver despite minimal blood test abnormalities and a lack of symptoms. In fact, it is possible for more than half of one's liver to be replaced by a tumor without causing significant blood test abnormalities or symptoms.

The only diagnostic test to detect HCC is a blood test known as *alpha-fetoprotein* (AFP). This test is one of the tumor markers (a blood test indicative of, but not diagnostic of, cancer). Normal adult level is less than 20 nanograms per milliliter (ng/ml). If the level in a person's blood is over 400 ng/ml, then it is pretty safe to say that liver cancer is present. Levels under 400 ng/ml are a little more confusing. This is due to the fact that AFP levels can also be elevated as a result of many other conditions (see bulleted list below), especially any conditions in which there may be liver damage, such as cirrhosis or acute hepatitis—although levels rarely exceed 100 ng/ml.

Other causes of an elevated AFP, other than HCC, include:

- Hepatitis—both acute and chronic

- Cirrhosis

- Liver metastases

- Pregnancy

- Cystic fibrosis

- Gastric cancer

- Pancreatic cancer

A rapidly rising AFP level, say from 60 ng/ml to 230 ng/ml within a few months—even if levels do not reach 400 ng/ml—is also suggestive of HCC. This abrupt increase signals the need to commence an intensive search for the tumor. It has been shown that initial AFP levels above 100 ng/ml in a person with chronic liver disease may foreshadow the development of HCC within the next five years. These people should be closely observed for tumor development. The degree of elevation of AFP is usually related to the size of the tumor—the larger the tumor, the higher the value. Thus, with very small lesions, AFP is often barely elevated.

After successful treatment of HCC, the level of AFP should normalize. It should rise again if there is a recurrence of the tumor. It can be seen that the AFP blood test is useful as a marker for the recurrence, as well as the initial detection of HCC. However, a person should not be lulled into a sense of total security if his AFP level is normal. Only about 67 percent of HCCs secrete AFP. This means that an HCC is actually present in about 33 percent of people whose AFP is normal. Therefore, while this marker is very useful, it does have limitations.

Des-gamma-carboxyprothrombin (DCP), an abnormal form of prothrombin (a protein produced by the liver involved in blood clotting), is found to be elevated in 60 to 90 percent of people with HCC. In some people with HCC whose AFP level is normal, DCP is often positive. The accuracy of this blood test is still being evaluated through research. Once statistical significance of DCP has been confirmed, the combination of both the AFP and the DCP blood tests will most likely lead to greatly improved percentages of HCC detection.

Imaging Studies

One or more imaging studies (discussed in Chapter 3) are usually performed on people suspected of having HCC. The first is usually a sonogram. Tumors less than 2 centimeters in size (and possibly less than 1 centimeter in size) can be detected by this imaging study. Also, sonograms are the study most commonly recommended for screening for HCC.

CT scan is often the next study obtained. A contrast dye is used to enhance the tumor, thus giving improved accuracy of diagnosis. A substance known as *lipiodal,* an iodinized poppy-seed oil contrast dye, is injected into the hepatic artery. This substance is promptly cleared from the rest of the liver, but remains in the HCC because it identifies abnormal tumor cells. This can be detected by a repeated CT scan at about two weeks time. This substance creates an obvious contrast between normal tissue and the tumor. Tumors as small as 0.2 to 0.3 centimeters can be identified using lipiodal-enhanced CT scans.

MRI is also being used with increasing frequency to detect liver masses but has an accuracy similar to that of an enhanced CT scan. Enhancing substance, such as gadolinium, improves diagnostic accuracy for some tumors as it enables there to be an obvious contrast between normal tissue and a tumor.

Hepatic angiography is also used to aid in the detection of an HCC. It is the most invasive and expensive of all the imaging techniques, and it is used primarily to determine operability. In this technique, a catheter is placed into the hepatic artery and contrast-enhancing dye is introduced into the vessels that feed the tumor. Since the tumor is *vascular* (contains an abundance of vessels) as compared with the surrounding liver tissue, the vessels present in the tumor will be directly seen, thereby enabling the doctor to successfully locate the tumor.

Liver Biopsy

Once a tumor has been detected, if the diagnosis is still in question, a liver biopsy is sometimes performed. The biopsy is usually performed by sonogram or CT scan guidance. Due to the fact that liver tumors are very vascular, the risk of bleeding increases. Also, there is a small risk of spreading the tumor along the track of the needle. Therefore, the use of a smaller size needle is generally recommended. However, since the tissue sample extracted using a small needle is often poor, diagnostic uncertainties typically result. Thus, for people with liver tumors, the role of liver biopsy is somewhat controversial. For a complete discussion of liver biopsies, see Chapter 5.

Screening and Surveillance for HCC

Screening and surveillance is done in order to detect HCC at an early enough stage so that surgery can either successfully remove the tumor in its entirety and thereby cure the condition or significantly improve the person's chances for long-term survival. The importance of screening people who are at risk for liver cancer cannot be overemphasized. The chances of successful treatment are far greater when a tumor is detected in its earliest stages than in an advanced stage, where it may have already spread to other areas of the body. Anyone with cirrhosis from any cause and people with chronic hepatitis B with or without cirrhosis are at risk of developing HCC. These people should be screened regularly for HCC. In this way, if a tumor forms, it is more likely to be detected in its earliest stages when it is most amenable to treatment.

While the exact method and interval of screening is subject to differing opinions, as a general rule, screening is advisable approximately every three to twelve months. Screening is simple, quick, relatively inexpensive, and painless. It generally consists of a sonogram at least once a year and the AFP blood test at least once every six months. With diligent surveillance, approximately 25 to 65 percent of tumors are detected when they are only 2 centimeters or smaller. Unfortunately, as previously noted, up to 37 percent of people with HCC will have normal levels of AFP. This underscores the importance of using both screening methods in anyone who is at risk of HCC.

The Long-Term Prognosis for Those With HCC

When small tumors (less than 5 centimeters) are detected by screening and surveillance techniques, there is a chance that they can be successfully removed in its entirety through surgery. Once the HCC has grown to greater than 5 centimeters, it is probably not curable as it will most likely have already spread to other areas of the body (metastasized)—most commonly nearby lymph nodes. Unless some form of therapy discussed on the following pages is initiated, only 1 percent of these people will survive two years from the time HCC is detected.

The Potential Treatment Options for HCC

While prolonged survival of people with HCC is possible for some, in general, long-term prognosis is somewhat poor. The most common treatment options for HCC include surgical resection, liver transplantation, and alcohol injection directly into the tumor. Other options include tumor embolization, chemotherapy, hormonal manipulation, radiotherapy, and immunotherapy. Sometimes, a combination of these therapies will maximize results. All of these options will be discussed in more detail below.

Options differ greatly for those tumors that are surgically correctable (that is, single tumors and those less than 5 centimeters in size) as compared with tumors that are not amenable to surgery (that is, tumors at multiple sites in the liver and those that are greater than 5 centimeters in size or that have metastasized to other organs). The size of the tumor, the number of tumors present in the liver, and the status of the underlying liver disease are the important variables looked at when deciding which therapy would provide the best long-term results in each particular case.

Surgical Resection

Surgical resection (the removal of the tumor through surgery) is usually the first option considered for people with HCC. In the absence of cirrhosis, up to 80 percent of a person's liver can be removed, and the remainder will "regenerate" to its former full size, as discussed in Chapter 1. Surgical resection, performed on people who meet specific criteria, can potentially cure a person of HCC. The best candidate for surgical resection is a person with a solitary tumor less than 5 centimeters in size in a liver without cirrhosis. The tumor should also be isolated just to the liver and not have spread to other sites. Other factors that increase the likelihood of positive results include people with compensated cirrhosis, people who are in otherwise good health, and people younger than fifty years old. Approximately half of people who are good surgical candidates will still be alive at least five years after surgery. The major disadvantage of surgical resection is that there remains a high risk of tumor recurrence because new tumors may develop.

Liver Transplantation

Only approximately 30 percent of people with liver cancer have surgically resectable tumors at the time they are diagnosed. The remaining people must consider liver transplantation. Liver transplantation has the potential for removing from the body not only the tumor, but also any underlying cirrhosis. The topic of liver transplantation is discussed in further detail in Chapter 21.

Therapy for Inoperable Tumors

Unfortunately, due to the clandestine nature of liver disease, by the time some tumors are recognized, they are already in advanced stages and are not amenable to any form of surgery. Other people are not candidates for surgery due to advanced age or poor general health. For these people, options include percutaneous alcohol injection, chemotherapy, radiation therapy, hormonal therapy, and gene therapy. The following is a discussion of these other options.

Percutaneous Alcohol Injection (PEI). Using this therapy, a small needle is inserted *percutaneously* (through the skin) into the liver, much in the same manner as a liver biopsy is performed. The exact location of the tumor is pinpointed using a sonogram. Alcohol is then injected directly into the tumor through the needle. The alcohol acts to kill the cancer cells. The most common complaints concerning this procedure include mild pain and low fever, but otherwise it is well-tolerated. People who do best with this treatment are those who have a tumor smaller than 5 centimeters, who have less than three tumors in the liver, and who do not have advanced cirrhosis. In fact, up to 90 percent of small, solitary tumors less than 3 centimeters in size have been reported to have been successfully killed using this method, and up to 70 percent of these people are alive up to four years later. People with larger tumors or advanced cirrhosis do not have as high a success rate, and the incidence of recurrence of the tumor in these people is high, even when the original tumor was successfully killed using this method. For these people, other options are offered. These alternatives include combining PEI with chemoembolization (see below), the use of solutions other than alcohol (such as hot saline or acetic acid) for injection into the tumor, and even the placement of a microwave electrode directly into the tumor. The success rate, incidence of recurrence, and number of years of prolonged life applicable to each of these therapies is currently being reviewed by researchers. Although definitive numbers have not been established, some preliminary studies involving these treatments have shown positive results.

Tumor Embolization and Chemoembolization (Embolization Using Chemotherapeutic Agents). When a cholesterol plaque becomes lodged in an artery that leads to the heart, blood flow to the heart stops. This blockage of blood flow causes part of the heart muscle to die. This is commonly referred to as a heart attack or *myocardial ischemia.* Extrapolating this principle, if the hepatic artery (the artery that leads to the liver) is clogged, liver cancer cells may die. This deliberate clogging process is known as *embolization.* Substances that are used to block blood flow to liver cancer cells include gelatin-sponges (Gelfoam) and metallic coils. In many cases, anticancer drugs, such as doxorubicin or cisplatin, are introduced through the hepatic artery at the same time as the Gelfoam or other substances. This is known as *chemoembolization.* This provides an increased concentration of the chemotherapy directly into the tumor—with less of the side effects of general chemotherapy. While this treatment method does appear to reduce tumor growth, especially when lipiodal solution is added to the regimen, long-term survival is only slightly improved.

Other Options. Chemotherapy, using agents such as 5-fluorouracil, doxorubicin, or mitomycin, whether introduced as a single agent or in combination with each other, has not been found to significantly prolong survival.

Radiation therapy is used primarily to reduce pain associated with the tumor. Promising research is being conducted on *proton irradiation* and *intraarterial irradiation,* discussions of which are beyond the scope of this book.

Hormonal therapy using substances that inhibit both male and female hormones has been attempted. *Antiandrogens* (male-hormone inhibitors) have had poor results.

Antiestrogens (female-hormone inhibitors), such as tamoxifen, have shown promising results in some, but not all, studies. Research continues to be conducted in this interesting area.

Interferons are proteins made naturally in the body. They play an important role in regulating the immune system. It has been shown that they have both antiviral and anti-tumor properties. One group of researchers has demonstrated that the administration of interferon can prolong survival in people with inoperable HCC. Additional research will need to be done in this area before definite conclusions can be established. Interferon was discussed in more detail in Chapters 11, 12, and 13.

The freezing of liver tumor cells, also known as *cryosurgery*, is another technique being studied. One drawback to this therapy is that it requires open surgery. Another promising treatment involves the burning of liver tumor cells. This is known as *thermal ablation* and consists of transferring energy, in the form of radiofrequency waves, directly to tumor cells. One advantage to this technique is that no surgery is needed. Delivery of this thermal energy is via a needle inserted directly into the tumor under sonogram or CT-scan guidance. In this manner, liver tumor cells are killed by actually being "fried" to death. Both of these therapies take advantage of the fact that cancer cells are sensitive to temperature extremes.

Preliminary studies in Japan with *polyprenoic acid*, a form of vitamin A, appear promising.

Gene therapy, while still in experimental stages, is a promising new area of research aimed at combating cancers. HCC seems to be well-suited for this treatment method, as some scientists believe that HCC involves a mutant gene—the p53 gene mutation. It is hoped that if the defective p53 gene could be replaced with a healthy copy of the p53 gene, the cancer process might be halted or even reversed.

Angiogenesis inhibitors are undergoing intensive research in mice. *Angiogenesis* is a term that means the development of new blood vessels. Just like all the organs in the body, cancers need a blood supply in order to live and grow. Angiogenesis inhibitors aim to block the signals that cancer cells release in order to entice new blood vessels. If this signaling process is blocked, tumor cells would die, as their blood supplies would be cut off. This most interesting area of research awaits study trials on humans with HCC.

CONCLUSION

This chapter underscores how important it is for all people with liver disease to be under the care of a knowledgeable liver specialist. With regular screening and monitoring, if a malignancy has formed, it can be detected in its earliest, most treatable stage. With the rapidly advancing new treatment regimens and the enforcement of implementation of preventive measures, we should be experiencing a substantial decrease in the incidence of HCC in years to come. This chapter also discussed how HCC manifests so differently in people from other parts of the world. We have seen from this chapter that there are numerous benign masses of the liver. It is important to remember this fact, because if a mass is detected on the liver, there is no need to automatically assume a fatal outcome.

This concludes Part Three of the book. In the next part, treatment options and lifestyle changes will be discussed. Part Four will also provide an in-depth look at liver transplantation.

PART FOUR

Treatment Options and Lifestyle Changes

20

Treatment of Common Symptoms and Complications

S ince liver disease often occurs without symptoms, it has the potential to go undetected for many years. During this time, a person may unknowingly progress to cirrhosis. There are, however, a significant number of people with liver disease who do have symptoms. These symptoms, which include fatigue, itching, and abdominal pain, can be relatively mild, or they may be so severe that they are even debilitating. Sometimes, it is specifically these symptoms that first bring a person to the attention of her doctor. As you've learned in previous chapters, the severity of symptoms does not always correlate with the severity of the liver disease. In other people, serious complications of liver disease—including ascites (fluid in the abdomen) and encephalopathy (coma)—initially bring a person to medical attention. These serious complications always indicate a severe liver disorder. In any case, symptoms and complications of liver disease tend to be similar no matter which liver disease a person has.

Getting medical treatment is the most important step a person with liver disease can take to improve her health. However, treatment is only complete when the symptoms and complications of liver disease are treated as well as the liver disease itself. This chapter discusses the treatment of some of the most common symptoms and complications that pertain to liver disease. Helpful tips and suggestions on the prevention and management of fatigue, sleep disturbances, depression and other psychological disorders, itching, flu-like symptoms, and abdominal pain and distention are discussed. Treatment options for some of the complications associated with chronic liver disease—ascites, variceal bleeding (bleeding blood vessels), encephalopathy, and bone loss—are also addressed.

TREATMENT OF SYMPTOMS

Some of the common symptoms that may occur in people with liver disease were discussed in Chapter 2. Here you will read about the treatments of these symptoms.

Read on to learn out about some medical treatments and some additional helpful ways to treat fatigue, insomnia and other sleep disturbances, psychiatric disorders, itching, flu-like symptoms, headaches, and abdominal pain and distention.

Treatment of Fatigue

One of the most common, relentless, and debilitating symptoms among people with liver disease is fatigue. This symptom is universal to all liver diseases. Some people do not experience fatigue until several years after they have been diagnosed with liver disease. In others, fatigue is the primary reason that they seek medical attention. Fatigue does not necessarily correlate with the severity of the disease, so it may be just as debilitating to a person in the early stages of liver disease as it is in a person with advanced cirrhosis.

The successful treatment of fatigue can be a challenge. First, all of the potential causes of a person's fatigue should be looked into. Some are easily managed. Some commonly occur in people with liver disease. These potential causes of, and/or contributors to, fatigue include the following:

- Thyroid disease (may be primary cause of, or contribute to, fatigue).

- Anemia (may be primary cause of, or contribute to, fatigue).

- Disorders of other organs, including the heart (for example, congestive heart failure) or the brain (for example, brain tumors).

- Nutritional deficiencies (for example, a lack of iron or a lack of protein).

- Disturbances in fluid and electrolyte balance (for example, a low sodium level).

- Depression that is not attributable to liver disease.

- Some medications and drugs (a doctor should review all medication, prescription and over-the-counter, and omit those that cause fatigue, if possible).

- Excessive use of caffeine.

- Excessive use of alcohol.

- Emotional stress.

- Lack of exercise.

- Lack of sleep.

- Overwork.

If fatigue continues to persist after ruling out or correcting any medical conditions, there are a few lifestyle changes that may be helpful. For example, eating a healthy, low-fat, well-balanced diet, quitting smoking, refraining from alcohol consumption, and exercising daily are all lifestyle changes that can have a beneficial effect on fatigue. Drinking plenty of water and limiting caffeine-containing beverages to one or two cups per day are also recommended. It goes without saying, but bears repeating: People with liver disease should avoid drinking alcohol, another cause of fatigue. It's also a good idea to begin a program to eliminate excess weight by following a healthy weight-reducing diet. (Never lose more than one to two pounds per week.) See Chapter 23 for more information on exercise and nutrition.

The demands of a hectic job or harried home life may need to be reduced—overwhelming stress may cause fatigue even in a person who is not suffering from liver disease. Excessive and/or emotional stress are often the cause of fatigue in people with liver disease. Therefore, friends and family should attempt to reduce any excessive or unnecessary obligations or expectations that they may normally have had of the person.

If possible, a thirty- to forty-five-minute daytime nap should be taken daily. This can help rejuvenate a person with liver disease. In some cases, it may be necessary for a person with liver disease to incorporate naps into her daily schedule. Often, a doctor's letter to the patient's employer or supervisor may be in order. A person with fatigue should feel free to ask her doctor for such a note.

Remember, the treatment for fatigue cannot be found in pill! Be especially wary of any product that boasts "improved energy levels" on its label. Because the liver is in charge of breaking down all supplements and medications, more harm than good may result from taking such a product. Also, be aware that taking excessive amounts of vitamins and minerals in an attempt to treat fatigue—especially vitamin A, niacin, and iron—can lead to a worsening of liver disease. This will be discussed in more detail in Chapter 23. It is essential that a person with liver disease consult a liver specialist prior to taking any supplements or products that promise to cure fatigue.

Treatment of Insomnia and Other Sleep Disturbances

People with liver disease often suffer from sleep disturbances. In fact, approximately 35 to 50 percent of people with cirrhosis report having sleep-related difficulties. Some people have trouble falling asleep and others have difficulty staying asleep. Many people complain of being tired all day and awake all night. Others complain of erratic sleeping habits characterized by days of excessive sleep (a condition known as *hypersomnia*) alternating with days of lack of sleep (a condition known as *insomnia*). Still others state that they experience delays of their usual bedtimes and wake-up times. For most people suffering from these sleep disorders, the sleep they do get is not refreshing.

The cause of sleeping disorders in people with liver disease is unclear, but most likely it relates to alterations in the body's production of *melatonin*—a hormone that is produced by the pineal gland and involved in the sleep cycle. Sometimes, sleep disturbances stem from medications used for the treatment of liver disease. For example, interferon, ribavirin, prednisone, and propanolol all can be associated with insomnia. Pruritus (itching) can sometimes cause a sleeping disorder. People suffering with intense itching (discussed on page 281) may find themselves awake half the night scratching. Also, caffeine, nicotine, and alcohol consumption may contribute to disturbed sleep habits and, as such, abstinence from these substances will likely assist in the quest for a good night's sleep. Note that sleep disturbances may also be a sign of impending encephalopathy (see page 288).

Treatment of sleeping disorders associated with liver disease consists of both behavioral modification and medical management. People should use their beds only for sleeping and never for other activities, such as reading, watching television, or eating. These activities should be performed in other areas of the home. If a person is unable to fall asleep within twenty minutes of retiring, she should get out of bed and read a book or perform another relaxing activity in another room. Lights should be kept low and the television turned off. Only after becoming tired should she return to bed. Also, people should make an effort to wake up at the same time each day—regardless of the amount time spent sleeping during the night. Although long naps of two to three hours during the day are not recommended to people with sleep disturbances, a twenty- to thirty-minute nap in the early afternoon, if it can be arranged, may have a helpful effect. In no circumstances should alcohol be used as a sleeping aid. Also, as most prescription and over-the-counter sleeping pills are broken down by the liver, they should be avoided unless their use (in low doses and for short periods) is okayed by a liver specialist. People with liver damage are at increased risk of prolonged sedative effects if these medications are used at their generally prescribed dosages. Although used primarily for the treatment of depression, selective serotonin reuptake inhibitors (SSRIs)—such as Paxil (manufactured by SmithKline Beecham), Zoloft (manufactured by Pfizer) and Prozac (manufactured by Dista/Eli Lilly)—are generally safe for most people with liver disease and may help treat insomnia. Supplemental melatonin, in dosages of 1 to 2 milligrams per day taken a half hour before going to bed, may be helpful; however, melatonin supplements are not regulated by the FDA and may therefore contain varying amounts of the active ingredient per pill depending on the brand.

Treatment of Psychological/Psychiatric Disorders

Any chronic illness, especially chronic liver disease, may cause a person to become anxious and depressed. Furthermore, many of the medications used to treat liver disease may also cause psychological symptoms or worsen a psychiatric disorder that already exists. Interferon, for example, has been associated with depression, irritability, confusion, emotional instability, insomnia, and lack of concentration. And prednisone has been associated with mood swings, personality changes, depression, and irritability.

People who do not have severe psychiatric problems but are prone to depression, anxiety, and/or emotional instability may benefit by taking antidepressant or antianxiety medications prior to starting interferon or prednisone therapy. People who already suffer from severe depression (especially when associated with suicidal thoughts or suicide attempts) or other serious psychiatric disorders should avoid interferon therapy until their underlying psychiatric problems have either stabilized or abated. Most important, a person should never feel reluctant or ashamed to seek support from a psychological counselor or psychiatric doctor. Obtaining as much additional help as possible is generally a good idea.

All drugs are metabolized, at least to some extent, through the liver. While people with a chronic liver disease should avoid any nonessential medications, this may be outweighed, in some cases, by the greater benefit of treatment with antidepressant or antianxiety medications. As discussed above, the safest antidepressants are the SSRIs. For people being treated with either interferon or prednisone, if depression or any other psychiatric problem becomes severe, a reduction in the dose of these medications is advised, if possible. People who already have a psychiatric condition or who experience side effects while on interferon or prednisone should be managed jointly by a liver specialist and a psychiatrist. If an alternative approach is chosen, the herb St. John's wort (*Hypericum perforatum*) can be tried. (See Chapter 21 for more information on herbs.)

A doctor should investigate all the possible causes of a patient's psychiatric symptoms, as certain symptoms may be readily remedied. For example, thyroid disorders (symptoms of which may mimic psychiatric disorders) are often associated with certain liver diseases and their treatments. Thyroid disorders are usually correctable with medications, and once treated, the associated psychiatric symptoms typically abate. Certain types of anemia may cause psychiatric symptoms, which may also be readily correctable with proper treatment. Moreover, excessive alcohol use has been associated with hallucinations and abnormal thoughts and behavior. This may be remedied by cessation of alcohol use and by hospitalization. Also, the beginning stages of encephalopathy (the treatment of which is discussed on page 288), which is associated with cirrhosis, may be the cause of altered mental status or psychotic behavior. Finally, negative lifestyle factors (including excessive stress, lack of sleep, and poor dietary habits, such as excessive caffeine consumption) may lead to, or contribute to, psychological or psychiatric symptoms. Therefore, certain lifestyle changes may have a corrective effect on certain psychiatric symptoms.

Treatment of Itching (Pruritus)

Pruritus is a localized or generalized intense sensation of itching that necessitates the need to scratch. The cause of pruritus associated with liver disease is unknown. It is most often found in people with cholestatic liver diseases, such as primary biliary cirrhosis (PBC), or in cases in which cholestasis complicates any liver disease—such as can occur in people with advanced cirrhosis who have jaundice. Pruritus occurs in approximately 80 percent of people with PBC, and in approximately 20 to 50 percent of people with jaundice. It is usually at its worst at night and often is most severe on the palms and soles. The intensity of this symptom varies—from mild itching, which does not interfere with a person's life, to intractable (incapable of being relieved) itching, which may severely interfere with normal daily activities. Pruritus can become so severe that it can lead to sleep deprivation and suicidal thoughts. In fact, intractable pruritus is sometimes so bad that liver transplantation may be the only way to relieve it.

The treatment of pruritus can be difficult and is often unsatisfactory. Scratching does not commonly relieve pruritus. In fact, some people with pruritus, having found their fingernails to be insufficient, have attempted to scratch themselves using sharp objects, such as knives and hair brushes. This can lead to chronic skin irritation, scarring, and infections and should be avoided. Treatment of infected skin involves the use of antibiotics and meticulous cleaning of wounds. It is important for people suffering with pruritus to wear loose fitting clothes made of soft, smooth material and to keep their skin as moisturized as possible. During hot and humid weather, these people are advised to stay indoors in air-conditioned places.

The medication that has been most successful for treating pruritus is *cholestyramine* (Questran). Cholestyramine is known as a bile-acid binder (also known medically as an anion-exchange resin). It captures bile acids and eliminates them from the body via the stools. This generally results in relief from itching. It is recommended to take one packet of cholestyramine immediately before and one immediately after breakfast in order to take advantage of the emptying of the bile-filled gallbladder after an overnight fast. If further doses are needed, they should be taken with meals. As cholestyramine may inhibit the absorption of other medications, it is crucial that any other medications be taken at least two hours before or after taking cholestyramine. Colestipol (Colestid) is another bile-acid binder that is also used to treat itching.

Antihistamines, such as diphenhydramine hydrochloride (Benadryl), may help reduce itching, but usually need to be taken in conjunction with cholestyramine. As people with PBC complicated by Sjögren's syndrome already suffer from a dry mouth, antihistamines should be avoided in these people since they can worsen this symptom.

Phenobarbital is a *barbiturate* (a central nervous system depressant) that has—in rare instances—been successfully used to treat pruritus. People should be particularly careful to avoid consuming alcohol when taking phenobarbital, as alcohol (another central nervous system depressant) will enhance the sedative effects of phenobarbital. This has the potential to lead to coma.

Rifampin is an antibiotic that has been shown to alleviate itching in some people with cholestasis. Since rifampin can be toxic to the liver, its use must be very closely monitored.

Opiate antagonists are medications capable of blocking the effects of narcotics. *Naloxone, naltrexone,* and *nalmefene* are examples of opiate antagonists that have been used in the treatment of pruritus. Naloxone works only if given intravenously. It may provide benefit where the itching is so severe that it is considered a medical emergency and/or in people with intense itching who are awaiting liver transplantation. Its use in the management of chronic itching is not practical, due the necessity of intravenous administration. Nalmefene and naltrexone may be administered orally, and some studies have shown that they can significantly reduce pruritus.

Nalmefene is awaiting FDA approval in the United States, and naltrexone is potentially hepatotoxic (toxic to the liver). Therefore, neither of these drugs can be recommended at the present time.

Methotrexate, a type of chemotherapy, has been reported to decrease scratching activity, but more study is needed to confirm this. Techniques such as *plasmapheresis* (removal of plasma without the removal of other cells—that is, red blood cells—from the body), *charcoal hemoperfusion* (a form of blood cleansing), and ultraviolet light, have been experimentally used to treat pruritus, although none of these techniques have clearly demonstrated their effectiveness. Numerous other medications have been tried or are under study, including serotonin antagonists (ondansetron [Zofran]) administered intravenously, codeine (a narcotic pain reliever), S-adenosylmethionine (SAMe; an anticholestatic substance), and the enzyme-inducer flumecinol. However, until further studies have been performed, none of these options can be recommended for use in the treatment of pruritus.

Treatment of Flu-Like Symptoms

Many people with liver disease experience flu-like symptoms, including low-grade fever, muscle and joint aches, nausea, and headaches. (Headaches will be discussed separately in the following section.) Usually these symptoms are intermittent (occurring occasionally), although for some people they are chronic. Sometimes, flu-like symptoms are a result of the treatment a person is undergoing, such as interferon therapy for chronic hepatitis B or C.

Acetaminophen, taken in moderation (1 to 2 tablets per day), may help alleviate some flu-like symptoms, especially if one stays well-hydrated by drinking about twelve 8-ounce glasses of water per day. (As will be discussed in Chapter 24, aspirin and other NSAIDs are worse for the liver than acetaminophen and should be avoided.) Taking a warm bath may also help relieve some flu-like symptoms. Never take an alcohol sponge bath, as the fumes from the alcohol are not good for the liver. Amantadine (Symmetrel) is an antiviral drug used in the treatment of the influenza A virus (the flu). It has also been used with varying success in the treatment of hepatitis C. Some people have reported a decrease of flu-like symptoms while taking this medication. Thus, amantadine may be of some benefit both for treating liver disease and for relieving its associated side effects. However, further study needs to be conducted before it becomes more routinely prescribed to treat the side effects of liver disease.

Treatment of Headaches

Headaches are common among the general population, and those with liver disease are no exception. However, persistent severe headaches need to be evaluated with an MRI (a type of imaging study) and, perhaps, with other tests as well. Many headaches associated with liver disease stem from treatment medications, such as interferon, or from immunosuppressive agents, such as cyclosporine or tacrolimus, used after a liver transplantation. Medication-induced headaches may be eased by reducing the dose of the medication. High blood pressure is also a common cause of headaches. Therefore, people experiencing frequent headaches should have their blood pressure routinely monitored. Sumatriptan (Imitrex) is very helpful in the treatment of migraine-type headaches. However, the dosage of Imitrex may need to be lowered in people with cirrhosis. Some people obtain relief of headaches with beta-blockers (such as propanolol [Inderal]), which have the added benefit of reducing portal pressure in people with portal hypertension (discussed under Treatment of Bleeding Varices on page 287). Finally, lifestyle changes, stress-reduction techniques, elimination of excessive caffeine, plenty of rest, regular exercise, and avoidance of all alcohol can also help reduce the frequency and severity of headaches.

Treatment of Abdominal Pain and Distention

Abdominal pain and/or pain over the liver (right upper quadrant pain) in a person with liver disease may have many causes. Therefore, this type of pain should not automatically be attributed to a liver disorder—other causes should be investigated. In fact, abdominal and right upper quadrant pain is rarely due to chronic liver disease. Right upper quadrant pain, when due to the liver, occurs most commonly in the acute stages of liver disease or during a flare-up of a chronic liver disease. In these circumstances, the cause of this pain is due to acute inflammation, irritation, and distention of the liver. Otherwise, the liver is rarely tender in people with chronic liver disease. Yet, many people with chronic liver disease state that although they do not actually experience pain, they do feel a vague sense of "fullness" or an "awareness" of the liver. The cause for this is unclear.

Gallstones, as the name suggests, are stones that form in the gallbladder. Approximately 20 million Americans have gallstones. Gallstones often occur in people with liver disease—especially those with primary biliary cirrhosis (PBC)—or those with cirrhosis due to any liver disease. Other risk factors for gallstones include female gender, obesity, a family history of gallstones, multiple pregnancies, rapid weight loss, and biliary-tract narrowing (known as *biliary strictures*). The typical pain from gallstones is a right upper quadrant discomfort that usually lasts from a half hour to six hours before abating. Pain is usually severe and usually recurs. Diagnosis of gallstones is made typically by obtaining an abdominal sonogram. People with symptomatic gallstones require surgical removal of the entire gallbladder, not just the gallstones. This is known as a *cholecystectomy* and is usually performed using a laparoscope (a type of endoscope inserted through a small incision in the abdominal wall). This is known as a laparoscopic cholescystectomy. *Ursodeoxycholic acid* may dissolve some small gallstones, but their recurrence is common, and in most cases, surgery is eventually required. Therefore, this medication cannot be recommended as a treatment for gallstones.

People with chronic liver disease from any cause are at risk for the development of liver cancer, which may also cause pain in the right upper quadrant. Diagnosis and treatment of liver cancer is discussed in Chapter 19.

Stomach disorders are also common among the American population and in people with liver disease. *Peptic ulcer disease* (PUD) and *gastritis* (inflammation of the stomach lining) may be the cause of abdominal pain in people with liver disease. An upper endoscopy (a procedure wherein a flexible tube with a light at the end is inserted down the esophagus into the stomach and then into the first part of the small intestine) is typically performed in order to diagnose these stomach disorders. During an upper endoscopy, a biopsy is typically performed for *Helicobacter pylori,* a bacteria that may cause gastritis and ulcers. These stomach ailments are readily treatable with medications, such as proton-pump inhibitors (omeprazole [Prilosec]) and lansoprazole [Prevacid]), either alone or in combination with antibiotics, depending upon the precise diagnosis.

Intestinal pain caused by irritable bowel syndrome (IBS) must also be considered as a cause of abdominal or right upper quadrant pain. The right side of the large intestine lies in close proximity to the liver, and the transverse colon lies in the middle of the abdomen (see Figure 1.1 on page 9). Therefore, spasms of the intestines, a symptom that characterizes IBS, are often mistakenly attributed to the liver by the person experiencing the symptom. The symptoms associated with IBS—abdominal pain and cramping, bloating, and excessive gas—can be treated with *anticholinergic* medications (such as clindinium [Librax] and hyoscyamine [Donnatal]), dietary restrictions, and stress reduction.

Other causes of abdominal and right upper quadrant pain that should be investigated in people with liver disease include scar tissue from prior abdominal surgery known as *adhesions* and inflammation of the pancreas (a condition known as *pancreatitis*), which may occur with increased frequency in people who drink excessive alcohol and in those with primary biliary cirrhosis.

If a person experiences abdominal pain along with distention and swelling of the abdomen, *ascites* must be considered as a cause. Ascites is associated with cirrhosis and is discussed on page 286. However, abdominal distention occurring in people with liver disease may be due to ailments other than ascites. Abdominal distention can result if the digestive tract fills with gas. When this happens, a person may experience the sensation of being bloated. This type of abdominal distention may be due to impaired or inadequate absorption (known as *malabsorption*) or digestion (known as *maldigestion*) of certain foods that can be associated with certain liver disorders (see Chapter 23 for more information). This is a controllable condition and may be treated by the avoidance of specific foods, such as dairy products or wheat (gluten) products. Fatty liver is another condition that can lead to abdominal distention and liver abnormalities. In people whose fatty liver stems from being overweight, a distended abdomen may occur due to excessive *adipose* (fatty) tissue. This condition, which was discussed in Chapter 16, is often reversible with weight reduction.

TREATMENT OF COMPLICATIONS

Complications associated with cirrhosis were covered in Chapter 6. The following section discusses the treatment of four complications of chronic liver disease: ascites, variceal bleeding, encephalopathy (which all can occur in people with cirrhosis and portal hypertension), and osteoporosis (which often occurs in people with chronic liver disease with or without cirrhosis and portal hypertension).

Treatment of Ascites (Fluid Accumulation)

Ascites is characterized by massive accumulation of fluid in the abdominal cavity. This results in abdominal swelling and distention. Treatment of ascites includes a low-sodium (low-salt) diet and fluid restriction to about one liter of fluid per day. Low-sodium diets are discussed in detail in Chapter 23. Treatment through sodium and fluid restriction alone adequately decreases ascites in only about 20 percent of people. Therefore, diuretics (water pills) are often added to dietary restrictions in an effort to maximize results. The most commonly used diuretics are furosemide (Lasix) and spironolactone (Aldactone). This type of therapy works well in approximately 90 percent of people. When medical therapy fails, a person is known as having *refractory ascites.*

Refractory ascites can be managed by physically removing the fluid by a process known as a *paracentesis.* A paracentesis involves the removal of large amounts of fluid through a needle inserted into the abdomen. A paracentesis should also be performed on all patients with ascites at the time when ascites first develops in order to examine the fluid for possible infection—a condition known as *spontaneous bacterial peritonitis* (SBP)—or for liver cancer or other cancers, such as ovarian. People with SBP commonly have a fever and abdominal pain, although these symptoms are sometimes absent. SBP requires hospitalization and treatment with intravenous antibiotics.

If the ascitic fluid is not infected, four to six liters of it can be safely removed once every two weeks. However, if multiple paracentesis procedures are repeatedly required over time in order to prevent fluid reaccumulation, a *transjugular intrahepatic portosystemic shunt* (TIPS) should be considered. TIPS is a procedure that creates a shunt (an alternative passageway) in the liver between the portal and hepatic veins. Creating this shunt has the effect of decreasing the portal pressure and diminishing the amount of ascitic fluid. Originally, TIPS procedures were performed strictly to control bleeding from esophageal and gastric varices (discussed below). Yet TIPS is now considered to be very useful in the control of refractory ascites.

TIPS is performed by a radiologist. The patient is given only a local anesthetic and a mild sedative. Neither a surgical operation nor general anesthesia is required. The radiologist inserts a needle into the jugular vein in the neck, passes the needle into the hepatic vein, and advances the needle into the portal vein. This creates a passageway for a catheter to be left in place between the hepatic and portal vein, creating a shunt. One complication of TIPS is encephalopathy in approximately 25 percent of people who undergo this procedure. Another complication is the potential for occlusion (blockage) of the shunt, thereby necessitating its replacement. While TIPS makes ascites much more manageable, this procedure has no effect on liver function, on the progression of disease, or on the patient's survival. Therefore, people with refractory ascites inevitably need to be evaluated for a liver transplant (see Chapter 22 for more information).

Treatment of Bleeding Varices (Bleeding Blood Vessels)

The most serious complication of cirrhosis is bleeding esophageal and gastric varices. This complication occurs when the blood pressure in these blood vessels becomes so high (a condition known as portal hypertension) that they dilate to such a degree that they literally explode. When this happens, profuse, life-threatening bleeding results. In fact, it is estimated that between 30 and 50 percent of people could die within one to two months of their first episode of bleeding varices.

Doctors can stop the bleeding during an endoscopy by injecting a clotting agent directly into the dilated blood vessel (also known as a *varix*). This procedure is known as *esophageal* and/or *gastric sclerotherapy.* Alternatively, the doctor can stop the bleeding during an endoscopy by strangling the bleeding varix with a miniature rubber band. This procedure is known as esophageal and/or gastric *variceal ligation.* Since these methods control the acute emergency but do not prevent recurrence, patients should be placed on a beta-blocker, such as propanolol (Inderal), a medication that acts to reduce portal pressure and to decrease blood flow through the varices, thereby ultimately reducing the risk of recurrent bleeding. Ideally, all people with evidence of varices should be placed on a beta-blocker, since this type of medication may prevent varices from bleeding in the first place. Sometimes another medication, isosorbide mononitrate (Isordil), is added to propanolol in an effort to further decrease portal pressure.

If the above-mentioned methods fail to stop recurrent bleeding, a man-made shunt should be considered. *Portal-systemic shunts* (PSS) were the first types of shunts used to control variceal bleeding. This procedure entails surgically joining the portal vein to the inferior vena cava. PSS are performed by a surgeon, and the patient must undergo general anesthesia. While this technique can successfully control variceal hemorrhage, portal blood flow is diverted away from the liver. Thus, the liver actually becomes starved for blood. This may lead to an increased incidence of encephalopathy and accelerated progression of the patient's underlying liver disorder. Another type of surgical shunt is known as the *distal splenorenal shunt* (DSRS). The DSRS procedure involves joining the splenic and kidney veins together. In this manner, blood flow to the liver is preserved, as blood is able to flow to the liver through the portal vein. As such, the incidence of encephalopathy and the rate of progression of liver disease is less among people undergoing DSRS than among those undergoing PSS. TIPS, as discussed above, creates a shunt connecting the hepatic and portal veins, thereby decreasing pressure in the esophagus and decreasing the risk of bleeding, while not requiring surgery or general anesthesia. While any of these man-made shunts may successfully control variceal bleeding, they do not prolong survival. Therefore, people with variceal bleeding, like those with refractory ascites, ultimately need to be evaluated for a liver transplant (see Chapter 22).

Treatment of Encephalopathy (Altered Mental Function)

Encephalopathy is an altered or impaired mental status in people with cirrhosis that typically leads to coma. Treatment should begin with eliminating the factor that started the encephalopathy. Factors that can cause encephalopathy include the following:

- Excessive use of diuretics (water pills), known as *overdiuresis.*

- Use of pain medications, sleeping pills, or tranquilizers.

- Excess consumption of animal protein.

- Infection.

- Constipation.

- Bleeding in the digestive tract (for example, bleeding esophageal varices).

- Electrolyte imbalances (for example, low potassium level, a condition known as *hypokalemia.*)

- Kidney dysfunction.

- Excessive alcohol consumption.

- Liver cancer.

Treatment includes the discontinuation and avoidance of all sedatives, tranquilizers, and pain medications; discontinuation or reduction in the dosage of all diuretics; treatment of infection (particularly SBP); elimination of constipation; control of gastrointestinal bleeding; and reduction or total elimination of the amount of animal protein in the diet. Vegetarian diets are thought by some liver experts to be more beneficial than animal-protein diets for improving encephalopathy.

Further management involves oral administration of an antibiotic, most commonly *neomycin.* Since bacteria that naturally live in the intestines produce ammonia, and ammonia has been linked to encephalopathy, treatment with neomycin (which reduces bacteria) should improve encephalopathy. People found to have *Helicobacter pylori* in their stomachs must be treated with antibiotics and a proton-pump inhibitor. Since this bacteria produces *urease* (an enzyme needed to produce ammonia), it may have a role in precipitating encephalopathy. *Lactulose* is a very sweet, synthetic sugar that acts as a powerful laxative. It acidifies the stool and thereby traps ammonia and drags it out of the body along with other fecal material. Therefore, lactulose can be quite useful in the management of encephalopathy. Moreover, zinc levels should be checked and supplemented if found to be deficient, as zinc deficiency may be a contributing factor to encephalopathy. Administration of branched-chain amino acids (leucine, isoleucine, and valine) may have some benefit; however, evidence supporting this is inconclusive. Two other drugs, *flumaze-*

nil and *bromocriptine,* may be useful in the treatment of encephalopathy, although further study is needed to confirm this. Fortunately, if the precipitating factor is promptly corrected and if treatment with lactulose is expeditiously started, encephalopathy, in most cases, will be reversed—at least on a temporary basis. In any case, people with encephalopathy should be evaluated for a liver transplant.

Treatment of Osteoporosis (Bone Loss)

Osteoporosis is a condition marked by decreased bone mass and decreased bone density. This leads to a weakening of bones, thereby increasing the risk of bone fractures. People with any chronic liver disease are at increased risk for the development of osteoporosis due to a lack of activity resulting from excessive fatigue, poor nutritional habits, reduced muscle mass, and disturbances in hormonal levels (a condition known as *hypogonadism*).

This complication of liver disease can be quite painful and debilitating. Furthermore, there often are no warning signs of osteoporosis until a fracture occurs. Since osteoporosis can be so incapacitating, prevention of this complication of liver disease is crucial. Therefore, as postmenopausal women are already at high risk for bone fractures, they should attempt to refrain from long-term treatment with prednisone or to use the lowest dose possible, as this medication can worsen osteoporosis. This especially applies to those postmenopausal women discovered to have autoimmune hepatitis, and those who underwent a liver transplant. In fact, it is especially important for all people prior to liver transplantation to attempt to avert osteoporosis, as liver transplant recipients, regardless of age and menopause status, inevitably lose bone mass during the three to six months immediately following transplantation.

All people with chronic liver disease should undergo bone-mineral-density testing in order to determine whether they have osteoporosis. This test is performed by a radiologist and should be repeated once every three to five years. Blood tests, by themselves, are an insufficient means to measure bone density and calcium requirements. People with chronic liver disease, especially women over the age of fifty, should have their bone density measured. If found to be low, these people are strongly advised to start on medication, such as Fosamax (alendronate sodium), that is aimed at inhibiting bone loss, in addition to a calcium and vitamin D supplement. In fact, people who are at a particularly high risk for osteoporosis (women with primary biliary cirrhosis, for example) should start taking Fosamax before the development of bone loss. See below for a further discussion of Fosamax and other biphosphonates.

There are some steps that people with liver disease can take to reduce the likelihood of osteoporosis. People should supplement their diets with calcium (1,000 to 2,000 milligrams per day) and vitamin D (400 to 800 IU per day). Also, an exercise routine, including weight-bearing exercises, must be incorporated into one's lifestyle. Weight-bearing exercises not only increase muscle size, but they increase underlying bone mass, thus, decreasing the likelihood of osteoporosis. These issues are discussed in more detail in Chapter 23. Smoking, alcohol, and excessive caffeine should be avoided. Since the incidence and severity of osteoporosis correlate with the dose and duration of prednisone therapy, people should attempt to taper off this medication as soon after transplantation as possible. Most transplant centers have begun to routinely decrease the dose of prednisone soon after transplant, and some transplant centers discontinue prednisone use altogether one year after transplant.

Estrogen-hormonal therapy has been demonstrated to increase bone mass. However, oral estrogen replacement should generally be avoided in people with liver disease, as it may cause additional liver problems, such as worsening of cholestasis. Furthermore, estrogen supplementation may prompt certain benign liver tumors, such as hemangiomas and/or hepatic adenomas to enlarge (see Chapter 19). Estrogen patches are generally a safer choice.

Biphosphonates (alendronate [Fosamax] and etidronate [Didronal]) have been shown to increase bone mass, to prevent bone loss, and to decrease the incidence of bone fractures. People with liver disease, especially those with cholestatic liver disease, may benefit from starting biphosphonate therapy before they develop osteoporosis. Any person who already has osteoporosis should begin biphosphonate therapy promptly. These medications may also prove to be protective if used after liver transplantation. However, people with esophageal varices should probably avoid alendronate because of the drug's capability to cause ulcers in the esophagus.

CONCLUSION

Often the symptoms and/or complications of chronic liver disease discussed in this chapter are what prompt people to see their doctors and lead to the diagnosis of liver disease. Treating the symptoms and complications of liver disease and cirrhosis can be as challenging as treating the underlying liver disorder. In fact, it is specifically the unresponsiveness of some symptoms and complications to therapy that typically leads a person to liver transplantation (which will be discussed in Chapter 22). While appropriate and effective treatment of the symptoms and complications of liver disease will not provide a cure, it is a crucial step towards improving a person's well-being. People with chronic liver disease who experience severe symptoms, such as fatigue, often seek out herbs and other alternatives to the conventional medical therapy discussed in this chapter. Therefore, the next chapter will discuss herbs and alternative therapies for liver disease—covering issues such as safety and effectiveness.

21

Herbs and Other Alternative Therapies

Current estimates show that Americans make more visits to doctors and other healthcare professionals who specialize in alternative medicine than to doctors who practice conventional medicine. (Alternative medicine is any therapy used to treat an illness that is not within the realm of conventional and/or accepted medical therapies.) People with liver disease are no exception to this trend. For example, most people with chronic hepatitis C have tried (or have at least inquired about) the herb milk thistle. Well, why not? It is now commonplace to find an entire aisle at the local drugstore or even the supermarket devoted to herbal remedies, some of which claim to help protect liver cells and help support liver function. Dozens of publications and books proclaim the proficiency of herbs for the treatment of hepatitis, cirrhosis, and other liver diseases. Some of these books have even made it to the *New York Times* bestseller list. On the Internet, numerous websites proclaim the effectiveness of herbs for treating liver disease. However, as you will learn, there is much more information to consider.

Some alternative therapies may be helpful if used properly under the guidance of a knowledgeable licensed healthcare professional and may also be beneficial when used as part of a total treatment regimen in conjunction with conventional medical therapies. Some medical insurance companies have started to cover the cost of visits to practitioners of alternative therapies. Many well-respected institutions and organizations, including the National Institutes of Health, have conducted seminars on complementary and alternative medicine. It appears that the worlds of conventional and alternative medicine may be moving in the direction of integration. In fact, there is a burgeoning field of medicine known as *integrative medicine*. However, be aware that some alternative therapies are simply a waste of time and money and can even be outright harmful and cause complications that can result in liver failure. This is why it is important for people with liver disease to obtain a clear understanding of both the pros and cons of using herbs and alternative therapies. This chapter will help you do just that. It discusses herbal remedies and some other

291

alternative therapies for chronic liver disease and hepatitis. It provides a guide to help you distinguish among empty promises, helpful therapies, and those treatments that are flat-out dangerous. What constitutes an alternative treatment, as well as what an herb is, is defined within this chapter. Also, the Dietary Supplement and Education Act of 1994 (DSHEA) and its implications are discussed. This chapter also explains how to research information concerning the efficacy and side effects of some of the most popular herbs being used in the treatment of liver disease. Milk thistle (silymarin) and other herbs that are claimed to benefit the liver, as well as herbs that have the potential to harm the liver are discussed in detail. In addition, alternative therapies other than herbs are discussed. Finally, conclusions on the safety and efficacy of various alternative remedies are drawn, and recommendations for the use of alternative therapies are made.

TAKING A CLOSER LOOK AT HERBS

Herbs are plants or plant parts that are used for healing purposes. These herbs, which generally have a bitter taste, are known as *medicinal herbs.* They are distinct from *culinary herbs,* which are tasty and used to season food. There has been a rebirth in the popularity of herbal remedies, as many people are desperately searching for alternatives to conventional synthetic medications. In fact, herbal products are estimated to be a multibillion-dollar-a-year industry, whose revenue has increased dramatically in recent years and continues to increase with each year. It's easy to understand why herbal remedies are becoming such a popular alternative to Western medicine. With each new advance, medical science seems ever more intimidating. The latest technological breakthroughs often alienate as much as they ameliorate. Herbs, on the other hand, are a much friendlier commodity—as comfortably familiar as the kitchen spice rack. They can be purchased over the counter (without a prescription) in drug stores, supermarkets, health food stores, by mail order, and over the Internet.

There are several things that people with liver disease in particular need to know about herbal medicines and how they differ from standard pharmaceuticals. The following information provides the facts—both good and bad.

A Brief History of Herbal Medicine

Herbs have been used throughout time by every culture to treat virtually every type of ailment—from the common cold to cancer, and yes, of course, liver disease. They can be consumed as teas, slices of root, and in modern pill or capsule form. The first written records describing treatment of disease with herbal remedies date back to about 1500 B.C. inscribed by the ancient Egyptians on papyrus. In China, the basis of traditional Chinese medicine was first recorded in the *Materia Medica,* which was written about 2,000 years ago. In fact, traditional herbal remedies continue to form the backbone of modern Chinese medicine. Many institutions in China are devoted to the controlled study of medicinal herbs, and the Chinese Ministry of Public

Health oversees the administration of new herbal products. Traditional Japanese medicine, known as kampo, is based on herbs. In 1988, regulations were established in Japan to regulate the manufacture and quality of kampo medicine and to insure compliance with the Japanese government's regulations for manufacturing control and quality control of drugs. In Germany, where herbal remedies are commonly used by people and often recommended by doctors, Commission E oversees the safety of these preparations and requires that certain standards of purity be met.

In the United States, much of our knowledge about herbs comes from the Native American Indians who had numerous uses for the plants that grew in abundance around them. Until the 1940s, medical textbooks often made reference to the medicinal uses of berries, bark, leaves, and roots. However, with the fantastic advances of modern technology during the twentieth century, these more natural remedies took a backseat to the scientifically developed synthetic medicines of today. Note, however, that approximately 10 to 20 percent of today's prescription drugs contain at least one active ingredient derived from plants or herbs. For example, digitalis, a popular drug used to treat certain heart conditions, is derived from the leaves of the herb *foxglove. Salicin,* which is used to make aspirin, was originally extracted from the bark of willow trees (now it is made synthetically). And some cough drops contain menthol, lemon, eucalyptus, or mint—all derived from herbs.

The Reasons Why Some People Are Turning to Herbal Medicine

There are many reasons why people with liver disease are turning to herbal remedies for answers. First, many people equate herbs with being safe because they are natural. Remember, however, that *natural* does not mean *harmless*. In fact, some herbs, which will be discussed on page 304, can be harmful to the liver. Second, some people who fail to respond to accepted medical treatments become disillusioned with conventional medicine and begin to look for alternatives. Third, many people with liver disease feel fine and may find it difficult to consider taking a medication that has the potential to make them feel ill—especially if they believe that herbal preparations can make them feel even better. Finally, while all herbs aren't inexpensive, they may still be cheaper than prescription medications over the course of long-term treatment. This is particularly true for people without medical coverage.

How to Evaluate the Research on Herbal Medicine

Walking through the aisles of a health food store or supermarket, it is common to see many frequently used everyday products—such as green tea, licorice, artichokes, dandelion root, peppers, and turmeric—claiming to be beneficial in the treatment of liver disease. Obviously, a person should and must research the herb more thoroughly before she takes it with the expectation that it will help her liver. Simply reading the label on a supplement bottle, reading the description in an herbal remedy book, or asking the owner of the health food store if a particular herb will help the liver may not be enough. There are many steps a person can take on her own to determine if the herbal product that she is considering taking is, in fact, effective.

Many libraries, as well as the Internet, have access to MEDLINE (an electronic catalog maintained by the National Library of Medicine), which contains thousands of medical research papers. It is important to get a copy of the original scientific article cited in a magazine, book, or journal in order to have an idea of what doses the investigators used and under what conditions they were used. Also, the first edition of the *Physicians' Desk Reference* (PDR) *for Herbal Medicines* was published in 1999. This book provides much needed information. It provides indications for an herb's use, including whether the indication is considered controversial; some of the known side effects of the herb; and some possible interactions with other drugs. Anyone contemplating the use of an herbal preparation is urged to purchase this book. Thanks to this book, people now have a good starting place for researching a particular herb or dietary supplement. In addition to the *PDR for Herbal Medicines,* the Office of Dietary Supplements (ODS) at the National Institutes of Health (NIH) has an up-to-date comprehensive website containing a database of scientific publications related to dietary supplements (see Appendix for website addresses). And, in 1998, the *Commission E Monographs* was translated into English—*The Complete German Commission E Monographs: Therapeutic Guide to Herbal Medicines.* This book describes which herbs have been approved or rejected in Germany for medicinal uses, the recommended dosages and uses of approximately 250 specific herbs, the contraindications, possible adverse reactions, and drug interactions that may occur with specific herbs.

As a general rule, there isn't as much scientific research on herbal remedies as there is on conventional therapies. Much of what does exist is usually based on a small number of test subjects who have taken the herb in question for a short duration. Still, it's worthwhile finding out exactly what sort of information exists. With the increased interest in herbal products, there are bound to be more and better controlled scientific studies in the future. In fact, a study is now being contemplated to evaluate the efficacy of milk thistle (silymarin) combined with Rebetron for people with chronic hepatitis C.

In order to evaluate a research study, a few guidelines must be kept in mind. First and foremost, no single study can be considered to truly prove anything. Find out if the results have been reproduced in other laboratories or by other researchers. Next, try to determine the study's credibility—has it been published in a well-respected medical journal (such as most of those appearing in the bibliography of this book) or has it only been self-published—as in a book or pamphlet that does not require any type of review. Look closely at the details of any study you are trying to evaluate. Did the investigators actually compare two groups of subjects (a control group and an experimental group) or had they simply performed an observational study, which simply involves looking at what happened to people taking the product in question? If they used a control group, how did they ensure that the two groups were indeed comparable in every way before the study began? Is there a possibility that the control group was actually sicker than the experimental group?

What criteria did they use to include people in their study? Have they made sure that there weren't other disorders or other medications that confounded their results? How long did the study last and what happened after the treatment was stopped?

After examining the methods that were used to conduct the experiment, look at the conclusions. Are they warranted by the evidence? Have the investigators taken into account the *placebo effect* (an improvement in response to treatment with a placebo, not the substance being tested)? Be particularly wary of research that does not include possible alternative explanations for its findings.

If a person can't find any useful information from independent sources on the efficacy of the particular herbal remedy in question, then it may be time to ask some tough questions, including: Do I want to be a guinea pig for an untested product? How do I know if the product is safe if I become pregnant? What guarantees do I have that the compound won't promote cancer, trigger ulcers, or contribute to liver failure? How do I know what dose I should use and how often? If the person still decides to take the compound, she should be sure to tell her doctor, so that the doctor can be on the lookout for any potential side effects or drug interactions.

What We Don't Know About Herbal Medicine

While the amount of information and research concerning herbs is increasing, there are still two important matters that have not been as clearly defined about herbs. First, due to the lack of controlled research on herbal remedies, the exact extent of drug-herb interaction is not entirely known. Thus, an herb that a person may be taking in an attempt to prevent liver damage may have a negative interaction with the medication that she is taking to control high blood pressure. For example, licorice—proclaimed to be beneficial in the treatment of viral hepatitis—may cause fluid retention and worsen high blood pressure. Furthermore, many herbs may increase or decrease the activity of conventional medicine. For example, the herb *cannabis sativa* (marijuana) has been demonstrated to diminish the effectiveness of interferon. Though potential drug-herb interactions can be looked up in the *PDR for Herbal Medicines,* this list may be incomplete.

Furthermore, the noted side effects of an herb, in general, may be incomplete. This is due to the fact that it can be very difficult to trace side effects to a particular herb. It may take weeks, months, or even years for problems to show up. By that point, people don't always remember that they have taken an herbal remedy or have become so accustomed to a particular side effect that they dismiss it. Complicating matters even further, many natural remedies contain dozens of active ingredients depending on exactly how they were prepared. Finally, there are no regulatory laws mandating that the manufacturer or distributor of an herbal preparation report possible adverse reactions of the herb to the FDA or other government agency (see "The Dietary Supplement Health and Education Act of 1994" on pages 296 and 297). So, in all likelihood, all the possible drug-herb interactions and other side effects associated with a given herb are not listed in *PDR for Herbal Medicine.*

Second, there is a lack of standardization among herbal products. It is impor-

The Dietary Supplement
Health and Education Act of 1994

For a synthetic drug to become available by prescription, it must undergo rigorous premarket scrutiny by the United States Food and Drug Administration (FDA). Similarly, foods must meet manufacturing standards before they are deemed safe to eat. Herbal remedies have always presented a problem for the FDA. Should they be classified as a food or a drug? Until 1994, the FDA pretty much resolved this dilemma by treating herbal products as food additives. The manufacturers refrained (for the most part) from making any medical claims about their products. And, if the FDA felt that an herbal product was unsafe, it could pull the product from the market and subject it to further testing.

In 1993, the FDA decided that herbal manufacturers would soon have to provide more scientific data about their products because more and more people were taking them. This decision was met with opposition. Members of Congress were bombarded with complaints from health food store owners, herbal medicine manufacturers, and the supplement-taking public.

The outcome of this upheaval was the Dietary Supplement Health and Education Act of 1994 (DSHEA). This legislation essentially declared that any herb, vitamin, mineral, or other botanical product (other than tobacco) that was marketed as a dietary supplement was exempt from further regulation by the FDA. The maker must simply provide "reasonable assurance" that no ingredient "presents a significant or unreasonable risk of illness or injury." Herb manufacturers still couldn't claim that their products prevented, treated, or cured disease, but they were allowed to make one claim that they had never before been allowed to make—they could advertise that their products "supported the structure or function" of various organs in the body. But in order to make such a claim, they had to include on the label the following disclaimer: *This statement has not been evaluated by the Food and Drug Administration. This product is not intended to diagnose, treat, cure, or prevent any disease.*

While there are still some rules about what can go on product labels, the FDA has no jurisdiction over what is written in books, said on videos, or writ-

tant to be aware that not all parts of the herb contain the active ingredient proclaimed to produce the beneficial effect. For example, one study compared ten different brands of the herb ginseng and found that the active ingredient *ginsenoside* varied drastically among different brands, although all were essentially similar in their descriptions of ingredients contained in the bottle. In fact, some pills or capsules contained almost none of the active ingredient. A different study found that ten on the Internet. As a result, claims about cures, treatment, and prevention of disease have proliferated. It is now totally up to the consumer to evaluate the validity of these claims.

How DSHEA Affects Consumers

Due to this law, no proof of safety or effectiveness of an herbal product needs to be submitted to any governmental regulatory agency before becoming available to the public. This means that side effects and toxic reactions caused by herbs or herbal products may be discovered only after they happen. Moreover, there is no regulatory process mandating that adverse reactions to herbs be reported. Therefore, the toxicity associated with herbal remedies may be underestimated. The Congressional Research Service reports that according to their analysis, many people believe that "any product that appears in pill form has been reviewed for safety by the FDA." Thus, many people who use herbal remedies incorrectly assume that these products are regulated by the FDA for safety and efficacy.

How DSHEA Affects the Labeling of Herbs

Although claims that an herbal product prevents, treats, or cures disease are not permitted to appear on a product label, claims can be made about the effect of the remedy on the body's structure or function. For instance, the label on a bottle of milk thistle can claim that the product "may support the liver" or "may inhibit factors responsible for liver damage," but it cannot state that it cures or prevents liver disease. However, though a label cannot make such blunt claims, other advertising venues are not prohibited from making them. This leads to confusion over exactly what claims manufacturers are making about their products. Also, since the labeling of herbs is unregulated, they may often lack crucial information—such as the exact ingredients and the amount and potency of the ingredients. Some herbal remedies contain only one ingredient, while other remedies contain a mixture of ingredients. Consumers should research the quality and efficacy of the herbs or herbal products and shouldn't rely solely on the manufacturers' claims.

up to one-quarter of the products on health food store shelves did not contain any of the listed ingredients.

Due to the absence of regulation, it is possible that a totally different herb can be substituted for the one on the label. Furthermore, there have been reports that some herbs have been spiked with steroids, painkillers, tranquilizers, or other substances to improve their effectiveness. Other substances, including lead and even powerful heart stimulants (such as digitalis), have been discovered adulterated in herbs. So how can someone determine whether the contents listed on the label of an herbal product accurately reflect its contents? First, it is important to determine whether the company manufacturing the herbal product is a well-known, legitimate company with a good track record of providing consumers with safe and effective products. Second, a person can request a "certificate of analysis" from the manufacturer concerning a particular herbal product. This ensures that the ingredients listed on the label have been analyzed by a laboratory and are accurately represented on the label. Or a sample of the herbal product can be sent to an herbalist, a nutritionist, or a compound pharmacist, all of whom are capable of performing an analysis of the ingredients contained in the herb. Lastly, a compound pharmacist—a pharmacist who prepares, mixes, assembles, packages, and labels medications from scratch—can prepare an herb in its active form. (See the Appendix for information on how to find a compound pharmacist.)

MILK THISTLE—THE MOST WIDELY USED HERB FOR LIVER DISEASE

Milk thistle (also known as silymarin and its scientific name *Silybum marianum*) is a tall plant, characterized by sharp spines that resemble artichokes and leaves that are riddled with distinctive white veins. It was originally discovered growing in the Kashmir region bordering India and Pakistan. It can now be found all over the temperate world, growing in dry and rocky soil. Its stems and leaves secrete a milky substance when crushed. The following sections contain important information regarding this popular herb. (Please note that some preparations of milk thistle may contain iron and should therefore be avoided by people with hemochromatosis or other liver diseases associated with iron overload.)

The History of Milk Thistle

As with so many other herbs, the medicinal claims for milk thistle have an ancient history. Originally believed to help nursing mothers produce milk, milk thistle became more well known for its effects on the liver. This can be traced back to ancient Roman times when Pliny the Elder (A.D. 23–79) referred to the milky juice of this plant as being excellent for "carrying off bile." John Gerard, a sixteenth century British herbalist, recommended milk thistle for "expelling melancholy," a symptom attributed to liver disease during that era. In Germany during the nineteenth century, doctors commonly treated jaundice and other liver diseases with an extract from milk thistle seeds. The scientific study of herbs continued to be concentrated in Europe, and in 1949, German researchers found that milk thistle appeared to protect the livers of animals exposed to high doses of carbon tetrachloride, a potent liver toxin.

In 1968, it was found that the active ingredient in milk thistle is located in the seed, and that it consists of three components *silybin, silydianin,* and *silychristin.* These components are now collectively referred to as the flavonoid *silymarin.* Silymarin is currently used mainly in Europe to treat all types of liver disorders. Due to the lack of FDA regulation, the actual percentage of biologically active silymarin in a given preparation of milk thistle is unknown.

The Benefits Claimed for Milk Thistle

The following claims have been made about milk thistle:

- Milk thistle may reverse liver damage in alcoholics.

- Milk thistle may reverse liver injury in patients with chronic hepatitis.

- Milk thistle may slow the advancement of cirrhosis.

- Milk thistle may improve the long-term survival rate among cirrhotic patients.

Herbalists claim that milk thistle achieves the above in three different ways: First, milk thistle is said to strengthen the outer protective membrane of liver cells so that they are better at deflecting toxins. Second, milk thistle is said to shield the liver from free radicals, which are potentially dangerous, yet inevitable byproducts of some of the body's basic metabolic functions. And finally, milk thistle is said to stimulate the production of new liver cells to replace old damaged ones. This section will examine some of the evidence that forms the basis for each of these alleged properties of milk thistle.

Ability to Inhibit Factors Responsible for Liver Damage by Strengthening the Outer Membrane of Liver Cells

This characteristic of milk thistle would prevent the entrance of potentially toxic substances into the liver. This property can be demonstrated if a person decides to go on a wild mushroom picking expedition and accidentally eats the deadly fungus *deathcap*. These mushrooms are found in North America and Europe and are part of the *Amanita phalloides* family of mushrooms. They are known for containing deadly toxins known as *phallotoxins* that are famous for causing liver failure or even death when consumed—thus the nickname "deathcap fungus." Unfortunately, a person would have to be a *mycophagist* (an expert mushroom picker) to tell the difference between a deathcap and other tasty amanita mushrooms that are edible and nontoxic. It doesn't take much for a poisonous mushroom to destroy the liver. Within about eight hours of ingestion, diarrhea, stomach pains, nausea, and vomiting will occur. About a week later, LFTs will elevate, and total liver failure, along with encephalopathy and death, is not too far off. That's where milk thistle comes in. Milk thistle has been shown to compete effectively with these mushroom toxins to occupy the same site on the liver cell membrane. If ingested in time, milk thistle may block the entrance of these mushroom toxins into the liver and prevent damage from occurring. Or, if taken soon after ingestion, milk thistle may actually displace the toxins from their sites and thereby stop any further damage.

It must be emphasized that most of the evidence of the liver-protective properties of milk thistle stems from experimental animal studies. For example, laboratory animals were experimentally poisoned with *Amanita phalloides.* The animals given milk thistle at five hours and twenty-four hours after poisoning displayed little evidence of liver damage and had normal levels of liver enzymes. Animals that did not receive milk thistle either died of liver damage or had elevated liver enzymes. Case reports of humans who ingested poisonous mushrooms revealed marked improvement of liver-related abnormalities and a successful outcome when treated with milk thistle. However, these results must be interpreted with caution. These are isolated incidences, consisting of only three people. Moreover, other treatments, such as antibiotics and steroids, were also administered along with the milk thistle. Therefore, whether the benefits achieved were due to milk thistle or other therapies is unclear.

As you can see from the above, there is some very suggestive, though not conclusive, evidence in favor of milk thistle's ability to help protect the liver from acute mushroom poisoning. Many people would consider the data to be good enough to warrant trying milk thistle, along with other medical treatments, especially in the event of such an emergency. But don't forget that most people who have been poisoned by mushrooms are otherwise in good health. Their liver cells have not been damaged. They have not lived with years of irreversible scarring of the liver. So even if milk thistle is one day proven to be the standard antidote for some kinds of mushroom poisoning, it doesn't necessarily mean that it will protect people with other forms of liver disease.

Protects Liver Cells From Free-Radical Damage

Free radicals are highly reactive molecules that the body creates as a natural consequence of just being alive. The number of free radicals produced often skyrockets under the influence of such factors as a high-fat diet, smoking, and exposure to the sun or excess radiation. Free radicals may result in severe damage of cells and tissues in the body. Most free radicals in the body consist of toxic oxygen molecules. Oxygen in its toxic state can oxidize molecules in the body, corroding them, similar to the formation of rust—which is simply oxidized iron. Since the body can't live without these rogue chemicals, it also produces antioxidants that gobble up any free radicals they can find and render them harmless. Probably one of the hardest working antioxidants produced by the liver is an enzyme called glutathione peroxidase, which protects the liver from free-radical damage. In fact, one of the ways that alcohol and liver toxins damage the liver is by interfering with the body's ability to create glutathione. A few tissue studies have suggested that milk thistle can boost the level of glutathione in liver cells, thus affording protection to the liver from these toxins. Commonly known antioxidants include vitamins A, C, and E. Milk thistle claims to possess ten times more antioxidant power on the liver than vitamin E.

Iron is a major catalyst of free-radical reactions and can be a potent toxin to the liver. Iron overload diseases are associated with liver damage and cirrhosis. Iron-induced oxidation of cellular membranes is known as *lipid peroxidation.* Lipid peroxidation byproducts, such as hydrogen peroxide, are thought to be the mediators of the toxic effects of iron on the liver. This is thought to be an important mechanism leading to iron toxicity. Milk thistle is believed to possess antioxidant activity and specifically scavenge *hydroxyl* and *peroxyl* radicals. Experimental studies done on rats who were fed high iron diets showed lack of iron-induced liver toxicity when administered milk thistle. Comparative studies will need to be done before conclusions can be made for humans. Additional experimental studies on animals given other liver toxins, such as carbontetrachloride (CCL4), alcohol, or acetaminophen, and on small groups of humans exposed to toluene and xylene vapors, showed similar protective effects of milk thistle. However, one study attempting to demonstrate the protective effect of milk thistle on acetaminophen-induced liver damage not only failed to show protection but actually demonstrated liver cell death.

The largest human studies with the longest follow-up time and that best demonstrate the beneficial effects of milk thistle on the liver have been conducted on people with alcoholic liver disease. Some of these studies have suggested that mortality in people with alcoholic cirrhosis may be reduced by treatment with milk thistle when compared to a group of people with similar alcohol-induced disease-related characteristics, who were not treated with milk thistle. However, many flaws can be found with these studies. For example, upon closer examination of one study, it was noted that patients in the nontreated group were slightly sicker and had higher bilirubin levels and more advanced stage of liver disease compared with people in the group treated with milk thistle. Some studies done on people with alcoholic cirrhosis have demonstrated a normalization of liver enzymes after one month of treatment with milk thistle. However, other large studies in which people with alcoholic liver disease were treated with milk thistle have shown no benefits to either liver enzymes or mortality.

Stimulates Production of New Liver Cells to Replace Old Damaged Ones

In experimental studies (not performed on human subjects), milk thistle was demonstrated to increase the production of ribonucleic acid (RNA). Since RNA is one of the building blocks of life, the production of protein is thereby increased, and therefore, theoretically, new liver cells may be formed replacing destroyed liver cells. Once again, it must be emphasized that this property of milk thistle has not been proven to occur in humans.

The Most Effective Way to Take Milk Thistle

So, if a person decides that she wants to try milk thistle, how should she take it in order to maximize its proclaimed effects on the liver? Well, since milk thistle does not easily dissolve in water, its proclaimed benefits cannot be reaped by drinking it as a tea or by eating the leaves. The best way to take milk thistle is either in capsule form, especially from concentrate, or from a form that contains other substances—such as beta-cyclodextrin or phosphatidylcholine (silipide)—that render milk thistle more soluble in water. In this way, milk thistle becomes more *bioavailable* to the body, and its effects are more pronounced. The concentration of silymarin is highest in the seeds of the plant, although it is also found in the fruit and leaves.

With milk thistle, as with all herbal remedies, there is no standard recommended dose schedule or length of time to take the herb in order to best achieve its proclaimed benefits. Recommendations made on labels and in herbal publications vary—from as low as 70 milligrams twice per day to as high as 420 milligrams three times per day. Recommendations for duration of use range from one month to as long as nine months. No recommendations are made concerning the best time of day to take the herb or whether to take it with food as opposed to on an empty stomach. The *PDR for Herbal Medicines* recommends 200 to 400 milligrams of silymarin daily, but there are no additional recommendations made regarding its use.

The Side Effects of Milk Thistle

Most reports on milk thistle claim that there is a total lack of side effects when taking this herb. However, on close review of the literature, the following side effects were noted: headache, irritability, minor intestinal upset, and, most commonly, diarrhea. These side effects are similar to those commonly encountered in connection with the use of interferon (the FDA-approved treatment for hepatitis B and C). One experimental study, which has not been duplicated, demonstrated that liver cell damage occurred as a result of exposure of milk thistle to liver cells. The long-term side effects of milk thistle usage are not known.

OTHER HERBS USED FOR HEPATITIS AND LIVER DISEASE

This section discusses six of the most common herbs used in the treatment of liver disease—licorice, green tea, dandelion, artichoke, turmeric, and black and long peppers. Read on to learn about some of the facts people with liver disease need to know before deciding to take these herbs.

Licorice

The word *licorice* tends to conjure up an image of chewy black or red candy. However, licorice (*Glycyrrhiza glabra*) is also a powerful herb that has been proclaimed to help the liver. The active ingredients of licorice come from its roots and are believed by some to be due to *glycyrrhizic acid,* which also accounts for licorice's sweet taste. This acid functions similarly to the body's own naturally occurring hormone, aldosterone, which regulates salt and water in the body. Thus, side effects of licorice may include high blood pressure, water retention, and potassium depletion. It is important to avoid licorice during pregnancy. Also, people who have glaucoma, heart disease, or high blood pressure should avoid licorice.

Licorice has been shown in some experimental studies to stimulate production of the body's natural supply of interferon. This may account for its popularity in

Japan where it is sometimes used in the treatment of chronic viral hepatitis. When used intravenously, licorice has been demonstrated to lower liver enzymes. However, these results have not been universally demonstrated, and some studies have revealed no beneficial effects on the liver in humans. Furthermore, it has been noted that if licorice is taken for more than one week, there is an increased risk of serious side effects, such as high blood pressure or dangerously low potassium levels. Sustained beneficial effects from licorice use have not been clearly demonstrated. Ironically, the *PDR for Herbal Medicines* states that licorice is contraindicated (use is inadvisable) in people with chronic hepatitis, cholestatic liver disease, and cirrhosis. (Please note, licorice may contain iron and should therefore be avoided by people with iron overload diseases.)

Green Tea

Green tea (*Camellia sinensis*), a popular tea in the Orient, contains a high dose of *catechin,* a plant chemical. By comparison, black tea, which is popular in the United States, has undergone the process of fermentation, resulting in a lower concentration of catechin. Catechin is a flavonoid with antioxidant properties that has the ability to stabilize cell membranes. Therefore, the proclaimed liver-protective properties of catechin are similar to those that are claimed for milk thistle.

Experimentally induced liver damage in rats and in liver cell cultures has demonstrated the protective effects on the liver afforded by catechin. However, most human studies have failed to show similar results. Side effects noted in one study included fever, hemolysis (breakdown of red blood cells), and urticaria (an allergic rash). Dosages used in humans were 20 to 40 milligrams per kilogram daily as opposed to 200 milligrams per kilogram daily used in rats. It has been suggested that higher dosages should be used on humans in order to reap the herb's benefit of liver protection. However, the side effects that accompany higher dosages render such an approach impractical.

Dandelion

Anecdotally, it has been claimed that dandelion (*Taraxacum officinale*) possesses liver-healing properties. In fact, dandelion has been purported to enhance bile flow and to improve both hepatitis and jaundice. However, actual studies involving dandelion are difficult to locate. Dandelion has an extremely high vitamin-A content, higher than that of carrots. Since high levels of vitamin A can lead to serious liver damage (which will be discussed in Chapter 23), it is not advisable to use any herbal preparation that contains dandelion. (Please note, dandelion may contain iron and should, therefore, be avoided by people with iron overload diseases.)

Artichoke

The active ingredient of artichoke is found in the leaves and is known as *caffeylquinic acid* or *cynara.* The alleged properties of artichoke are similar to those alleged for milk thistle. Studies using artichoke on people with liver disease are difficult to locate.

Turmeric

Turmeric (*Curcuma domestica*) is the main ingredient in Indian curry powder. Going back thousands of years, this herb has been commonly used by India's practitioners of traditional Ayurvedic medicine as a cure for liver disease. The herb's active component is the yellow pigment *curcumin*. This herb is proclaimed to have antioxidant properties. In experimental animal studies, it has been shown to inhibit liver damage from aflatoxin and other liver toxins. It might, therefore, be concluded that the Indian population has a lower incidence of liver disease than the rest of the world, but this has not been demonstrated.

Black Peppers and Long Peppers

Piperine is the active ingredient of black peppers (*Piper nigrum*) and long peppers (*Piper longum*), which are among the most commonly used spices. In cases of experimentally induced liver disease in mice, piperine reduced the damaging effects of toxins on the liver. These studies explained such a beneficial effect on the liver by claiming that piperine had the ability to prevent depletion of glutathione, the liver's own protective antioxidant. There are no known studies comparing the occurrence of liver disease in people who consume these peppers with those who don't.

HERBS THAT MAY HARM THE LIVER

As mentioned previously, the mere fact that herbs are natural does not mean that they are harmless. In fact, there have been many reports of people suffering serious health problems and even dying as a result of their use of herbal remedies. Since everything that enters the mouth is metabolized through the liver, the liver is a prime target for the toxic effects of some herbs. People with normal functioning livers without a history of prior liver disease have experienced the adverse effects of certain herbs on the liver. Obviously, the potential for adverse consequences in people with liver disease is greatly increased. Remember, it is the liver's job to rid the body of potentially harmful substances. A liver that is already damaged will have to work overtime to clear a toxic herb from the body. Quite obviously, it is inadvisable to subject a poorly functioning liver to this type of stress. A doctor, unaware that a patient has taken herbal remedies, or unaware of the hepatotoxic effects of certain herbal remedies, may attribute any worsening of the patient's condition as a natural course of the disease.

Below is a brief discussion of some of the herbs that have been determined to be dangerous to the liver along with an extensive list of various herbs that have been linked to hepatitis, liver damage, and liver failure. In general, a key point to keep in mind is that any herb containing *pyrrolizidine alkaloids* is potentially hepatotoxic

(toxic to the liver). Hepatotoxicity due to pyrrolizidine-containing herbs can result from either small amounts ingested over long periods of time or from large amounts ingested over a short period of time. Pyrrolizidine alkaloids have been found in approximately 350 different plant species. The most toxic of these has been noted to be from the *senecio, heliotropium, crotalaria,* and *symphytium* species. Pyrrolizidine poisoning is common in Africa and Jamaica, two areas of the world where herbal teas containing this substance are consumed as folk remedies for a number of ailments. The pyrrolizidine alkaloids have been associated with a severe type of liver disorder known as *veno-occlusive disease.* In this disease, the hepatic vein becomes clogged, blocking off the blood supply to the liver. This can result in abdominal pain, vomiting, ascites, hepatomegaly (an enlarged liver), edema (leg swelling), cirrhosis, liver failure, and even death due to extensive liver damage.

The most well-established example of a liver-toxic pyrrolizidine alkaloid-containing herb is comfrey (*Symphytum officinale*). Comfrey has been used to relieve joint and stomach aches and is commercially available as a tea or in tablet or capsule form in the United States. Many herbal preparations that contain a mixture of herbs include comfrey, but due to the lack of labeling regulations of herbal products, comfrey may or may not be listed as an ingredient on these products.

Germander, an herb marketed as safe and natural, was at one time widely used in France as a weight-loss remedy. Since 1992, this herb has been banned from the French market because it was discovered to be the cause of twenty-six cases of severe hepatitis. Additional cases of hepatitis due to germander were also reported in Canada. It is thought that the *diterpenoid* content of germander is the culprit causing hepatotoxicity.

Chaparral, an herb proclaimed to be an aging retardant, has been reported to cause jaundice, fulminant hepatitis, and liver damage. In one reported case, the damage was so extensive that the patient required a liver transplant. *Jin Bu Huan,* typically used as an herbal sedative, has been reported to cause acute hepatitis. Some herbs may be dangerous to ingest while pregnant. In fact, death of a newborn baby was reported in a woman who consumed a hepatotoxic herbal preparation during pregnancy.

The above are just a few brief examples of herbs that have led to liver damage, which is often permanent and occasionally fatal, though sometimes reversible. Though the following list of herbs that are known to have caused liver problems is long, it cannot be considered complete due to unreported data. Herbs that have been associated with liver disease include the following:

- Buckthorn (*Rhamnus cathartica*).

- Chaparral (also known as creosote bush or greasewood) (*Larrea taridentata*).

- Comfrey and other herbs containing pyrrolizidine alkaloids (*heliotropium, senecio, crotalaria, symphytum*).

- Germander (*Teucrium chamaedrys*).

- Groundsel (*Senecio vulgaris*).

- Jin Bu Huan.

- Lobelia (*Lobelia inflata*).

- Ma huang (*ephedra*).

- Mate (also known as paraquay tea) (*Ilex paraguariensis*).

- Mistletoe (*Viscum album*).

- Nutmeg (*Myristica fragrans*).

- Pau d'arco (*La pachol*).

- Pennyroyal (*Mentha pulegium*).

- Poke root (*Phytolacca americana*).

- Ragwort (*Senecio jacoboea*).

- Sarsparilla (*Smilax species*).

- Sassafras (*Sassafras albidum*).

- Senna (*Casio acutifolia*).

- Skullcap (*Scutellaria laterifolia*).

- Sweet clover (*Melilotus officinalis*).

- Tansy (*Tanacetum vulgare*).

- T'u-san-chi.

- Valerian (*Valeriana offinalis*).

- Woodruff (*Galium odorata*).

- Certain Chinese herbal formulas—a complex mixture of a variety of different herbs.

- Herbal preparations containing "ecstasy" (3,4-Methylenedioxymetamphetamine).

- Herbal preparation known as "Prostata," which contains saw palmetto.

OTHER ALTERNATIVE TREATMENTS FOR LIVER DISEASE

It is important for people to explore the feasibility of all options that are available to treat hepatitis and liver disease. However, it is also important that they not allow themselves to be fooled into trying therapies that simply do not work or that may exacerbate their liver conditions. Conventional medical therapies have proved their ability to save the lives of many people with liver disease. It is important to keep this point in mind when considering alternative treatments as a substitute for the time-tested conventional therapies. This section discusses some alternative therapies other than herbs that people with hepatitis or other liver diseases may be tempted to try.

Ozone Therapy

Most people are somewhat familiar with the ozone layer. This protective layer in the atmosphere is responsible for absorbing toxic forms of radiation emitted from the sun. Without this protective layer, all forms of life on the earth would die. Proponents of ozone therapy theorize that because ozone is, in essence, saving our lives, administering it directly into the body can cure a whole host of diseases, including cancer, AIDS, and hepatitis. Advocates of ozone therapy contend that viruses (such as the hepatitis B and C viruses) and other microorganisms that are responsible for causing disease survive and actually flourish in a low oxygen environment. Consequently, they believe that if an oxygen-rich environment (such as ozone, which is made of three oxygen molecules) is substituted for the oxygen-poor environment of the body (oxygen is comprised of two oxygen molecules) that viruses, such as the hepatitis viruses, would die. To date, no study has confirmed this hypothesis. In fact, there have been a few reported cases of people who acquired hepatitis C (and also HIV) as a result of poorly sterilized ozone-therapy equipment. Finally, if ozone can actually kill viral cells, it would also have the potential to kill healthy human cells. Therefore, ozone therapy for people with hepatitis or other liver diseases cannot be recommended at this time.

Alpha-Lipoic Acid Therapy

Alpha-lipoic acid, also known as thioctic acid, is a coenzyme (an enzyme helper) manufactured by the body, which functions as an antioxidant. It also helps cells in the body to produce energy. Alpha-lipoic acid has been proclaimed to be a substance that can protect the liver from toxins. In people with acute liver poisoning (such as from toxic mushrooms or from an acetaminophen overdose), alpha-lipoic acid (administered intravenously) may protect the liver when administered soon after such poisoning. It probably functions similar to the herb milk thistle. However, these findings are based on anecdotal reports. In people with chronic liver disease, there is no conclusive evidence that alpha-lipoic acid protects the liver, slows progression of disease, reverses cirrhosis, or eradicates chronic hepatitis B or C. Therefore, until further research establishes the efficacy of this coenzyme, it cannot be recommended to people with chronic liver disease.

Thymosin Therapy

The thymus is a gland located in the neck that secretes hormones (*thymosin, thymopoietin,* and *serum thymic factor*) involved in the regulation of the immune system. These hormones may stimulate the body's production of interferon. People with low levels of these hormones are often susceptible to infection. Thus, some researchers have suggested that people with hepatitis B and C possibly can benefit from the administration of thymus gland hormones, either by mouth (Complete Thymic Formula manufactured by Preventive Therapeutics, Inc.) or by injection (Thymosin-alfa 1 manufactured by SciClone Pharmaceuticals).

A study conducted on people with chronic hepatitis C who did not respond to, or who could not tolerate, interferon failed to show any benefits from taking Complete Thymic Formula (an over-the-counter supplement containing thymosin, thymopoietin, thymic humoral factors, herbs, vitamins, minerals, and enzymes). Studies investigating the benefits of injectable thymosin (Thymosin-alfa 1) have yielded mixed results. Used alone, it did not appear to help people with chronic hepatitis C. However, when injectable thymosin was used in combination with interferon, some people experienced a sustained eradication of the virus. Therefore, thymosin-alfa 1 used in combination with interferon may provide some benefit for people with chronic hepatitis C. Further study with a larger group of people is required to confirm the findings of these studies, each of which used a small group of patients. This will be necessary before therapy combining thymosin-alfa 1 with interferon can be recommended for people with chronic hepatitis C.

Metabolic Therapies

Metabolic therapies are based on the belief that harmful substances that accumulate in the body are the cause of disease. These therapies vary, but often include a combination of high-dose vitamins, dietary restrictions, and coffee enemas. For people with liver disease, metabolic therapies can be especially harmful. Metabolic therapy diets usually include high doses of carrot juice. Carrot juice, consumed in excess, may lead to elevated levels of vitamin A, a vitamin that can potentially cause liver damage if taken in extreme dosages. Coffee enemas are purported to stimulate the secretion of bile, eliminate poisons from the liver, and remove these poisons from the body. However, excessive use of enemas may lead to a serious dehydration problem, dangerous electrolyte imbalances, and a loss of muscle tone in the colon leading to chronic constipation. Furthermore, this form of treatment has not been proven to be beneficial for people with liver disease and should be avoided.

Megadose Vitamin Therapy

Some alternative practitioners believe that megadoses of vitamins (in the case of hepatitis, megadoses of vitamin C) can cure disease. This belief is unsubstantiated. Furthermore, megadose vitamin therapy is potentially harmful. Since vitamin C promotes the absorption of iron, toxic levels of iron may accumulate in the liver, leading to additional damage. Also, as discussed in Chapter 23, megadoses of vitamin A can lead to severe liver damage. Therefore, megadose vitamin therapy is not recommended.

Other Alternative Therapies

There are numerous (too numerous to describe in this book) alternative therapies that, although they have no proven merit, are being touted as being beneficial to the liver. These therapies include placing hot and cold castor oil packs on the skin over the area of the liver (supposedly to draw poisons out of the body) and using medicinal mushrooms, such as reishi, which can be deadly if confused with the liver-toxic mushroom amanita. Any alternative therapy that a person may be considering should first be discussed with her liver specialist.

Supportive Therapy

Supportive therapy from friends, loved ones, religious groups, and other organizations is an important part of getting better, no matter what liver disease a person has. Some people find that joining a local support group is also helpful. In fact, it has been medically proven that psychological and moral support can help people get better faster and live longer lives. So, while supportive therapy is technically not a form of alternative therapy, it should be considered an important adjunctive therapy for all people with liver disease.

RECOMMENDATIONS CONCERNING THE USE OF ALTERNATIVE THERAPIES

The role of alternative therapies for the treatment of people with liver disease and hepatitis remains to be conclusively established. Many studies performed to date and their conclusions are based on animal subjects, and most of the clinical trials conducted on humans lasted only a short period of time (approximately one to two months in many studies) and involved small numbers of people. Many studies with encouraging results unfortunately used generalized terms such as "liver disease" or "hepatitis." So, which liver diseases actually improved as a result of the alternative therapy utilized in the study is unclear. Therefore, any benefits to the liver achieved with an alternative therapy may not be equally applicable to all liver diseases. Furthermore, follow-up observation time was too short to attribute any long-term benefit to most alternative therapies studied.

While a decrease in liver enzymes was demonstrated in many people treated with a given alternative therapy (such as people with hepatitis C treated with milk thistle), the therapy's effect on other parameters (such as HCV RNA viral loads in the case of people with hepatitis C treated with milk thistle) was typically not addressed. Furthermore, whether liver enzyme normalization was sustained once the alternative therapy was discontinued was also not addressed in all studies. Finally, the effect of the alternative therapy on inflammation and/or scarring (as per liver biopsy samples before and after therapy) was not addressed in any alternative therapy study. So, taking these issues into consideration, the following list contains some guidelines that a person interested in exploring alternative therapies for liver disease and hepatitis should follow:

- If a person decides to try an alternative treatment regimen, her liver specialist should be informed of this. This will allow the doctor to monitor the results of the alternative therapy through blood tests and physical exams. Furthermore, the doctor will be able to observe the patient with an eye towards possible adverse effects. The patient should keep a diary of symptoms, side effects, and laboratory reports. This is necessary in order to assess the degree of improvement and to track adverse reactions.

- The patient should be jointly managed by the conventional medical doctor and the alternative healthcare practitioner. This will help minimize any conflicting therapies and will facilitate prompt recognition of an adverse reaction due to therapy.

- Licensure laws and practice guidelines for alternative healthcare practitioners vary from state to state. It is important for a person to review the credentials of the alternative healthcare provider who she is considering seeing. Some helpful information concerning questions to ask a prospective doctor can be found in Chapter 4.

- Any alternative therapy that the patient intends to use should be fully researched by both the patient and the conventional medical doctor prior to commencement of therapy. There are numerous reference books and resources that will enable a person to investigate a particular alternative remedy or find the most knowledgeable alternative medicine practitioners (see the Appendix for a list of these resources).

- If an herb is being used, start with the lowest dose recommended. Do not exceed usage for over six month's time or for longer than any of the study periods. Also, since most studies on the benefits of milk thistle observed positive results within one month, it is probably advisable to discontinue its use if benefits are not experienced within this time period. The same holds true for any herbal preparation.

- Do not use herbal mixtures that contain a variety of herbs and other components.

- If at any time side effects are experienced, or if a woman discovers that she is pregnant, the alternative therapy should be discontinued immediately. Under such circumstances, the patient should promptly alert her doctor of her pregnancy or of the side effects experienced.

- It is important to keep in mind that any form of alternative therapy, no matter how harmless, no matter how safe, may still have the effect of endangering a person if its use delays the commencement of a proven therapy. No matter how effective an alternative therapy claims to be, it should never be substituted for proven medical therapies. It is essential that all people discuss the full range of conventional options with their doctors before starting alternative remedies.

• The validity of some alternative therapies for people with liver disease or hepatitis may ultimately be established through controlled medical studies. Standardized double-blinded, placebo-controlled studies must be conducted before any alternative therapy can be recommended for use in the treatment of liver disease. Research in this area is ongoing, but needs to be conducted in large numbers of people in a reproducible manner.

CONCLUSION

Disillusionment with conventional medicine (especially in light of the less-than-optimal success rate in the treatment of chronic hepatitis C) has led many people with hepatitis and other liver diseases to seek out alternative treatments—the majority of which do not have sufficient research backing them. The surge of interest in the area of alternative medicine will undoubtedly spark some rigorously conducted research protocols that will hopefully provide the answers to exactly what and how much benefit an alternative therapy has on the liver. Such studies should be aimed at clearly defining those groups of people who can benefit from herbal remedies and/or other alternative treatments. Furthermore, these studies should provide guidance on whether to administer such remedies alone or in combination with more conventional treatments. Medical therapy for liver disease may eventually see a mutually beneficial partnership between conventional and alternative therapy. Certainly, this appears to be the outlook for the future.

When all therapies, whether conventional, alternative, or a combination of the two fail in a person suffering from complications of liver disease, liver transplantation is the only viable option. The next chapter discusses this operation.

22

Liver Transplantation

Fortunately, most people with chronic liver disease will never need a liver transplant. So why read this chapter? Well, all people who have chronic liver disease are at risk (which varies depending upon a multitude of factors) for the associated complications of chronic liver disease. These include cirrhosis, liver failure, liver cancer, and intolerable symptoms, such as severe itching and fatigue. If one or more of these complications occur, a person may become a candidate for a liver transplant. Therefore, all people with chronic liver disease and their family members can benefit by reading this chapter to increase their understanding of liver transplantation. More important, it is crucial for people to be aware that liver transplantation is an accepted standard treatment option for those with liver failure and that it is a quite successful, life-saving operation.

Only people who have the greatest likelihood of survival should undergo a liver transplant; therefore, this chapter discusses those people who make good candidates and those people who make poor candidates for transplantation. This chapter also discusses the evaluation process that leads to a person becoming listed for a liver transplant. General indications for transplantation and specific indications based on individual liver disorders are detailed. The biggest problem in the field of liver transplantation is that there is an ever growing scarcity of available livers for donation. This issue and some potential solutions to this problem are also discussed in this chapter. Issues of post-transplant medications and what to expect after a liver transplant conclude this chapter.

THE HISTORY AND SUCCESS RATE OF LIVER TRANSPLANTS

The first successful human-to-human liver transplant was performed by Dr. Thomas Starzl in 1968. (The first attempt at liver transplantation occurred in 1963 but was unsuccessful.) Liver transplantation is now a routinely successful operation. The high success rate is due to the many advances that have occurred since the early days of transplantation, when the one-year survival rate after a liver transplant was less than 30 percent. Now, approximately 85 to 90 percent of people will survive at least one year, and approximately 75 to 85 percent of people will survive at least five years after receiving a new liver. Not only can people live a long life after a liver transplant (one person has been living with a transplanted liver for over twenty-eight years!), but the quality of life is typically excellent. Most people can return to their regular jobs and daily routines without limitations.

According to the website maintained by United Network for Organ Sharing (UNOS), there are currently 123 transplant centers in the United States. In 1997, there were 4,167 liver transplants performed in the United States—out of a transplant waiting list that numbered 11,745. In 1999, 12,487 people were on the liver transplant waiting list.

DETERMINING WHO NEEDS A LIVER TRANSPLANT

Simply having chronic liver disease or even cirrhosis does not automatically indicate or qualify a person for a liver transplant. Certainly, a person does not want to wait until it is too late to be evaluated for a transplant. On the other hand, it is not necessary that everybody with chronic liver disease be evaluated for a liver transplant as soon as a liver problem is discovered. So, is there some kind of special gauge hidden on the body that only an experienced liver specialist can see that tells her when it is time to send her patient for a transplant evaluation? Well, not exactly. However, there are some specific criteria that are used when making this decision. Depending on the underlying liver disease, specific indications for liver transplantation vary somewhat. Indications for a transplant that are specific to the cause of liver disease will be addressed on page 316. The following section is a brief discussion of some general indications for liver transplant independent of the cause of liver disease.

GENERAL INDICATIONS FOR LIVER TRANSPLANT

A person is referred for a liver transplant when it is estimated that she will not live more than two years without a new liver. Accordingly, evidence of decompensated cirrhosis (such as ascites, variceal bleeding, or encephalopathy) is an indication for liver transplantation. Any manifestation of liver failure, whether due to acute or chronic liver disease (such as persistent jaundice or coagulopathy) is an indication for liver transplantation. People who have developed liver cancer due to chronic liver disease should also be evaluated for a transplant. People with intolerable symptoms due to chronic liver disease, such as relentless fatigue or intractable itching, that significantly diminish the quality of life, may also be candidates for a liver transplant evaluation. Finally, some people who had liver transplants in which the newly transplanted liver is not functioning are candidates for transplantation. While it is crucial that a patient be evaluated by a liver transplant center once one of the above-mentioned conditions have developed, medical treatment should be the first line of therapy and should be utilized to stabilize the patient until a new liver is available.

THOSE WHO ARE POOR CANDIDATES FOR LIVER TRANSPLANTATION

A liver transplant is obviously a very serious undertaking for everyone involved— the transplant surgeon and the transplant team, the patient, and the patient's loved ones. It is of utmost importance that the decision to go ahead with a liver transplant takes into consideration the probability that a successful outcome will be achieved. There is a shortage of donor livers available for transplantation, and this problem continues to worsen. It stems, in large part, from the improved success rate of liver transplantation. Therefore, when dealing with such a valuable, scarce commodity as a donor liver, the transplant team will always carefully assess whether a person is a good candidate for the operation.

There is a list of conditions that disqualify someone from undergoing a liver transplant because a successful outcome is unlikely. These conditions are known as *absolute contraindications* and include the following:

- HIV positivity.

- Cancer presently existing in an organ other than the liver.

- Severe active infection.

- Active substance abuse (for example, alcohol or heroin).

- Irreversible brain dysfunction.

- Advanced heart or lung disease.

- Pychosocial assessment indicating an inability to adhere to post-liver transplant medication regimen and instructions.

There are many other conditions that are less than optimal for a liver transplant, but do not rule out the possibility. These conditions, which are known as *relative contraindications,* include:

- Age (approximately seventy years old or older).

- Previous cancer in an organ other than the liver. (A two-year or more waiting period is required between treatment of the cancer and liver transplantation. This is due to the high incidence of cancer recurrence when a person is subjected to transplant immunosuppression drugs prior to this two-year plus waiting period.)

- Kidney failure.

- Morbid obesity.

- Malnutrition.

- Prior portosystemic shunts (see page 286).

- A blood clot in the portal vein, known as portal vein thrombosis.

EVALUATING A PATIENT FOR A LIVER TRANSPLANT

Once the doctor has determined that a patient should be evaluated for a liver transplant, many diagnostic tests will need to be performed. First, the patient must meet with, and be evaluated by, the entire liver transplantation team. This team generally consists of a transplant surgeon, liver specialist, psychiatrist, and social worker. Other specialists, such as a cardiologist (heart doctor) or pulmonologist (lung doctor) may also need to be consulted. The opinions of each of these people concerning the patient's suitability for a liver transplant is crucial to reach a final decision. The extent of additional testing required will depend upon the evaluation of these healthcare professionals. Such testing may include special imaging studies of the liver, heart exams such as a stress test, and further blood tests. Finally, financial issues are considered.

Since the evaluation process can seem scary and overwhelming, it's always a good idea for the patient to bring a family member, loved one, or close friend along to the appointment. Not only will this person serve as emotional support, but she will assist in recalling and sorting through all the details of the day and in helping to arrange future testing.

Once the transplant team determines that a person is a candidate for a liver transplant, she is placed on a waiting list and is ranked according to how urgent the need for transplantation is. Her status on the list will change as her health changes. The most current United Network for Organ Sharing status-ranking system appears in Table 22.1 on page 317. The rankings are based on the points accumulated when assessed for severity of liver disease based on the Child-Turcotte-Pugh (CTP) scoring system, which appears in Table 22.2 on page 318. The more points accumulated, the higher the status on the transplant list. Patients are also listed according to their blood type and donor size requirements—height, weight, chest circumference, and liver volume. It should be noted, however, that these current criteria are subject to change by UNOS and have been altered over the years.

TRANSPLANTATION FOR SPECIFIC LIVER DISEASES

Regardless of the cause of chronic liver disease, when all medical therapies have failed or if complications from cirrhosis have developed, liver transplantation must be considered. The general indications for liver transplantation were discussed on page 314. This section discusses liver transplantation for specific liver diseases, all of which were discussed in detail in either Part Two or Part Three.

Hepatitis A

People with hepatitis A (discussed in Chapter 8) do not progress to chronic liver dis-

Table 22. 1. United Network for Organ Sharing Criteria for Liver Transplantation

STATUS	CONDITION
Status 1	Patient has fulminant liver failure, or patient has dysfunction of a newly transplanted liver within seven days of transplantation.
Status 2A	Patient is hospitalized in intensive care unit (ICU) for chronic liver failure with a life expectancy of less than seven days and CTP score greater than 10.
Status 2B	CTP score of greater than 10 or CTP score of greater than 7 and one of the following: 1) Active variceal bleed that continues after adequate therapy (for example, endoscopic sclerotherapy) and patient requires blood transfusions. Surgical shunts either contraindicated or failed. 2) Hepatorenal syndrome (HRS) (see Chapter 6) 3) Spontaneous bacterial peritonitis (SBP) (see Chapter 6) 4) Refractory ascites (ascites nonresponsive to medical therapy). Surgical shunts either contraindicated or failed.
Status 3	Patient requires continuous medical care either in a hospital (for less than five days) or at home. CTP score greater than 7.
Status 7	Patient is stable and is temporarily unsuitable for transplant.

ease. Therefore, the usual indications for liver transplantation, which were discussed on page 314, do not apply to people with hepatitis A. However, in very rare instances (about 100 cases per year), people with hepatitis A develop a particularly severe form of acute hepatitis known as fulminant hepatitis A, which was discussed in Chapters 7 and 8. These people become extremely ill, developing severe jaundice (yellow tint to the skin and eyes), encephalopathy (mental confusion leading to coma), and coagulopathy (bleeding tendency noted by a prolonged prothrombin time). Liver failure develops abruptly—usually within eight weeks from the onset of symptoms or within two weeks from the onset of jaundice. Everyone with fulminant hepatitis A needs immediate hospitalization in an intensive care unit and prompt referral for a liver transplant. People who receive liver transplants due to fulminant liver failure have approximately a 70-percent chance of surviving one year, which is much lower for people who receive a liver transplant due to complications of cirrhosis.

Hepatitis B

Approximately 5,000 people die each year in the United States from liver failure due to hepatitis B (discussed in Chapter 9). Therefore, liver transplantation can be a potentially life-saving option for people with complications due to hepatitis B.

Table 22.2. Severity of Liver Disease According to the Child-Turcotte-Pugh Scoring System

Points	1	2	3
Encephalopathy	None	Grade 1–2	Grade 3–4
Ascites	Absent	Controlled by diuretics	Present despite diuretics
Albumin (g/dl)	Less than 3.5	2.8–3.5	Greater than 2.8
Prothrombin time (PT) (seconds prolonged)	Less than 4	4–6	Greater than 6
Bilirubin	Less than 2	2–3	Greater than 3
Bilirubin for PBC only	Less than 4	4–10	Greater than 10

However, as compared with transplantation due to other liver diseases, initial results for people who received transplants due to hepatitis B-related liver failure were very poor. Prior to current preventive therapies, the chance that the hepatitis B virus (HBV) would reinfect the newly transplanted liver was approximately 80 percent. And in people who had high levels of HBV DNA prior to transplantation, reinfection was almost universal. Some of these people developed severe acute hepatitis B after transplantation, which led to immediate retransplantation. Others developed rapidly progressive liver damage leading to liver failure and/or death. In fact, cirrhosis has been seen to occur in people reinfected with HBV after transplantation in as little as one year! Whereas the five-year survival rate after transplantation is approximately 80 to 85 percent for all other liver diseases, until recently, the five-year survival rate for people who received a liver transplant due to hepatitis B was only 48 percent. Fortunately, many new treatment modalities (discussed below) have been devised that not only decrease the patient's chance of reinfecting the new liver with HBV, but can also significantly prolong the lives of those who receive a transplant due to hepatitis B.

Administration of the hepatitis B immune globulin (HBIG) has been proven to be effective in preventing, or at least delaying, reinfection of the new liver in many people. When HBIG is given both before and after transplantation, the risk of recurrence of hepatitis B may be reduced to between 10 and 40 percent. And the five-year survival rate after transplantation for people with hepatitis B who receive HBIG is now equivalent to that of people undergoing transplantation for other liver diseases! However, since recurrence of hepatitis B may still occur even with HBIG therapy, other treatment options are being evaluated.

Alfa interferon (discussed in Chapters 11, 12, and 13) given in small doses—1.5 million units, three times per week—may be beneficial for some people with decompensated cirrhosis due to hepatitis B in that it may lessen or possibly eradicate HBV DNA prior to transplantation. This may decrease the likelihood of post-transplant reinfection with HBV. However, alfa interferon may prompt rejection of the new liver, and therefore, after transplant it should be used with extreme caution.

Lamivudine (an oral antiviral medication discussed in Chapter 12) has also been proven to be beneficial in preventing reinfection when given before and after transplantation. In fact, lamivudine has eradicated detectable HBV DNA levels in people who suffered a recurrence of HBV after a transplant, despite having received preventive therapy with HBIG. Whether people will need to continue lamivudine therapy lifelong is being evaluated. The biggest challenge to lamivudine therapy appears to be the development of mutations of HBV DNA that are resistant to further therapy. Possibly, lamivudine in combination with HBIG may be the optimal regimen for the prevention of hepatitis B after liver transplantation.

Ganciclovir (an intravenously administered nucleoside analogue) and famciclovir (an oral nucleoside analogue) appear to decrease HBV DNA levels after transplantation in some people. (These drugs were discussed in Chapter 12.) While these treatments may cause an improvement in liver inflammation due to recurrent hepatitis B, HBV DNA levels may return after these agents are discontinued. Further study on these drugs is necessary in order to determine optimum dose and duration of use.

Combination therapy using HBIG and lamivudine appears to be very promising and may be the therapy of choice if further study confirms existing results. Other combinations, such as the simultaneous use of two nucleoside analogues, are currently being investigated.

In conclusion, all people with hepatitis B, especially those with high HBV DNA levels, need to be treated with some form of viral suppressive therapy prior to undergoing liver transplantation.

Hepatitis D

People who are coinfected with the hepatitis B virus (HBV) and the hepatitis delta virus (HDV) have a lower incidence of reinfection of the new liver compared with people infected with HBV alone. (Coinfection with HBV and HDV was discussed in Chapter 9) If reinfection does occur, it is usually mild. When these coinfected people receive HBIG prior to undergoing liver transplantation, the incidence of reinfection is only approximately 13 percent.

Hepatitis C

Liver failure due to chronic hepatitis C is the most common reason for liver transplantation in the United States. Recurrence of the hepatitis C virus (HCV) in the newly transplanted liver occurs in practically all cases. Reinfection with HCV can lead to cirrhosis, liver failure, or death. Accordingly, retransplantation (a second transplant) is often necessary. Despite this fact, five-year survival rates among people who receive a transplant due to hepatitis C are comparable to survival rates for people who receive transplants for other liver diseases. However, there is clearly a small group of people who fare poorly after transplantation. Most (but not all) studies have identified this group as having high pretransplant HCV RNA loads and genotype 1b (see Chapter 10). In fact, approximately 15 to 20 percent of people with hepatitis C have a rapidly progressive course within five years after transplantation. Cirrhosis may occur in less than two years from transplantation in some people, and approximately 10 percent of people develop failure of the new liver, making retransplantation necessary. Unfortunately, retransplantation for people with hepatitis C has been associated with a poor outcome. Less than 40 percent of these people survive one year. Therefore, the focus is on prevention, or at least suppression, of viral replication after transplantation.

Levels of HCV RNA are generally higher after transplantation than before transplantation—to the tune of approximately 10 to 200 times the pretransplant level. This is due presumably to the fact that the immunosuppresive therapy (such as the corticosteroid prednisone) that is administered after a liver transplant, increases viral replication and thereby enhances the risk of recurrent hepatitis C. Therefore, if the amount of immunosuppression is either decreased or discontinued soon after transplantation, the HCV RNA load should decrease. This approach is currently being evaluated. In fact, some transplant centers routinely discontinue corticosteroid therapy within six months after transplantation. Furthermore, the use of the antirejection immunosuppresive agent tacrolimus as opposed to the antirejection immunosuppressive agent cyclosporine (see After the Transplant on page 328) requires significantly lower doses of prednisone to achieve adequate immunosuppression. Therefore, it is recommended that people who undergo transplantation due to chronic hepatitis C be placed on tacrolimus for immunosuppression.

Prevention of reinfection with HCV of the new liver has been the target of much research. Unfortunately, interferon therapy for recurrent hepatitis C after transplantation has had minimal success. Furthermore, it has been associated with an increased rate of rejection of the new liver. However, if given soon after transplant when HCV RNA load is still low, interferon therapy has been shown to have some benefit in reducing the incidence of recurrent hepatitis C. Studies using interferon combined with ribavirin (Rebetron) administered after the transplant appear to be very promising, and this may become the treatment regimen of choice. Further studies are being conducted to confirm the efficacy of this treatment regimen and to determine if all people or strictly those at high risk for a poor outcome should routinely start this after transplant.

Autoimmune Hepatitis

Despite the availability of successful medical therapy, approximately 20 percent of people with autoimmune hepatitis (AIH; discussed in Chapter 14) become candidates for a liver transplant. This may be due to the development of complications of cirrhosis or to failure to respond to medical therapy (for example, corticosteroids and azathioprine) after attempting treatment for approximately four years. The success rate of transplantation in people with AIH is excellent, with approximately 92 percent of people living at least five years after liver transplantation. Autoantibodies generally disappear within two years from the time of transplantation. Although it is uncommon, the disease may recur after transplantation. Recurrence can usually be managed successfully by adjustment of immunosuppressive drug dosages. Although dosages of immunosuppressive drugs may be decreased after transplantation, total discontinuation is not recommended.

Primary Biliary Cirrhosis

People with primary biliary cirrhosis (PBC; discussed in Chapter 15) have a very slow, yet relentlessly progressive disease course that spans approximately twenty years. Medical therapy (ursodeoxycholic acid, for example) has been shown to slow the progression of disease, thus delaying the need for a liver transplant in some people. Nonetheless, these people continue to advance to cirrhosis and its complications or to have symptoms associated with PBC, such as osteoporosis (bone loss), severe fatigue, or uncontrollable pruritus (itching), any of which may necessitate liver transplantation. In fact, between 5 and 18 percent of people who undergo liver transplantation for PBC do so because fatigue or pruritus has significantly diminished their quality of life. Liver transplantation ultimately leads to improvement in bone strength. However, this benefit is not seen until a year after the transplant due to the use of high doses of corticosteroids and the initial period of inactivity after transplantation, each of which weakens bones.

Five variables should be taken into consideration when the decision is being made to refer a person with PBC for a liver transplant. These variables are the person's age, the bilirubin level, the albumin level, the prothrombin time, and the presence or absence of edema (leg swelling). When these five variables are applied to a special formula—known as the "Mayo Clinic risk score or natural history model for PBC"—it can be calculated approximately how many more years a person with PBC is expected to live. This formula may be used to optimally estimate the point at which a person should be referred for transplantation. Of the variables, it appears that a persistently rising bilirubin level is the most significant indicator of the need for a liver transplant. In fact, it has been shown that once the bilirubin level rises above 10 milligrams per deciliter, the person has slightly more than one year to live. Therefore, some transplantation centers use a bilirubin level of approximately 6.0 milligrams per deciliter as a criterion for listing a person with PBC for a transplant.

PBC accounts for about 10 percent of liver transplantations in the United States. People with PBC do very well after liver transplantation. Approximately 88 percent of them survive at least five years. Typically, these people enjoy a good quality of life and can return to their normal lifestyles.

Unlike the disappearance of the antinuclear antibody after transplant in people with AIH, the antimitochondrial antibody remains elevated in people who receive transplants due to PBC. It appears that PBC can recur in the new liver. However, since the disease is so slowly progressive, it will take many years for any significant symptoms to occur, if they occur at all.

Nonalcoholic Steatohepatitis

Statistics peg nonalcoholic steatohepatitis (NASH; discussed in Chapter 16) as accounting for approximately 1 percent of transplants in the United States. However, this percentage is probably underestimated, since many of the cases of cirrhosis referred for liver transplantation that have no definable cause are most likely due to NASH. NASH may recur in the new liver and may cause a rapid progression to cirrhosis. The likelihood of this happening, however, is unknown. Since NASH is a relatively newly defined syndrome, research on all aspects of this disease is ongoing.

Alcoholic Liver Disease

The subject of liver transplantation for people with alcoholic liver disease (ALD; discussed in Chapter 17) has been an ongoing area of controversy. Some have argued that since livers are such a scarce resource, a person who consciously caused her liver failure by deliberately abusing alcohol should not be given the chance to be listed for a transplant. Others have argued that alcoholism is a disease, and as such, it is not a person's "fault" that she has liver failure due to excessive alcohol use and should therefore be given the same chance at a new liver as anyone else with liver disease.

A viewpoint somewhere in the middle currently prevails on the issue of transplantation for people with ALD. Once the patient is aware of the consequences that have occurred due to her alcohol abuse, it is then considered to be her responsibility to successfully complete a rehabilitation process and to adhere to lifelong abstinence. The rehabilitation process may include Alcoholics Anonymous (AA), an inpatient rehabilitation program, and psychiatric treatment. After sobriety has been achieved for a sustained duration, the person may then be considered a candidate for a liver transplant. While UNOS does not utilize a defined abstinence interval, the length of time of documented abstinence has been arbitrarily chosen to be six months by many transplantation centers. The person with ALD must also demonstrate that she has a stable social support system in the form of a loved one or a friend, and that she does not have other substance abuse problems or psychiatric disorders. A patient is removed from the list if she does not comply with medication instructions, office visits, medical advice, dietary restrictions, or, of course, if she returns to alcohol use.

Numerous people with ALD have undergone successful liver transplants. In fact, transplantation for ALD makes up approximately 20 percent of transplants performed in the United States. Survival rates after transplant are excellent and are similar to that of people transplanted for other causes of liver failure.

After transplantation, people have lived active and productive lives, without recidivism (relapsing back to old bad behavior, in this case, drinking alcohol). Return to alcohol abuse after transplantation occurs in approximately 15 to 20 percent of people within three years. After transplantation, the patient is advised to continue Alcoholics Anonymous (AA) meetings until a psychiatrist determines that the risk of recidivism is unlikely.

Hemochromatosis

When the diagnosis of hemochromatosis (discussed in Chapter 18) is made early and treatment is begun promptly prior to the development of cirrhosis, people with hemochromatosis usually have a normal life-expectancy. However, when hemochromatosis is not discovered until after cirrhosis has already developed or if a person does not adhere to a strict phlebotomy schedule, long-term complications of liver disease may occur, necessitating liver transplantation.

Liver transplantation for people with hemochromatosis has not been as successful as transplantation for other liver diseases. People with hemochromatosis appear to have an increased incidence of developing infections and heart failure after transplantation. This accounts for the poor survival rates of people with hemochromatosis after transplant. In fact, the chance of surviving one year after transplant is only approximately 60 percent, and the chance of surviving five years after transplant is approximately 55 percent. Survival after transplant is significantly improved if iron depletion is performed prior to transplant. In these cases, there is a one-year survival rate of 75 to 83 percent.

People with both hemochromatosis and cirrhosis are 200 times more likely to develop liver cancer compared with the general population. In fact, approximately 27 percent of people who receive transplants due to hemochromatosis have been found to have liver cancer, and approximately 19 percent of these liver cancers were not even diagnosed until the time of transplant. Surprisingly, the discovery of an incidental liver cancer found during transplantation in people with hemochromatosis does not appear to significantly decrease the chances of living for one year beyond transplant.

It is unknown whether hemochromatosis recurs in the new liver. Since iron stores increase slowly in people with hemochromatosis, a study monitoring a large number of people for ten to twenty years after transplantation is needed to accurately answer this question.

Liver Tumors

People discovered to have a malignant liver tumor (discussed in Chapter 19) should consider surgical resection (the removal of the tumor) as the first option. Unfortunately, only approximately 30 percent of people with liver cancer have surgically resectable tumors at the time they are diagnosed. When the tumor's size or location prevents resection, or if cirrhosis is present, liver transplantation should be considered. Liver transplantation has the potential to remove not only the tumor, but also the underlying cirrhosis, since the entire liver is replaced. Unfortunately, most people in the United States with liver cancer who undergo transplantation have cirrhosis due to hepatitis C or B, and these viruses invariably recur in the newly transplanted liver. Thus, the underlying disease usually recurs, thereby setting the stage for another tumor to grow.

The same prognostic factors that are associated with survival that apply to transplantation apply to surgical resection. The best outcomes normally occur in young, otherwise healthy people, who have one small tumor (less than 5 centimeters in size) or two to three tiny tumors (all less than 3 centimeters in size) limited to the liver alone—meaning that the cancer has not spread to lymph nodes, surrounding vessels, or other organs. In fact, survival after liver transplantation performed on otherwise healthy people with small, isolated tumors is approximately 75 percent at four years. Similarly, 90 percent of people who undergo liver transplantation, and who are incidentally discovered to have a small tumor, survive for at least five years.

For people who do not possess the above-mentioned ideal characteristics, recurrence of liver cancer is high, and long-term survival after transplantation is low. Much research is being conducted in the hope of decreasing recurrence and improving survival times for these people. One promising therapy involves the use of chemotherapy drugs at various intervals before, during, and/or after transplantation. Other studies utilizing different types of therapies, such as cryosurgery or ethanol injections in combination, are also being conducted.

LIVER DONORS

Despite the growing success and acceptance by doctors and patients alike of liver transplantation, the average number of donor organs available at any given time has continued to remain the same. The result has been that the demand for livers far outweighs the supply. In this respect, liver transplantation has become a victim of its own success. And each year the gap widens further. The number of people placed on the transplant list continues to grow at a faster rate than the number of available donor organs. Approximately 12,500 to 27,000 potential organ donors die each year in the United States. That's a lot of livers—enough to cover the amount of people on a waiting list. So, why is there a shortage of livers? Well, unfortunately only 15 to 20 percent of suitable organ donors become actual organ donors for various reasons. This section discusses some issues associated with organ donation, and some ways that have been devised to increase the number of livers available for transplantation.

General Criteria for Organ Donation

One of the most important steps toward a successful outcome of a liver transplant is choosing an appropriate donor liver. Thus, it is crucial to eliminate those donors whose livers have a poor chance of functioning properly.

The major source of livers for donation comes from brain-dead people with a functioning heart and circulatory system. A designated family member must sign a witnessed consent form allowing donation. If the potential donor has AIDS, is infected with HIV, has cancer (except of the skin or brain), or has evidence of active hepatitis B, the liver may not be used as a donor under any circumstances. Ideally, the donor's liver function tests (LFTs) should be normal, and the donor's liver should contain no more than 30-percent fat. It has been shown that donor fatty livers (see Chapter 16) function quite poorly and are often rejected soon after transplantation. The body size and blood type of the donor and the recipient should be compatible. The donor's age should preferably be under fifty.

In an effort to increase the number of suitable donor livers available for transplantation, the above criteria have become somewhat less stringent. Livers from donors over the age of fifty, and sometimes even those as old as seventy, have been used with favorable results. Livers from donors who have hepatitis C have been utilized in cases where the patient undergoing the transplant also has hepatitis C.

Education and promotion of organ donation among lay people and healthcare professionals is needed to help to expand the donor pool. In the United States, in order for a person to donate an organ, she must obtain and sign an organ donor card. This card must be carried at all times. Finally, it is important for the potential donor to notify family members concerning her wishes about organ donation. This will eliminate any confusion or uncertainty regarding this issue at the time of death.

Split-Liver Transplantation

Sometimes, one viable donor liver is split in two, with each half being transplanted into a separate person. This procedure, known as *split-liver transplantation,* would obviously double the number of livers available for donation. Usually, an adult receives the larger right side of the liver, and a child or small adult receives the smaller left side of the liver. However, newer techniques are enabling a more even split, so that one donor liver can be utilized for two adult patients. The first split-liver operation was performed in 1988. Since that time, major advances in surgical and technical expertise and experience have occurred, allowing this procedure to be employed with increasing frequency and success. So far, this procedure appears to be very promising. Patients appear to have a survival rate after transplant that approximates the survival rate after conventional whole liver transplantation.

Living Donors

Living liver donation involves the removal of the left lobe of the liver from an adult, and its transplantation typically into a child. This technique offers another means of expanding the existing liver donor pool. The adult may be either related to the recipient (*living-related liver donor*) or not related (*live-unrelated liver donor*). In either case, the donor must have a compatible blood type with the recipient. Approximately 30 percent of parents are not suitable donors for their children. The first successful living-related liver transplantation in the United States occurred in 1989. The success rate of this type of liver transplantation appears to be excellent, with approximately 94 percent of children still alive one year after transplantation.

Mortality rate among the living donor is exceptionally low, approximately 0.05 percent. With time, the donor's liver will regenerate the segment that was donated.

While living-donor transplantation has significantly helped the liver-donor shortage in the pediatric age group, it has not solved the donor shortage in adults. A major stumbling block to this procedure in adults has been the quantity of the donor's liver that needs to be removed. Obviously, a larger percentage of liver needs to be removed from the living donor if an adult is the recipient compared with the amount required to be removed if a child is the recipient. This adds additional risk, both to the living donor and to the recipient. Often, ethical issues arise, such as whether an adult patient's parent is too old to safely become a donor, or whether an adult patient's child is too young to safely become a donor. Further study on living liver donor transplantation for adult patients will hopefully resolve some of these issues in the years to come.

Auxiliary Transplants

An auxiliary liver transplant involves placing a small portion of a functioning liver from a donor into the body of a person with liver failure, without removing the patient's own liver. Since this procedure would require only part of a liver, either a living donor or the small half of a split liver could be used for an adult. This technique has been used in people with chronic irreversible liver failure, in addition to people with fulminant, potentially reversible, liver failure. Experience with auxiliary transplants in people with chronic irreversible liver failure has been somewhat limited. With more experience, this technique may prove to be helpful for some people for whom a whole liver is unavailable for transplant. For some people with fulminant liver failure, an auxiliary liver may be used temporarily until the patient's own liver recovers (for example, from liver failure due to a drug overdose, which is potentially reversible), then the auxiliary liver can be removed. While there have been some isolated reports of success with this procedure, further study is needed to confirm its efficacy.

Animal Livers

One potential way to solve the dilemma of the shortage of human livers available for transplantation is to not use livers from humans, but to use livers from animals. Known as *xenotransplantation,* this idea is far from new. In ancient times, animal parts were sometimes juxtaposed with human body parts in an attempt to either save the life of the human or in an attempt to create a super-human who would subsequently be worshipped as a god. In the early 1900s, medical experimentation with the concept of xenotransplantation took the form of transplanting kidneys from various animals (pig, goat, lamb, and baboons) into humans. Continued failure of xenotransplantation due to the human body's rejection of the animal organ, combined with increasing knowledge and advances in the field of immunosuppression, led to a decreased interest in xenotransplantation and an increased interest in human-to-human transplantation. However, we have now come full circle as the overwhelming success of human transplantation has resulted in a shortage of human organs. So, once again, scientists have turned to the concept of xenotransplantation in an attempt to resolve or at least significantly reduce the existent problem of liver-donor shortage. Theoretically, xenotransplantation should eliminate the problem of post-transplant recurrence of viral hepatitis in the new liver, as the livers of animals resistant to infection with human viruses would be used for transplantation. Three liver xenotransplants (one pig-to-human and two baboon-to-human) were attempted in the early 1990s, but were unsuccessful.

Problems concerning rejection of the animal organ may potentially be resolved by introducing human "anti-rejection-like" genes into the animal prior to transplantation. While this is a simplified description of what is actually done, this strategy has been attempted using pigs—the so-called "transgenic pig"—with some success. However, one serious problem that must be overcome, which has dampened enthusiasm for this approach, has been the potential for transmission of animal diseases—such as the porcine endogenous retrovirus (PERV)—into humans and the possible consequences that this might entail.

Continued interest and investigation into the area of xenotransplantation continues. One potential use for xenotransplantation may be as a temporary measure—as a means of keeping the patient alive until such time as a suitable human liver becomes available. However, in addition to ironing out the difficulties involving compatibility and rejection of the animal's organ by the human body, certain ethical and safety issues must be resolved before xenotransplantation can become a widely accepted option.

Hepatocyte Transplantation and Gene Therapy

Hepatocyte transplantation involves the infusion of a small number of liver cells (hepatocytes) from a donor liver into a person who has either a genetic defect of the liver (such as Crigler-Najjar syndrome) or fulminant liver failure. The use of hepatocyte transplantation might even eliminate the need for transplantation in some people with fulminant liver failure by enhancing spontaneous recovery. While there have been only limited attempts to implement this procedure in humans, the results appear promising.

Another exciting procedure that is still in the experimental stage is one that involves actually altering the genetic material within the liver cell and then reconstituting it back into the genetically defective liver. Known as *gene therapy,* it is also being evaluated for the potential use in preventing rejection of the donor liver, thereby eliminating the need for post-transplant immunosuppressant medications. These promising techniques are undergoing extensive evaluation.

Liver Dialysis—The Bioartificial Liver

Whereas people with chronic kidney failure can be maintained on dialysis for long periods of time until a donor kidney is located, a comparable form of long-term dialysis for people with liver failure has not been devised. However, there is a method of temporarily treating people with fulminant irreversible liver failure who are awaiting an immediate liver transplant (within a few days) or who have fulminant, potentially reversible, liver failure. These forms of liver dialysis are known as *liver assist devices*. These devices are designed to remove toxins from the blood of people with liver failure. Preliminary results show that this type of device may be effective in improving the liver function and mental status of some patients with reversible fulminant liver failure, thereby allowing the injured liver sufficient time to completely recover. Furthermore, this device may serve as a time-sparing method—by keeping people who are awaiting immediate liver transplantation alive for several extra days.

A further advance in this type of device is to provide entire liver function instead of simply removing toxins. This is achieved by adding functioning liver cells into the liver device. There are a few such devices currently in use. Some promising results have been reported. Additional data is required before recommendations on these types of devices can be made.

AFTER THE TRANSPLANT

The major hurdle that a person faces after a liver transplant is whether or not her body will accept the new liver as if it were its own. Rejection of the liver occurs if the patient's body does not recognize the new liver as belonging to itself. Therefore, similar to the situation that occurs in people with autoimmune hepatitis (AIH; discussed in Chapter 14), the body's immune system may attack the new liver in an attempt to reject it from the body. When this happens, the new liver may become damaged, or, even worse, it may become totally nonfunctional (rejected by the body).

This dilemma was the major stumbling block to successful liver transplantation prior to 1983. Since 1983, however, a powerful group of effective medications have become available to help reduce the likelihood of rejection. These medications are known as *immunosuppressants*. Beyond the first year after transplantation, rejection of the new liver is very uncommon. And, within the first year of transplantation, the incidence of rejection has been on the decline. While rejection rates were once approximately 15 to 20 percent, they are now as low as 2 percent in many transplant centers. (People with primary biliary cirrhosis and autoimmune hepatitis have a higher incidence of rejection).

The following is a discussion of the medications that a person may need to take after a transplant in order to prevent rejection, including potential side effects. In addition, this section also discusses what to expect after a transplant. Most people have a totally normal lifestyle and an excellent quality of life after a transplant. This section will also discuss specific issues regarding living with a new liver—such as pregnancy, sexual function, and returning to work.

Post-Transplant Medications and Their Side Effects

After transplantation, a person's immune system needs to be blunted or else the new liver will be rejected by the body. There are now a number of medications available to achieve this goal. These are known as antirejection, immunosuppressive agents. The regimen of post-transplant immunosuppression usually includes a corticosteroid (such as prednisone) combined with either cyclosporine or tacrolimus. Sometimes a third immunosuppressive drug is used—either azathioprine or mycophenelate mofetil. These medications are not without side effects. Furthermore, cyclosporine and tacrolimus may interact with other drugs, which can lead to either toxic levels or less than therapeutic levels of these immunosuppressants. See Table 22.3 on page 330 for a list of drugs that can interfere with an optimal dose of these immunosuppressants. Fortunately, due to the number of immunosuppresive agents now available, each patient may have a regimen individually tailored to minimize side effects and maximize potency, while maintaining a good quality of life.

Cyclosporine (Neoral)

The immunosuppressive properties of cyclosporine were discovered in 1972, and, as of 1983, cyclosporine was routinely used as an antirejection drug. Sandimmune (manufactured by Sandoz Pharmaceuticals) was the original oral form of cyclosporine, but was poorly and erratically absorbed in the digestive tract, leading to difficulties in achieving optimal dosing after transplantation. In 1996, Sandimmune was replaced with Neoral, an improved form of cyclosporine that displayed better gastrointestinal tract absorption, and as such, easier management of dosing.

There are many side effects associated with cyclosporine. Kidney failure may occur, but is readily reversible upon lowering the dosage. Due to changes in sugar (glucose) and fat (lipid) metabolism caused by cyclosporine, the patient may be at increased risk of hypertension (high blood pressure) and heart disease (also known as coronary artery disease). Cyclosporine may also affect the central nervous system—seizures, numbness, confusion, and hallucinations have been experienced by some people while on therapy. Increased hair growth, especially in brunettes, is common. Enlargement of the gums may occur, often necessitating surgical correction. There also appears to be an increased risk of cancer associated with cyclosporine use. Cyclosporine is generally used in combination with corticosteroids. However, some transplant centers add a third immunosuppresive agent, either azathioprine (discussed in Chapter 14) or mycophenolate (discussed on page 331).

Tacrolimus (FK 506 or Prograf)

The immunosuppressive properties of tacrolimus was discovered in 1984, and ten years later it was approved by the FDA specifically for antirejection therapy. Side effects associated with tacrolimus are similar to those of cyclosporine. Tacrolimus has been associated with greater kidney and neurological damage, as compared with

Table 22.3. Drugs That Interact With Cyclosporine and Tacrolimus

Drugs That Increase Levels (may cause toxic levels)	Drugs That Decrease Levels (may cause subtherapeutic levels)
• Erythromycin/Clarithramycin	• Phenytoin
• Ketoconazole	• Barbiturates
• Cimetidine (Tagamet)	• Rifampin
• Corticosteroids	• Alcohol
• Verapamil/Diltiazem	
• Oral contraceptives	
• Nonsteroidal anti-inflammatories	

cyclosporine, according to some, but not all, studies. People may experience insomnia, headache, and decreased alertness while taking tacrolimus. A high glucose level or even the development of diabetes may occur, thereby requiring an adjustment of dosage. Hypertension and high cholesterol levels can occur while on treatment, but this occurs less frequently than with cyclosporine. Less weight gain after transplantation has been noted in patients who were placed on tacrolimus compared with those on cyclosporine. It has been noted that people on tacrolimus may experience an increased incidence of infections. Other associated symptoms that can occur while on tacrolimus include stomach upset, hair loss, and itching.

Which immunosuppressant medications are used is determined on a case-by-case basis, and depends, as well, upon the preference of the transplantation center. Tacrolimus has some advantages over cyclosporine (as noted above) and is the primary immunosuppression drug in most large liver transplant programs in the United States. In fact, some studies have shown that a higher percentage of people may live longer after transplantation if placed on tacrolimus. (Approximately 80 percent of people treated with tacrolimus are alive three years after transplant versus approximately 73 percent of people treated with cyclosporine.) Tacrolimus is generally used in combination with corticosteroids alone; however, some transplant centers use a third immunosuppresive agent (either azathioprine or mycophenolate) as noted above.

Corticosteroids (Prednisone)

Prednisone is a corticosteroid (steroid) that possesses both anti-inflammatory and immunosuppressive actions. (Prednisone was discussed in detail in Chapter 14.) This medication is routinely used after a liver transplant in all patients as part of the antirejection regimen. Steroids were originally part of lifelong immunosuppressive therapy after liver transplantation. However, there is now a growing trend toward discontinuation of steroids after transplantation. This is advantageous, as there are numerous side effects of long-term prednisone use, and the discontinuation of steroids will minimize, or totally eliminate, the potential for developing these side effects. The major question is how soon after transplant is it safe to discontinue steroid use? While some centers are stopping steroids as early as two weeks after transplantation, most centers are more comfortable with discontinuation after at least three months to one year.

Results of people taken off steroids approximately three months after liver transplantation have been excellent. It does not appear that the discontinuation of steroids adversely affects either patient survival or the likelihood of rejection of the new liver. Furthermore, the incidence of medication-induced side effects is significantly less among people taken off prednisone three months after transplantation. After transplantation, high blood pressure occurs only half as much in people taken off steroids as it does in people continuing steroid therapy. And the incidence of developing diabetes appears to be negligible when steroids are discontinued approximately three months post-transplant.

The underlying liver disease leading to transplantation must also be taken into consideration when making a decision concerning withdrawal of steroids. For instance, since steroids stimulate the replication of both the hepatitis B and C viruses, early steroid withdrawal is quite advantageous for people with either hepatitis B or hepatitis C. However, people with autoimmune hepatitis (AIH) may not benefit from early withdrawal of steroids due to the potential for recurrence of AIH in the new liver. In general, determining the best time to withdraw the administration of steroids is done on a case-by-case basis.

Azathioprine

Azathioprine is an immunosuppressive drug with anti-inflammatory properties. It is commonly used to treat people with autoimmune hepatitis (AIH), typically in combination with prednisone, since it possesses "steroid-sparing properties." (Azathioprine was discussed in detail in Chapter 14.) However, use of azathioprine after transplantation has been supplanted by a similar agent known as *mycophenolate mofetil* discussed below.

Mycophenolate Mofetil

Mycophenolate mofetil (CellCept manufactured by Roche Laboratories), a new antirejection drug, works like azathioprine. It is now being used as an immunosuppressant in place of azathioprine. Mycophenolate mofetil has been shown to be effective for people experiencing rejection of a new liver despite the use of prednisone and other immunosuppressive agents. It is also used as an alternative immunosuppressant for people experiencing intolerable side effects from cyclosporine and/or tacrolimus.

Side effects of mycophenolate mofetil include digestive disturbances and bone marrow suppression (decreased white and red cell levels).

Living With a New Liver

If the liver transplant was a success, and if the patient's new liver continues to function well in the immediate aftermath of the procedure, the patient can usually be released from the hospital about a week or two after the operation. However, it is important for the patient to remain close to the transplant center for at least one month after the procedure, as close monitoring of post-transplant medications and the function of the new liver is necessary. Additional care may be required in the form of nutritional supplementation and/or the expedient management of any infections that may occur. Initially, the patient will be required to return to the transplant clinic once or twice a week, depending upon how well she is doing medically and upon how well she is adjusting to the new lifestyle. Visits to the transplant clinic will be required lifelong, but at decreasing frequency over time.

After several months have elapsed since the time of the transplant, the patient can follow up with her local doctor or preferably a liver specialist, instead of traveling to the transplant center. These visits should consist of a physical exam, a discussion of any symptoms or physical complaints the patient may have, and an evaluation of how compliant the patient is with her medication routine. In addition, a battery of blood tests will need to be taken in order to assess how well the new liver is functioning, to check for potential side effects of medications, and to assess whether the optimum dose of immunosuppressive medication is being provided.

As discussed on page 330, there is a trend favoring the discontinuation of steroids shortly after transplantation. The decision concerning when to discontinue steroids depends upon many factors, which can be discussed with the transplant team both before and after surgery. Many transplant centers are presently evaluating the possibility of discontinuing all medication after transplantation. So far, results look promising, but much more research is needed before this becomes a standard procedure.

Most people have a normal lifestyle and a good quality of life after a liver transplant. In women who underwent a transplant, menstruation typically returned within the first year. Therefore, women usually can become pregnant one year after transplantation (see Chapter 24 for more information concerning this matter). Social functioning, sexual activity, and mental health of people who underwent a transplant are usually reported to be equal to that of healthy people. Most people are able to return to work, either with no, or only a minor, decrease in workload. While some people occasionally experience some degree of physical limitation, overall, there appears to be a significantly improved quality of life after transplantation.

CONCLUSION

The advances made in the field of liver transplantation have been truly miraculous. Better surgical skills, better choice of transplant candidates, and improved immunosuppressive medication regimens are just some of the reasons liver transplantation has become so successful, and why it has become the accepted standard treatment for people with liver failure. People usually return to a normal lifestyle after the transplant and typically enjoy a good quality of life.

Future advances in the field of liver transplantation may allow the discontinuation of all medications after a transplant. This would be truly remarkable.

Unfortunately, the major impediment to the miracle of transplantation is the severe shortage of donor livers. While public opinion polls indicate that there is popular support for organ donation, family members commonly refuse to allow an organ to be removed from a recently deceased relative. It is estimated that only about 40 percent of potential organ donors become actual organ donors. The tragic truth is that many people die each year while waiting for a liver to become available, and the number of these deaths (some of which could have been prevented) continues to increase. Therefore, the need to increase public awareness of the importance of organ donation is urgent. In 1999, Pennsylvania became the first state in the United States to offer a monetary stipend of approximately $300 to assist the families of organ donors with the cost of the funeral. It is hoped that this method of providing financial reward for an organ will entice others to become organ donors.

The next chapter discusses ways that people can take active roles in improving their health and possibly prevent some complications of liver disease through diet, nutrition, and exercise.

23

Diet, Nutrition, and Exercise

After being diagnosed with liver disease, some of the first questions that a person typically asks concern nutrition and exercise. Commonly asked questions include: What foods are good for the liver? Are there foods that can harm the liver? Are vitamin supplements helpful? How much protein should I get in my diet? Is it a good idea to exercise? Should certain exercises be avoided? Unfortunately, many doctors lack the expertise to supply knowledgeable answers to these and similar questions. One reason for this is that most medical schools do not spend enough time on the topics of diet, nutrition, and exercise.

As you learned in Chapter 1, everything that enters the body must pass through the liver to be processed. The liver functions as a filter to protect the body from harmful substances and is responsible for the production and use of most nutrients. Therefore, everything that is ingested has an effect on the liver—some positive, some negative. That's why it is advisable for people to eat foods with an eye towards promoting liver health. This is especially true when the liver is damaged. Understanding the basics of nutrition is necessary in order to make intelligent food choices that will benefit the liver. Due to FDA regulations, food labels contain nutritional information. A person with liver disease should always read these labels carefully. Also, most people with liver disease need to restrict some foods from their diets. This should not be viewed as a punishment, but rather as a step in the direction of a healthier liver. Exercise is also an important practice in the fight against liver disease. Regular exercise will increase energy levels, decrease stress on the liver, and, in many cases, will even delay the onset of certain complications associated with liver disease.

The more people know about nutrition and exercise, the more likely they will be to institute and adhere to lifestyles that maximize health and minimize disease. That's why this chapter discusses these important issues. It provides pertinent details concerning protein, carbohydrates, fats, vitamins, and minerals and discusses how nutritional requirements differ depending upon the particular liver disease. Of course, a person—in accordance with her own specific dietary needs and limitations—may vary the recommendations contained in this chapter. This chapter also provides other nutritional information, such as tips on how to dine out while on a restricted diet. Finally, the importance of exercise, both aerobic and weight-bearing, for people with liver disease is discussed.

IS THERE AN OPTIMAL DIET FOR THOSE WITH LIVER DISEASE?

Unfortunately, a person cannot expect to walk into the doctor's office and request "a diet for liver disease." Such an across-the-board diet simply does not exist. Many factors account for the unfeasibility of a standardized liver diet, including variations among the different types of liver disease (for example, alcoholic liver disease versus primary biliary cirrhosis) and the stage of the liver disease (for example, stable liver disease without much damage versus unstable decompensated cirrhosis). Other medical disorders unrelated to liver disease, such as diabetes or heart disease, must also be factored into any diet. Each person has her own individual nutritional requirements, and these requirements may change over time.

It is also important to keep in mind the difference in calorie content among different food groups. While protein and carbohydrate each supply 4 calories per gram, fat supplies 9 calories per gram. It is also important to know that 1 gram of alcohol is equivalent to 7 calories. So alcohol actually supplies more energy in the form of calories to the body than protein and carbohydrates, and just slightly less than that supplied by fat. However, while alcohol may provide a person with some degree of energy, it has absolutely no nutritional value. Therefore, alcohol has been said to provide "empty calories."

GENERAL NUTRITIONAL GUIDELINES FOR LIVER DISEASE

Notwithstanding the above information, an example of an optimal diet for a person with stable liver disease (modifications to be made as per individualized needs) might contain all of the factors listed below. (You'll note that this diet resembles a generalized healthy diet for all people—even those without liver disease. And, in fact, that's exactly what it is!)

- 60- to 70-percent carbohydrates—primarily complex carbohydrates, such as pasta and whole-grain breads.

- 20- to 30-percent protein—only lean animal protein and/or vegetable protein.

- 10- to 20-percent polyunsaturated fat.

- 8- to 12 eight-ounce glasses of water per day.

- 1,000 to 1,500 milligrams of sodium per day.

- Avoidance of excessive amounts of vitamins and minerals, especially vitamin A, vitamin B_3, and iron.

- No alcohol.

- Avoidance of processed food.

- Liberal consumption of fresh organic fruits and vegetables.

- Avoidance of excessive caffeine consumption—no more than 1 to 3 cups of caffeine-containing beverages per day.

- Vitamin D and calcium supplement.

Since everyone eats a wide variety of foods, the liver must constantly be engaged in an intricate balancing act to ensure that the right nutrients get to the right parts of the body in the right amounts. In a healthy person, this balancing act occurs automatically. But when the liver has been weakened or damaged, it has trouble juggling the various nutrients. This is where the person with a liver problem comes in. If she eats the right balance of foods, her already burdened liver won't have to work as hard. Nutrition is one aspect of disease where a person has some degree of control and can actively participate in speeding recovery and minimizing the likelihood of additional injury. The following sections discuss different nutrients in detail.

Protein

Proteins are the major building blocks that the body uses to make body components, such as muscles, hair, nails, skin, and blood. Proteins also make up important parts of the immune system called *antibodies,* which help fight off disease. Proteins are themselves made up of smaller building blocks called *amino acids.* The liver bears primary responsibility for making sure that old proteins get broken down and recycled and that new proteins are always available. Thus, an adequate protein intake is important to build and maintain muscle mass and to assist in healing and repair. Proteins can also be used as an energy source, although they are not as efficient as carbohydrates and fat. They are used as an energy source only under extreme circumstances, such as during starvation or at the end stages of liver disease, when the body begins breaking down its own muscles in a desperate attempt to stay alive. Known as *muscle wasting,* this is manifested on the body as decreased, and sometimes even almost total lack of, muscle. People with muscle wasting are often referred to looking like just "skin and bones."

Since protein is such a vital component of the body, many people mistakenly believe that the more protein they consume, the better. Not only is this belief misguided, but for someone with liver damage such an approach to nutrition can actually be downright dangerous. The trouble is that a damaged liver cannot process as much protein as a healthy liver. And when a damaged liver gets unduly overloaded with protein, encephalopathy (a state of mental confusion that can lead to coma) may occur. Finally, diets high in protein have been demonstrated to enhance the activity of the *cytochrome P450 enzyme system,* which is responsible for drug metabolism. This enhanced activity increases the likelihood that a drug may be converted into a toxic byproduct capable of causing liver injury. This is discussed in more detail in Chapter 24.

Dietary Recommendations for Protein

When a person thinks of protein, a juicy hamburger or a roast chicken may come to mind. However, remember that protein has vegetable sources as well as animal sources. (See Table 23.1 on page 339 for the protein content of certain foods.) Protein intake must be adjusted in accordance with a person's body weight and the degree of liver damage present. Approximately 0.8 grams of protein per kilogram (2.2 pounds) of body weight is recommended in the diet each day for someone with stable liver disease. As such, total protein intake would range between about 40 and 100 grams per day—equaling the approximate 20 to 30 percent of daily calories derived from protein that a person should ideally consume.

When choosing animal protein, it is important to choose lean (low-fat) cuts of meat. However, keep in mind that even the leanest cuts of red meat are high in fat content. In fact, approximately 50 to 75 percent of calories from most red meats actually come from fat! Even a carefully trimmed cut of fine lean red meat probably derives about 50 percent of its calories from fat. This becomes especially significant for people with liver disease due to being overweight, as a diet high in fat may contribute to such a person's liver-related abnormalities. (See Fat on page 342 for more information.)

People with unstable liver disease or decompensated cirrhosis need to lower the percentage of protein content in their diets so that it falls between approximately 10 and 15 percent; and they need to eat only vegetable sources of protein. A diet high in animal protein (which contains a lot of ammonia) may precipitate an episode of encephalopathy among these people. Researchers aren't exactly sure what causes encephalopathy, but they suspect that an excess of ammonia in the body may be one of the triggers. Some popular weight-loss diets involve the consumption of a very high animal protein content. People with cirrhosis are advised to avoid any such diets.

Vegetarian diets, on the other hand, have a low ammonia content and have been shown to be much less likely than animal protein diets to induce encephalopathy. Also, vegetable fiber plays a role in helping to eliminate harmful waste substances, such as ammonia, from the body. Therefore, people prone to encephalopathy are advised to maintain a high intake of vegetable protein and a low intake of animal protein, or even better, to become vegetarians. Also, high-fiber, vegetable protein diets may reduce sugar levels in some people and may, therefore, be especially useful to diabetic people with cirrhosis. However, even vegetable proteins are not perfect and also may be subject to dietary restriction. For instance, if a person suddenly develops encephalopathy, it may be necessary to limit protein consumption to 20 grams or less per day. Permanent protein restriction is needed to help control mental symptoms in people suffering from some degree of chronic encephalopathy— that is, those who have some degree of mental confusion and/or memory loss all the time.

Table 23.1. Protein Content of Common Foods

Food	Portion Size	Protein Content
Bread (whole wheat)	1 slice	2.5 g
Broccoli (boiled, drained)	4 ounces	3.4 g
Cheese (Cheddar)	1 ounce	7.1 g
Chicken (dark meat, roasted without skin)	4 ounces	31.0 g
Chicken (white meat, roasted, without skin)	4 ounces	35.1 g
Egg (hard-boiled)	1 large	6.0 g
Flounder (baked, broiled, or microwaved)	4 ounces	27.4 g
Ham (roast)	4 ounces	28.4 g
Hamburger (cooked medium)	4 ounces	27.3 g
Lamb (cooked)	4 ounces	27.8 g
Milk (whole)	1 cup	8.0 g
Peas (frozen, boiled)	4 ounces	4.0 g
Potato (baked, with skin)	4 ounces	2.6 g
Rice (white, cooked)	4 ounces	3.1 g
Shrimp (steamed)	4 ounces	23.7 g
Spaghetti (cooked)	4 ounces	5.4 g
Steak (sirloin broiled)	4 ounces	34.4 g
Tuna (chunk light in vegetable oil, drained)	6 ounces	49.8 g

The Importance of Avoiding Protein and Amino Acid Supplements

It's very easy for people with liver disease to consume too much protein. It's just as important to realize that the ingestion of protein supplements, such as those commonly found in health food stores and groceries, can similarly be dangerous to people with a liver condition. Protein supplements force the liver and kidneys to work overtime in order to get rid of the excess protein ingested. Furthermore, excess protein supplements can increase the risk of dehydration, as extra fluid is required to eliminate the byproducts of protein metabolism from the body. Protein supplements are only required for people who are malnourished and unable to supply adequate protein intake through their regular diets.

Amino acid supplementation is another potentially dangerous fad for people with liver disease. Although amino acids are indeed natural, it doesn't mean that they're always safe, especially for people with liver disease. Most of the amino acid supplements that are available over the counter come in quantities that are far greater than the amount the body needs. Consumption of excessive amounts of amino acids may cause serious side effects. Probably the best known example of this is *L-tryptophan,* an aromatic amino acid (AAA) used as a supplement to aid sleeping. Initially promoted as safe and natural, L-tryptophan was eventually banned for sale by the FDA in 1990 because many people who consumed this amino acid developed a serious muscle disorder. Death even occurred in some people as a result of L-tryptophan ingestion. Some other amino acid supplements are high in AAA (for example, phenylalanine, tyrosine, and tryptophan), which have been demonstrated to be detrimental to some people with liver disease. Another amino acid, methionine, may induce encephalopathy in people with liver disease. Vegetables contain very little methionine, yet have a high content of the branched-chain amino acids (BCAAs; such as leucine, isoleucine, and valine). Some experts believe BCAAs are beneficial to people with encephalopathy. However, under no circumstances should any form of amino acid supplement be added to the diet of a person with liver disease.

Carbohydrates

The major function of carbohydrates is to provide a ready supply of energy to the body. Carbohydrates supply this energy in the form of glucose (blood sugar). There are two separate categories of carbohydrates. The first category is known as *simple carbohydrates* (sugars that can be easily broken down by digestion). Simple carbohydrates may consist of only one sugar unit, known as a *monosaccharide,* including glucose, fructose (fruit sugar), and galactose (a component of milk products). Or they may consist of two sugar units, known as a *disaccharide,* including maltose (used in the fermentation of beer), sucrose (table sugar), and lactose (milk sugar).

Complex carbohydrates consist of *polysaccharides* (hundreds of simple sugars linked together) and are commonly known as starches and fibers. Complex carbohydrates cannot be immediately used by the body as energy. They first must be broken down into glucose, either by cooking or by the digestive process. Examples of complex carbohydrates include grains, nuts, seeds, breads, pasta, rice, cereals, and potatoes.

Dietary Recommendations for Carbohydrates

People with liver disease should strive for a diet consisting of approximately 60- to 70-percent carbohydrates, with complex carbohydrates predominating. For such people, a well-balanced diet will include at least 400 grams of carbohydrates. (See Table 23.2 for the carbohydrate content of some common foods.) If there are too few carbohydrates in a person's diet, this will likely result in excessive protein and fat intake. If too much protein is consumed and not enough carbohydrates, the liver will be forced to use protein as an energy source. This is an inefficient use of protein, as protein will be diverted from its primary job of building cells and tissues. Furthermore, this will put undo stress on the liver, as it is more taxing for the liver to convert protein into energy than it is to convert carbohydrates into energy. If too much fat and not enough carbohydrates are consumed, many health disorders,

Table 23.2. Carbohydrate Content of Common Foods

Food	Portion	Carbohydrate Content
Apple	1 medium	21.1 g
Banana	1 medium	26.7 g
Bread (pumpernickel)	1 slice	14.7 g
Bread (wheat)	1 slice	10.6 g
Bread (white)	1 slice	13.0 g
Milk	1 cup	11.7 g
Peanut butter	2 tablespoons	5.7 g
Potato (baked with skin)	1 medium	51.0 g
Potato (mashed)	$\frac{1}{2}$ cup	18.4 g

including obesity, may result. This may eventually lead to fatty liver or nonalcoholic steatohepatitis (NASH). (See Fat on page 342.) It is also important to keep in mind that a meal of a complex carbohydrates, such as pasta, should not be drowned in sauces loaded with cream or butter. Doing so introduces too much fat into an otherwise healthy dish. Keep in mind that excessive complex carbohydrates, on the other hand, may lead to bloating and malabsorption of certain vitamins and minerals. This underscores the importance of adhering to the recommended balance of nutrients listed on page 336.

Simple carbohydrates, such as raisins, hard candy, or honey, may stick to teeth, thereby increasing the likelihood of cavities. Therefore, it is especially important that people suffering from dry mouth (sometimes present as a symptom in people with primary biliary cirrhosis or in people with chronic hepatitis B or C on interferon treatment) brush their teeth immediately after eating and snacking. This may require that these people bring a toothbrush, toothpaste, and floss to restaurants, work, and school. Also, these people may want to use a prescription dental cream specifically made for people prone to dental caries.

People with alcoholic liver disease (ALD) often suffer from abnormal carbohydrate metabolism. Approximately one-third of them have diabetes. A diet rich in high-fiber, complex-carbohydrate foods may improve their condition somewhat.

Carbohydrate and the Liver

The liver plays a crucial role in carbohydrate metabolism. Before sugars are able to supply energy to the body, they are routed to the liver, which is in charge of deciding their fate. The liver makes every effort to correct any nutritional imbalances attributable to poor eating habits. Thus, it may immediately send sugar (in the form of glucose) into the bloodstream to provide an instant energy boost to a person who needs it. Or the liver may send glucose to the brain or muscles, depending upon what activities are being performed at the time (for example, taking a test versus exercising). Or it may decide to store glucose (in the form of the starch *glycogen*) for later use when the body requires more energy. If too much carbohydrate is consumed, the liver transforms it into fat (in the form of triglycerides). In this case, excess fat becomes deposited on the body—usually in places where it is least wanted. Excess fat may be deposited directly into the liver, resulting in fatty liver or NASH (see Fat below).

Converting foods other than carbohydrates into energy is stressful even to a normal liver. By eating an unbalanced diet that is low in complex carbohydrates, a person with liver disease will add to the stress that the disease has already caused her liver. In fact, this is one reason why so many people with liver disease feel fatigued. Simply put, their diets are working against them. A well-balanced diet can help combat the fatigue associated with liver disease. (See Exercise for Those With Liver Disease on page 361 for other tips on combating fatigue.) Eating multiple small meals throughout the day instead of three large meals is recommended. Each meal should focus on complex carbohydrates, such as a plain baked potato or high-grain breads. By using such an eating strategy, a healthy energy source will be constantly supplied to the body. A diet rich in complex carbohydrates as opposed to one focused on simple sugars will provide a person with more sustained energy. For example, eating a candy bar provides a quick burst of energy because the body easily converts all those simple sugars into glucose. But the pick-me-up doesn't last long and is often followed by a swift energy drop as the liver tries to readjust energy levels. A plate of pasta, on the other hand, is a good source of complex carbohydrates. It takes more time to digest, and so provides a slower, more sustained release of energy.

Fat

Fats are the body's most efficient means for storing excess energy. They are a very concentrated source of calories. Gram for gram, fats contain more than double the amount of calories of other nutrients. Thus, a diet high in calories from fat is likely to result in more weight gain than a diet high in calories from protein or carbohydrates.

It is important for people with liver disease to minimize their fat intake by avoiding foods that are high in fat. (See Table 23.3 for the percentage of fat found in some common foods.) Excess fat on the body can result in fatty liver or nonalcoholic steatohepatitis (NASH). (See Chapter 16 for a full discussion of these disorders). Although it is uncommon, it is possible for someone with NASH to develop cirrhosis and liver failure. Fatty livers are so unhealthy that they are not even considered viable for use in transplantation. A fatty liver may cause liver disease or may contribute to the worsening of other liver diseases. People with alcoholic liver disease who are obese appear to be particularly prone to developing cirrhosis. And people with hepatitis C and a fatty liver are likely to develop scarring in the liver at an accelerated rate. Fortunately, most cases of fatty liver due to being overweight can be reversed with a low-fat diet, exercise, and weight loss. Some people with liver disease don't have to worry about obesity. Some are even underweight. But even

Table 23.3. Percentage of Fat Found in Some Common Foods

Food	Percentage of Fat	Food	Percentage of Fat
Avocado	86	Hotdog	83
Bacon	92	Margarine	100
Butter	100	Mayonnaise	98
Chicken (with skin)	56	Milk (whole)	49
Chicken (without skin)	35	Peanut butter	75
Egg	69	Pecans	89
Hamburger	61		

these people should not feel free to eat excessive amounts of fats, since fat deposits can accumulate in the liver no matter how much, or how little, a person weighs.

People with primary biliary cirrhosis (PBC) often have difficulty absorbing fats. This is due to the fact that the destruction of the bile ducts within the liver leads to a failure to secrete bile salts necessary to absorb fats. This can result in *steatorrhea,* a condition of fat malabsorption. Therefore, people with PBC should also adhere to a diet low in fat (see Chapter 15 for more information on this disorder).

Dietary Recommendations for Fat

As a general rule, no more than 30 percent of a person's caloric intake should come from fat. That's the absolute maximum. Ideally, a person should aim for something in the neighborhood of 10 to 20 percent. People who are overweight should aim for 10 percent. While it is important to eat as little fat as possible, eating a small amount of the more healthy fats does have some benefit. Fat supplies the body with a source of reserve energy. In emergency situations, stored body fat is transformed into energy. It is this stored fat that keeps people warm on cold winter days. Also, certain fatty acids are necessary for the normal functioning of some bodily processes. These fats, which are known as *essential fatty acids,* perform (as the name suggests) a variety of duties that are essential to the proper functioning of the body. However, it should be pointed out that as little as a tablespoon of polyunsaturated fat a day can provide all of the essential fatty acids that the body needs. In addition, people need some fat in order to properly absorb the four fat-soluble vitamins—A, D, E, and K. Without some fat, these vitamins may become deficient in the body, even if they are taken in supplemental form. This type of vitamin deficiency sometimes occurs in people with cholestatic diseases, such as primary biliary cirrhosis. Lastly, fat helps make food tastier. This is important for people who suffer from a suppressed appetite due to chronic liver disease.

Most people are familiar with the fact that saturated fats are less healthy than unsaturated fats. What accounts for this? Well, most saturated fats tend to be hard or solid at room temperature. Therefore, they have the ability to clog arteries and boost cholesterol levels. Polyunsaturated fats, which are liquid at room temperature, don't do this. So, it's best to stay on a diet that is low in saturated fats. (Keep in mind that fish fat is more liquid than chicken fat, which is more liquid than beef fat.)

Cholesterol and the Liver

Cholesterol is related to, but not synonymous with, fat. Cholesterol, which is found only in animal products, is not all bad. In fact, in some respects, it is essential to maintaining life. Cholesterol is needed to build sex hormones and bile salts. In the skin, it is made into vitamin D with the help of sunlight. However, people do not need to consume any cholesterol in order to facilitate these processes. The liver is capable of making most of the cholesterol required by the body—only about 15 percent of blood cholesterol comes from the diet. Yet many factors other than diet may account for high blood cholesterol levels. These include cigarette smoking, lack of exercise, and a genetic susceptibility for this condition. Triglyceride levels are a measurement of how much fat is circulating in the bloodstream.

High-density lipoprotein (HDL) is often referred to as the "good cholesterol," and low-density lipoprotein (LDL) is often referred to as the "bad cholesterol." HDL cholesterol seems to be responsible for sending cholesterol to the liver to be broken down and then either recycled or excreted from the body. Overweight people tend to have low levels of HDL and high levels of LDL. Excess fat located around the abdomen (more so than fat deposited elsewhere in the body) seems to be related to elevated blood-cholesterol levels. While not established with certainty, it is believed that the fatty acids released by abdominal fat tend to flow directly into the portal vein and from there directly into the liver. The liver then receives a signal to increase cholesterol output.

People with primary biliary cirrhosis (PBC) generally have high cholesterol levels (sometimes in the range of 500 to 1,000 milligrams per deciliter) that are not attributable to dietary indiscretions. However, they are not at increased risk for heart disease or heart attacks due to these elevated levels.

VITAMINS AND MINERALS

The liver is the body's main warehouse for storing nutrients. It absorbs and stores excess vitamins and minerals from the blood. If a person's diet does not supply an adequate amount of these nutrients on a given day, the liver releases just the right amount of them into the bloodstream. However, the liver has only a limited capacity for processing vitamins and minerals. Any excess amounts that the liver is unable to process are generally eliminated from the body. Yet, at some point, the liver can become damaged due to the strain of processing an overabundance of certain vitamins and minerals.

If a person eats a healthy, well-balanced diet, all the vitamins and minerals required for her daily needs and activities should be amply supplied. Despite this, many people feel that they should take vitamin and/or mineral supplements just to be on the safe side. While this may be fine for an overall healthy person, it may be

downright dangerous for someone with liver disease. Thus, excessive doses of vitamin and mineral supplements may do much more harm than good to an already
damaged liver.

However, there are exceptions to this rule: First, not everyone eats a healthy,
well-balanced diet. Also, some people follow strict vegetarian diets. Under these circumstances, vitamin and mineral supplementation may be necessary. People with
certain liver diseases, especially cholestatic diseases, such as primary biliary cirrhosis, absorb some vitamins poorly. Thus, these people may also require supplementation. Moreover, people with alcoholic liver disease have a need for vitamin
supplementation due to the nutrient-depleting effects of alcohol on the body. On the
other hand, some liver diseases actually result in an overload of a certain vitamin
or mineral. An example of this is hemochromatosis (discussed in Chapter 18), which
is a liver disease of iron overload. Alternatively, there are liver diseases that may be
associated with iron deficiency. This may be due to internal bleeding, which can
occur in people with bleeding esophageal varices due to decompensated cirrhosis.
Therefore, the requirements of vitamins and minerals in the diet of a person with
liver disease must be evaluated on an individualized basis.

Vitamins

Vitamins are organic substances that come from animals and plants. They are essential to human development, growth, and functioning. Vitamins are also known as
micronutrients because they are required by the body only in small amounts to
maintain health. Normally, the required amount is supplied by eating a well-rounded diet.

Just like foods and medications, vitamins must pass through the liver to be
metabolized. If taken to excess, any vitamin has the potential to cause serious health
problems. This is true even for people with normally functioning livers. However,
for people with liver disease, the potential for damage is much greater. Depending
upon the severity of liver damage, certain people may even need to eliminate from
their diets foods that have been fortified with certain vitamins. These may include
commonly consumed foods, such as some breakfast cereals.

Vitamins can be categorized based on their solubility characteristics—fat soluble and water soluble. This difference has important implications for people with
liver disease, and will be covered in the following sections on the different types of
vitamins.

Fat-Soluble Vitamins

Fat-soluble vitamins include vitamins A, D, E, and K. They are absorbed by the
body only with the help of fats or bile. These vitamins are stored in fat cells. In people with cholestatic liver disease, they are poorly absorbed by the body. In such
cases, vitamin supplementation is necessary. The best type of vitamin to take, in this
case, is a baby vitamin. Since infants have immature digestive tracts, supplements

designed specifically for them are often easier to digest. Each of the fat-soluble vitamins is discussed in more detail below.

Vitamin A. Vitamin A is needed to maintain normal vision, especially night vision, and is essential to the immune system. It also plays a vital role in building and maintaining healthy skin, bones, and teeth. Vitamin A belongs to a group of compounds known as *retinoids* (also referred to as retinol, retinoic acid, or retinyl esters). About 80 to 90 percent of the total body stores of retinoids are found in the liver. The liver makes the ultimate decision as to where vitamin A is needed most in the body.

For people without liver disease, 1,000 micrograms per day (3,333 IU per day) for men and 800 micrograms per day (2,667 IU per day) for women should be the maximum amount of vitamin A consumed. This can easily be obtained from a well-balanced diet. Still, approximately one-quarter of American adults take supplements that contain vitamin A. This vitamin is found in abundance in the following foods: liver, egg yolks, fortified milk and other dairy products, margarine, liver oil, and fish oil. A person with advanced liver disease should never take vitamin A supplements and should not consume excessive quantities of these foods.

Plant forms of vitamin A are known as *carotenoids* (also called carotene). Carotene is also referred to as *pro*-vitamin A, because the body must convert this substance to vitamin A before it can be utilized by the body as active vitamin A. The most common carotenoid found in food is beta-carotene. Foods high in beta-carotene include cantaloupes, carrots, sweet potatoes, and green leafy vegetables such as spinach.

Excessive consumption of vitamin A (doses of approximately 25,000 to 50,000 IU per day) is extremely dangerous to the liver as it may cause a liver disease known as *hypervitaminosis A*. In fact, this condition can lead to cirrhosis. Hypervitaminosis A may result from excessive vitamin A supplementation or from unusual dietary habits, such as excessive consumption of liver, eggs yolks, or dairy products. People with liver disease should avoid eating liver since it contains a superabundance of vitamin A, more than any other organ meat. Interestingly, hundreds of years ago, doctors believed that some eye disorders could be cured by applying a piece of liver directly to a patient's eye, due to its high vitamin A content. Medications, such as Accutane (isoretinoin) and Retin-A (tretinoin), both which are used in the treatment of acne, are derived from vitamin A and, therefore, should not be used by people with advanced liver disease.

Vitamin A's potential to cause liver toxicity may be enhanced by alcohol consumption or by excessive intake of other fat-soluble vitamins (such as vitamin E) or by a vitamin-C deficiency. Time wise, vitamin-A toxicity may manifest only a few hours after a person has taken a massive dose. However, hypervitaminosis A can also develop slowly in a person taking moderate doses of vitamin A over a long period of time. Symptoms of vitamin-A overload may include nausea, vomiting, visual disorientation, headaches, and bone and joint pain. The liver can become enlarged and scarred, eventually leading to cirrhosis. Even portal hypertension, accompanied by jaundice and ascites can occur (see Chapter 6). Vitamin-A toxicity is often, but not always, reversible with a cessation of vitamin A, if, of course, cirrhosis has not already developed.

The bottom line is that people with liver disease are advised to minimize their intake of this vitamin. An exception to this rule applies only to people in advanced stages of cholestasis who are suffering from night blindness. An example would include a person with stage four primary biliary cirrhosis (PBC), who is also taking cholestyramine, a medication used to control itching that further impairs absorption of vitamin A. It has been noted that approximately 20 percent of people with PBC are deficient in vitamin A. Most of these people show no obvious symptoms of a vitamin-A deficiency. Therefore, people with PBC should have their vitamin A levels checked. If found to be deficient, only those people experiencing difficulty with night vision should receive vitamin A supplements. (See Chapter 15 for more information on PBC.)

Contrary to retinoids, carotenoids are not toxic to the liver and cannot cause hypervitaminosis A. However, beta-carotene can turn a person's skin an orange-yellow color, giving her the mistaken appearance of being jaundiced and in danger of liver failure.

Vitamin D. Vitamin D, a fat-soluble vitamin, is often referred to as the sunshine vitamin. This is because sunlight is required to transform cholesterol into vitamin D. In order to insure an adequate supply of vitamin D, most people only need to expose themselves to approximately fifteen minutes of sunlight several times a week. Vitamin D is essential for the absorption and metabolism of calcium. This vitamin enables calcium to be available to bones. Thus, vitamin D is especially important for people with chronic liver disease who are prone to osteoporosis (bone loss) or osteomalacia (bone softening). These conditions were discussed in Chapters 2 and 20. People prone to these disorders include those with primary biliary cirrhosis, those with cirrhosis complicated by cholestasis, and those taking an immunosuppressive medication, such as prednisone. These people are advised to take a vitamin D supplement or to eat foods high in vitamin D. This is especially important if a person's sun exposure is limited due to weather conditions. Probably all people with chronic liver disease should supplement their diets with calcium and vitamin D to be on the safe side.

Food containing an abundant amount of vitamin D include milk (which is fortified with vitamin D), cold-water fish, fish oil, cod liver oil, and egg yolks. The United States recommended daily intake of vitamin D is 5 micrograms (200 IU). People with liver disease found to be deficient in vitamin D should take between 400 and 800 IU per day. Keep in mind that excessive supplementation with vitamin D can lead to dangerous deposits of calcium in the kidneys, heart, and blood vessels.

Vitamin E. Vitamin E, also known as tocopherol, acts as an antioxidant in the body. It protects red blood cells and other bodily tissues against damage. Some studies indicate that supplementation with vitamin E may serve to protect the liver from free-radical-mediated injury arising from excessive alcohol intake. Therefore, people who regularly drink alcohol, and, in particular, people with alcoholic liver disease, may benefit from supplementation with vitamin E. Since vitamin E requires bile for absorption, people with cholestasis may also benefit from supplementation with vitamin E (especially when the bilirubin rises above 3 mg/dl and alkaline phosphatase (AP) is above 1,000 IU/L). A vitamin-E deficiency may lead to a disturbance or a feeling of imbalance in walking.

The United States recommended daily allowance of vitamin E is most commonly 100 international units (IU) per day (although it can range from 30 to 400 IU per day) and can usually be obtained through the diet. Foods containing abundant amounts of vitamin E include vegetable oils, whole grains, dark leafy vegetables, nuts, and legumes. These foods fall under the category of polyunsaturated fatty acids. Most vitamin E supplements contain only alpha-tocopherol, which is the most potent form of vitamin E. To get full benefit from a vitamin E supplement, it should contain both alpha- and gamma-tocopherol and should be taken with zinc. If possible, try to obtain the water-soluble ester of vitamin E (d-alpha-tocopheryl-polyethylene glycol succinate). People with cholestasis can best absorb vitamin E when it is in this form.

Some researchers believe that vitamin E therapy may be a beneficial addition to the treatment of viral hepatitis. Further study is needed before this can be recommended.

Vitamin K. Vitamin K is used by the liver to manufacture the protein prothrombin. Prothrombin, as discussed in Chapter 3, is essential for proper blood clotting. Without vitamin K, people would hemorrhage (continue bleeding) as the result of a cut. Vitamin K also helps keep bones strong. Half of the vitamin K in the body is made by the bacteria that naturally lives in the intestines. The remainder comes from dietary sources. Abusing certain laxatives, such as mineral oil, or taking antibiotics for prolonged periods of time may result in a depletion of vitamin K.

When vitamin-K deficiency is due to poor absorption, the deficiency may be corrected by taking water-soluble vitamin K orally (5 to 10 milligrams per day) until the cause for malabsorption has been eliminated. People with cholestatic liver disease tend to have a vitamin-K deficiency that is impossible to correct with oral replacement. In situations where bleeding is a potential risk (such as for those people requiring surgery), intravenous infusions of fresh frozen plasma (FFP) must be given to the patient to temporarily correct this problem. In people with obstruction of the bile ducts outside the liver, the deficiency can often be corrected with an injection of vitamin K.

Foods containing an abundance of vitamin K include spinach and other leafy green vegetables, carrots, potatoes, cereals, and liver. There is no recommended daily allowance of vitamin K.

Water-Soluble Vitamins

Water-soluble vitamins include vitamin C and vitamin B complex, consisting of eight different B vitamins. Neither fat nor bile is needed to absorb water-soluble vitamins from the digestive tract, and therefore, a deficiency of these vitamins does not normally occur in people with cholestatic liver diseases. Water-soluble vitamins are stored in the body or are used to meet its daily requirements. Reserves of these vitamins can last many months. Therefore, people with liver disease rarely develop a deficiency of a water-soluble vitamin. One exception to this rule is people with alcoholic liver disease. This group often requires water-soluble vitamin supplementation due to the nutrient-depleting effects of alcohol on the body. Toxicity due to water-soluble vitamins is uncommon, as excessive doses of these vitamins can easily exit the body through perspiration or in the urine.

Vitamin C. Vitamin C, also known as ascorbic acid, aids in the healing of cuts and bruises. It also strengthens bones, cartilage, teeth, and skin. In addition, vitamin C enhances the absorption of iron. Therefore, people suffering from an iron overload disease, such as hemochromatosis, and people with chronic hepatitis C who have elevated iron levels, must be careful not to consume excessive amounts of this vitamin.

Most fresh fruits and vegetables contain abundant amounts of vitamin C. The recommended amount of vitamin C per day, which is approximately 60 to 72 milligrams per day, is easily obtained through a healthy diet. An exception to this rule occasionally occurs in people with alcoholic liver disease whose primary intake of calories in the diet is from alcohol. These people need to take vitamin C supplements. For all other people with liver disease, supplementing with vitamin C is generally not necessary.

Vitamin B Complex. The B complex vitamins consist of eight different vitamins: thiamine (vitamin B_1), riboflavin (vitamin B_2), niacin (vitamin B_3), pantothenic acid (vitamin B_5), pyridoxine (vitamin B_6), cyanocobalamin (vitamin B_{12}), folate, and biotin. All of these, with the exception of excessive doses of niacin (vitamin B_3), are safe for people with liver disease. The following is a discussion of each individual B vitamin.

- Thiamine (vitamin B_1) is essential for metabolizing carbohydrates into energy to be used by the brain and the nervous system. It also aids appetite and digestion. Symptoms of a thiamine deficiency include a loss of appetite, confusion, and disequilibrium (a feeling of imbalance). This vitamin is frequently deficient in people with alcoholic liver disease. When neurological signs of a thiamine deficiency occur in people with alcoholic liver disease, hospitalization and immediate intravenous thiamine replacement are often required.

  Thiamine can be found in whole-grain or enriched cereals, breads, brown rice, pork, liver, and soybeans. About 5 milligrams is the maximum amount of thiamine that can be absorbed per day from supplementation. Some "stress tablets" that purport to boost energy levels contain more than 5 milligrams of thiamine. The excess is simply eliminated from the body unused.

- Riboflavin (vitamin B_2) is also important in energy production. It helps promote the growth and repair of tissues and organs, specifically the skin, mucous membranes, eyes, and nerves. It is also essential to proper digestion. Deficiency can lead to mouth sores and visual problems. Riboflavin can be found in both whole-grain and enriched-grain products, as well as in liver, milk, and leafy green vegetables. If too much riboflavin is ingested, urine will turn a bright yellow color.

- Niacin (vitamin B_3), which is also known as nicotinic acid or nicotinamide, helps transform carbohydrates and fats into energy. It is also needed for healthy skin. Large doses of niacin are sometimes prescribed for people with high cholesterol. This can be very dangerous for people with liver disease, as dosages exceeding 3 grams per day can cause liver damage. Thus, people with liver disease are advised to refrain from excessive consumption of this vitamin. Good sources of niacin are milk, eggs, meats, vegetable, and peanuts.

- Pantothenic acid (vitamin B_5) is needed to convert proteins, carbohydrates, and fats into energy. Pantothenic acid also promotes immune function. Deficiency is uncommon, since pantothenic acid is synthesized by microorganisms that live in the small intestine. However, deficiency does occur occasionally in people who drink alcohol excessively. Megadoses of this vitamin can produce severe diarrhea. Deficiency can produce fatigue and depression. Food sources of this vitamin include fresh vegetables, brewer's yeast, eggs, nuts, and meat.

- Pyridoxine (vitamin B_6) is needed for proper protein, carbohydrate, and fat metabolism. It also aids in the production of hormones and red blood cells. Vitamin B_6 is found in so many foods (for example, liver, salmon, nuts, brown rice, most vegetable, and meats) that a deficiency is rare, except among people with alcoholic liver disease. Excessive doses of pyridoxine can lead to nerve damage.

- Cyanocobalamin (vitamin B_{12}) is needed to make blood cells. Therefore, a deficiency of this vitamin often leads to anemia and associated fatigue. This explains why people with liver disease who suffer from excessive fatigue often ask about vitamin B_{12} injections. However, the expectation that such an injection will provide an "extra boost" of energy is misguided. Since this vitamin is commonly found in animal food products such as meat, fish, milk, and eggs, a vitamin-B_{12} deficiency is a very uncommon cause of fatigue in people with liver disease.

    A few exceptions to the above statement exist. One exception applies to people with alcoholic liver disease (ALD) for whom the bulk of nutrients are obtained from alcohol. A vitamin-B_{12} deficiency may develop among these people. Furthermore, since alcohol interferes with absorption of vitamin B_{12}, a vitamin-B_{12} deficiency may develop if a person consumes an excessive amount of alcohol even if she maintains a well-balanced diet. (See Chapter 17 for more information on ALD.) A deficiency of this vitamin may also occur in people with chronic liver disease who maintain a strict vegetarian diet for long periods, such as is the case for those suffering with chronic encephalopathy. Finally, the older a person is, the more likely a vitamin B_{12} deficiency is to develop. This is because stomach acid is needed to absorb this vitamin from food, and as a person ages, the amount of acid in the stomach diminishes. Therefore, people with liver disease who are over the age of sixty should be checked for a vitamin-B_{12} deficiency. Also, people with liver disease who are chronically on medications that block stomach acid—such as H2 blockers (for example, Pepcid, Axid, Tagamet, and Zantac) or proton-pump inhibitors (for example, Prilosec and Prevacid)—should be checked as well. Symptoms of a vitamin-B_{12} deficiency include mood swings, irritability, rapid heart rate, fatigue, short-term memory loss, and severe psychosis.

- Folate is needed for proper brain functioning and is crucial to the formation of red blood cells. As with vitamin B_{12}, a folate deficiency can also produce anemia. In fact, vitamin B_{12} must be present in order to activate folate, which accounts for the fact that a deficiency of one tends to simultaneously cause a deficiency of the other. Folate deficiency is very common in people with alcoholic liver disease. Symptoms of folate deficiency include a sore red tongue, fatigue, and memory loss. Megadoses of folate can interfere with the absorption of certain medications and zinc absorption, and can mask signs of a vitamin-B_{12} deficiency. Sources of folate include leafy green vegetables, oranges, barley, brown rice, cheese, and whole grains.

- Biotin is needed for healthy hair, nails, and skin. It is produced by microorganisms living in the small intestines. Therefore, deficiency is uncommon unless excessive quantities of raw egg whites are eaten, as they may prevent the body's absorption of biotin. Biotin may be helpful while on interferon therapy for chronic hepatitis B and C to prevent or diminish hair loss sometimes associated with this treatment although this has not been proven. Good sources of biotin include brewer's yeast, poultry, and milk.

Minerals

Minerals are inorganic substances, which means that they are not manufactured by either plants or animals. They originate in soil and water and become incorporated, in varying degrees, in all plant and animal life. Minerals are essential for almost all of the body's functions. They play a crucial role in energy production, heartbeat regulation, and control of muscle tone. A well-rounded diet should provide ample amounts of all the minerals needed to carry out daily activities. *Macrominerals* include those minerals that the body needs in large quantities. Macrominerals that are of special relevance to people with liver disease include calcium and sodium. *Microminerals* are those minerals that the body needs in trace (small) amounts. Examples of microminerals that specifically concern people with liver disease include iron, zinc, and copper. The following is a discussion of these relevant minerals.

Calcium (Ca)

Calcium is essential for healthy teeth and bones, for normal muscle contraction, and for blood clotting. Almost all of the calcium in the body resides in the bones. Without an adequate amount of calcium, the bones become soft and brittle. Osteoporosis is characterized by reduced bone mass and the resulting increased risk for bone fractures. Osteoporosis is common to many liver diseases, especially cholestatic liver diseases, such as primary biliary cirrhosis (see Chapters 2 and 20). It is important for all people with chronic liver disease to consume foods rich in calcium and/or to supplement their diets with this mineral. However, it is important to remember that calcium supplementation alone will not prevent osteoporosis. Other factors, such as cigarette smoking, lack of exercise, excessive alcohol consumption, and abnormal hormone levels also play roles in the development of bone loss. Alcohol has been shown to be directly toxic to bone cells and may impair calcium absorption. Thus, it is especially important for people with alcoholic liver disease to take calcium supplementation. In fact, as stated above, it is a good idea for all people with chronic liver disease to take a calcium and vitamin D supplement.

Good sources of calcium include dairy products, leafy dark green vegetables (except spinach), tofu, canned sardines with bones, and salmon with bones. Excessive calcium consumption may interfere with the absorption of iron in addition to causing many medical problems, including kidney stones, constipation, and fatigue. Furthermore, as with all supplements, regardless of how much is consumed, the body will only use the amount needed. Any surplus will be eliminated from the body unused or will accumulate and perhaps cause medical problems. If calcium supplementation is taken, it should be limited to no more than 1,000 to 2,000 milligrams per day and should be taken with a vitamin D supplement (which is usually included in the calcium tablet). Since stomach acid is needed to properly absorb calcium, antacids, such as Tums, which reduce stomach acid, are poor sources of this mineral.

Sodium (Na)

Sodium is a mineral that the body requires to maintain precise water balance. Sodium occurs in nature only in combination with *chloride,* another mineral. Sodium chloride is commonly known as salt. The body requires about 50 to 400 milligrams of sodium per day. Yet the average American consumes about 25 to 35 times that amount! While this overconsumption of salt is not necessarily dangerous for most healthy people, it can create problems for a person with advanced liver disease.

Decompensated cirrhosis may lead to ascites (an abnormal accumulation of fluid in the abdomen). If not treated in a timely manner, this ascitic fluid may become infected (a condition known as *spontaneous bacterial peritonitis* or SBP). People with ascites must be placed on a severely salt-restricted diet. For every gram of sodium consumed, the accumulation of 200 milliliters of fluid results. The lower the consumption of sodium in the diet, the better controlled this excessive fluid accumulation is. For people with ascites, sodium intake should be restricted to under

1,000 milligrams per day and preferably under 500 milligrams. This goal is difficult, yet attainable.

In order to successfully adhere to a salt-restricted diet, it is important to become a knowledgeable food shopper and diligently read all food labels. People are often surprised to discover which foods are high in sodium. (See Table 23.5 for the sodium content of some common foods.) General guidelines regarding sodium consumption are as follows: the amount of sodium in fresh foods is significantly less than that in the same foods after they have been processed, cured, canned, or frozen; therefore, choose fresh foods whenever possible. Table salt and salt used for cooking should be totally eliminated from the diet. One teaspoon of table salt contains 2,325 milligrams of sodium! All canned foods and food from fast food restaurants should be avoided. Some over-the-counter medications have high sodium contents. For example, one tablet of Rolaids contains 53 milligrams of sodium, two tablets of Alka-Seltzer contains 567 milligrams of sodium, and one serving of Bromo-Seltzer contains 717 milligrams of sodium. These medications should be substituted with products that have a lower sodium content. If the label on a medication or other product does not clearly state the sodium content, a pharmacist should be able to supply such information or offer a way to obtain it. Meats, especially red meats, have a high sodium content. Consequently, adherence to a vegetarian diet may become necessary for people who develop severe ascites. Spices, such as basil, dill

Table 23.5. Sodium Content of Common Foods

Food	Portion	Sodium Content
Alka-Seltzer	2 tablets	567 mg
Anchovies (canned)	5	734 mg
Baking soda	1 teaspoon	821 mg
Big Mac	1	1,510 mg
Butter	1 tablespoon	116 mg
Chicken noodle soup (some types)	1 cup	1,106 mg
Corn (canned)	$\frac{1}{2}$ cup	285 mg
Corn flakes	1 ounce	351 mg
English muffin	1	378 mg
Frankfurter	1	504 mg
Ketchup	1 tablespoon	156 mg
Margarine	1 tablespoon	132 mg
Milk	1 cup	121 mg
Sauerkraut	$\frac{1}{2}$ cup	780 mg
Soy sauce	1 tablespoon	1,029 mg

pepper, and vinegar, to name a few, may be used in place of salt as a food season-ing. Salt substitutes containing potassium chloride should be avoided. These sub-stitutes tend to raise potassium levels in the body. This can be especially dangerous to people taking *spironolactone* (Aldactone), a potassium-sparing diuretic (water pill) used in the management of ascites.

It is fortunate that there are many foods on the market that have been specifi-cally manufactured as low sodium products. Furthermore, as of 1986, the FDA has required that the sodium content of all processed foods be listed on the package label. This regulation has been a boon to the consumer. People with liver disease without ascites are advised to refrain from excessive salt intake, although they need not limit their consumption as severely.

Iron (Fe)

There are two types of dietary iron. *Heme* (animal) iron found in animal foods, such as red meat, is well absorbed from the diet. *Nonheme* (plant) iron found in plant foods, such as spinach, is poorly absorbed into the body. (Popeye was wrong: spinach is not a good source of iron.) In fact, only about 15 percent of ingested ani-mal iron and only 3 percent of ingested plant iron is actually absorbed by the body. The average American consumes about 10 to 20 milligrams of iron per day. In order to increase the absorption of plant iron into the body, a vitamin C supplement should be consumed at the same time. On the other hand, tea, which contains tannins (a plant substance), inhibits the amount of iron absorbed from the diet.

The amount of the iron in the body usually amounts to about 3 to 4 grams (50 milligrams per kilogram in men and 40 milligrams per kilogram in women). The body has a limited ability to eliminate excess iron from the body. In fact, only about 1 to 2 milligrams of iron is capable of being excreted each day. Therefore, if too much iron is ingested (whether in the form of food or supplements), excess iron is stored in body tissues, primarily the liver. As such, the liver is the part of body that is most susceptible to the toxicity of iron.

Iron is an essential component of hemoglobin, a protein responsible for deliv-ering oxygen to the body's cells and organs. (One red blood cell carries approxi-mately 270 hemoglobin molecules, each of which contains 4 iron molecules). Iron is also a component of *myoglobin,* a protein responsible for delivering oxygen to the muscles. Finally, iron helps make *adenosine triphosphate* (ATP), an important component of energy. Thus, it is common to associate iron with energy and strength. (Interestingly, the link between fatigue and iron deficiency was brought to the atten-tion of the American public by a 1960s commercial for the supplement Geritol, which popularized the term "iron-poor blood.") People with liver disease often assume that when they feel weak and tired, they need to take iron supplements. But taking iron supplements under such circumstances is not always a wise move and may, in fact, be dangerous. The symptoms of iron deficiency and iron overload can be quite similar—fatigue, headaches, and shortness of breath. Also, the fatigue asso-ciated with liver disease is more likely to be due to something other than the amount of iron in the body. Therefore, prior to taking an iron supplement, it is crucial that a person with liver disease get her blood tested to obtain her iron profile. (See Chapter 18 for more information on iron studies.)

Excessive iron in the body of a liver patient can be extremely dangerous. In extreme excess, iron is toxic to the liver and can lead to cirrhosis, liver failure, and liver cancer. Furthermore, there is growing evidence that even mildly increased (or sometimes even normal) amounts of iron may cause or enhance the amount of injury to the liver in the presence of other liver diseases. This applies especially to people with alcoholic liver disease and chronic hepatitis C. In fact, iron overload is commonly seen in people with alcoholic liver disease and chronic hepatitis C, and has been found to worsen the outcome and to decrease the responsiveness to treatment. Liver scarring and liver cell damage are directly related to the iron content of the liver cell. Since a person's body is unable to eliminate an overabundance of iron, neither iron supplements nor vitamins containing iron should be included in the diet of a person with liver disease (unless it has been determined that she has an iron deficiency).

Hemochromatosis is an inherited disease of iron overload (see Chapter 18). People with this disease and those with high iron levels due to other liver disorders should avoid cooking with cast-iron laden cookware and should avoid eating with cast-iron laden utensils. These people should consume only moderate amounts of those foods that are high in iron content. (See Table 23.6 for the iron content of some common foods.) Furthermore, some herbs commonly taken to treat liver disease (for example, milk thistle, dandelion, and licorice) may contain iron. Therefore, people with hemochromatosis or other diseases associated with iron overload should avoid these herbs.

Zinc (Zn)

Zinc is essential to the normal functioning of the immune system and is important for the senses of taste and smell. Zinc is also necessary for vitamin-A activity. Therefore, quite often people who are discovered to be deficient in zinc are also deficient in vitamin A. A zinc deficiency may occur in people with cirrhosis, especially when cirrhosis is due to excessive alcohol use. This may stem from insufficient dietary intake of zinc or from a reduced intestinal absorption of zinc. Such a defi-

Table 23.6. Iron Content of Some Common Foods

Food	Portion	Iron Content
Beef	3 ounces	6.1 mg
Cereals (iron-fortified)	1 ounce	4.5 mg
Chicken	3.5 ounces	1.1 mg
Liver	3.5 ounces	14.2 mg
Shrimp	3 ounces	2.5 mg
Spinach	1 cup	0.8 mg

ciency may also be due to an increased excretion of zinc in the urine. A zinc deficiency may contribute to a decreased appetite, fatigue, and poor wound healing.
These symptoms are experienced by some people with alcoholic liver disease.
Replacement of zinc in the diet is important if a deficiency is discovered. Some studies show that zinc may help improve mental status in people with encephalopathy.

Good sources of zinc include beef, liver, brewer's yeast, seafood, egg yolks,
fish, and lima beans. People without a deficiency should not supplement their diets
with zinc, as an excess may lead to nausea, vomiting, and diarrhea.

OTHER DIETARY CONCERNS

Some foods and supplements have been associated with hepatitis and liver disorders. Therefore, it is recommended that people with liver disease avoid the foods
and supplements discussed in this section. Other nutritional concerns that people
often have include the adequate consumption of water and caffeine's effect on the
liver. These concerns will also be addressed in this section. Gas-related problems,
thoughts on gluten intolerance, and final nutritional tips will conclude this section
on nutrition.

Foods and Supplements to Avoid

Raw shellfish has been the source of many outbreaks of hepatitis A. People with
chronic liver disease are at increased risk of complications and poor outcomes if
they become infected with hepatitis A. Therefore, all people with chronic liver disease who intend to eat shellfish should get the hepatitis A vaccination. In fact, it is
urged that everyone with chronic liver disease, whether they plan to eat shellfish or
not, get the vaccination against hepatitis A (see Chapter 24 for more information on
vaccinations).

Many wild mushrooms found in North America and Europe contain deadly toxins known as *phallotoxins* (phalloidin and alpha amanitin). These mushrooms are
renowned for causing liver failure, or even death, when consumed. As a precaution,
all patients with liver disease are advised to avoid eating wild mushrooms, especially
if self-picked. See Chapter 21 for more information concerning these mushrooms.

Shark cartilage is a nutritional supplement that has been said to be of benefit to
some people with cancer. There is a possible, although unproven, association between shark cartilage and drug-induced hepatitis. People with chronic liver disease
are best advised to avoid this supplement until further evaluation is conducted.

Aflatoxin, a hepatotoxin (common in Asia and Southern Africa, but uncommon
in the United States), is produced by a fungus (*Aspergillus*). This fungus is a potential contaminant of foods that have been stored for prolonged periods of time in
damp, warm conditions. The most commonly infected foods are peanuts and corn.
Aflatoxins have been linked to hepatitis, cirrhosis, and liver cancer in some countries. This was discussed in more detail in Chapter 19.

Saccharin, a sweetener, has been associated with, although not proven as a cause of, acute hepatitis. People with liver disease are best advised to avoid it.

Adequate Water Consumption

The body requires water in order to carry out its essential functions. It is important for people to drink at least six to eight 8-ounce glasses of water per day. It is especially important for people with chronic hepatitis B or C who are on interferon therapy to stay well-hydrated. These people should probably increase their water intake beyond the recommended amount. People with liver disease often find that drinking abundant amounts of water helps give them an improved sense of well-being. And people on interferon often find that liberal water consumption helps them with some of side effects of the medication. On the other hand, people with ascites are prone to excessive water retention. These people are advised to restrict their water intake to approximately three to four 8-ounce glasses of water per day, depending upon the degree of fluid accumulation present. When drinking bottled mineral water, it is important to take note of the water's sodium content. In some instances, the sodium content may present a problem for people on sodium-restricted diets. (See page 352.)

Caffeine's Effect on Those With Liver Disease

Caffeine is present in coffee, tea, chocolate, cola, and some over-the-counter medications. Caffeine itself is not directly harmful to the liver. In fact, in moderation (one to two cups of a caffeine-containing beverage per day), caffeine may suppress the fatigue associated with liver disease to some extent. However, higher amounts of caffeine may contribute to irritability, restlessness, and insomnia. Some people even experience a rapid heartbeat and/or palpitations from caffeine consumption. Excessive intake of caffeine may put people with chronic liver disease at increased risk for osteoporosis and bone fractures. Therefore, it is best to consume caffeine in moderation. This is especially important for people taking interferon, as this medication may also cause symptoms similar to those caused by caffeine.

Gas-Related Problems

Some people with liver disease complain of increased gas production (flatulence), abdominal bloating, and abdominal distention. These symptoms may stem from *malabsorption* (impaired absorption) and/or *maldigestion* (impaired digestion) of certain nutrients by the body. These symptoms are especially likely to occur in people with alcoholic liver disease and cholestatic liver diseases, such as primary biliary cirrhosis. Such symptoms may also be caused by the medications used in the treatment of liver disease. Cholestyramine (Questran) is one example of a medication that is likely to cause increased gas production. Alternatively, flatulence may not be related to a liver disorder at all, but instead may stem from increased consumption of foods that have a tendency to cause gas (see the list on page 358) or from the development of a food intolerance, such as lactose intolerance.

To remedy these symptoms, people can try decreasing their consumption of gas-containing foods and of foods that they are having difficulty digesting. Often, elimination diets are helpful. An elimination diet involves eliminating one food at a time from the diet to determine whether that food is solely responsible for the gas production. It is usually best to begin by eliminating milk and milk products, as they are the foods most commonly not tolerated. One approach that will cut down on the gas-producing potential of fruits is to peel off the skins. Another is to cook fruits and vegetables until they are soft and soggy. Unfortunately, these methods of preparation also significantly reduce the nutritional value of these foods. Finally, taking an anti-gas remedy (typically containing simethicone) can sometimes help.

Foods that can cause gas include:

- Dairy products, such as milk (including skim and low-fat), yogurt, milk chocolate, cheese, and cheese pizza.

- Raw vegetables, especially onions, carrots, cabbage, lettuce, broccoli, cauliflower.

- Beans.

- Bagels.

- Pretzels.

- Soups.

- Fruits with skins.

- Dried fruits, such as raisins and prunes.

- Fatty foods.

- Artificial sweeteners, such as sorbitol.

- Carbonated beverages, such as soda.

- Chewing gum.

Gluten's Effect on the Liver

Gluten, a protein found in wheat, oats, barley, and rye, is often unable to be absorbed in people with primary biliary cirrhosis. This autoimmune disease is known as celiac sprue, and typically causes diarrhea and weight loss. Celiac sprue is approximately ten times more likely to occur in people with PBC than among the general population. Treatment consists of eliminating all gluten products from the diet. Both PBC and celiac sprue are discussed in Chapter 15.

Final Tips on Diet

Dining out can present a challenging situation for a person on a special or restricted diet. The fat, sodium, and calorie content of restaurant foods is not included on the menu. For this reason, it is best to steer clear of fast-food establishments completely. When dining out, food should be ordered cooked "dry," meaning it should be prepared with butter, margarine, or oil. It is important for a person with liver disease who is following a certain diet to stress to the waitperson that she is on a restricted diet and must have the food served in such a manner.

Most people with liver disease find that eating multiple small meals throughout the day is the best approach, as it maximizes energy levels and the ability to digest and absorb food. And, if a person's appetite is very poor, she can try eating baby food. That's right—baby food. Baby food is a good nutritious source of calories that is easy to digest.

Finally, once again, it must be stressed that all alcohol consumption should be avoided. This includes hidden alcohol contained in desserts, especially cakes and certain coffees.

WEIGHT PROBLEMS AND LIVER DISEASE

Most people have problems related to weight. Commonly heard comments among the general public include: I'm too fat! I'm too skinny! I'm not muscular enough! I have fat in all the wrong places! Well, people with liver disease are no different, but with one exception: weight problems are often related to their liver diseases. Therefore, it is important for anyone with liver disease who is experiencing an unexpected weight gain or weight loss to consult a doctor about this change. The following sections provide information about weight loss and weight gain in people with liver disease.

The Causes of Weight Gain and Weight Loss

If a person with liver disease experiences weight gain, it is important to determine the underlying cause. This is because the cause of the weight gain may have significant implications. While fat is the most common cause of weight gain, weight gain can also be due to ascites (fluid retention). Ascites is a sign of worsening liver disease. Weight gain may also be due to protein gain in the form of enlarged muscle mass. This should be construed as a healthy development. Muscle weighs more than fat, and therefore, if bodybuilding has been incorporated into a person's lifestyle, this type of weight gain is the reward. It is advisable to be evaluated by a specialist if unexpected weight gain occurs. The specialist will determine what treatment, if any, is necessary under the circumstances.

As with weight gain, weight loss can be due to a variety of factors. If one is on a fat- and/or calorie-restricted diet, then any weight loss is probably attributable to the diet. However, weight loss, especially if unsuspected, can be due to protein or muscle loss. This can be a sign of worsening liver disease or of liver cancer. It is important to consult with a doctor before starting a weight-reduction diet, and to remain under a doctor's supervision while the diet is ongoing. It is especially important to inform the doctor if an unexpected weight loss occurs.

The Reason Why People With Liver Disease Have a Hard Time Losing Weight

Many people with liver disease have a difficult time losing weight. This may be attributable to any of the following factors. First, some medications used in the treatment of liver disease can actually cause weight gain. The most common example of this is the medication prednisone. Prednisone is used to treat autoimmune hepatitis (AIH; discussed in Chapter 14) and is part of the panoply of antirejection medications used after a liver transplant. Prednisone is notorious for causing weight gain, both by increasing the percentage of body fat and through its tendency to promote fluid retention.

Second, people with liver disease often have hypothyroidism (a slow thyroid condition). This leads to a sluggish metabolism typically resulting in weight gain. Thyroid abnormalities are often seen in people with AIH and in people on interferon treatment for chronic hepatitis B or C. Thyroid abnormalities are easily correctable with medications.

Third, many people with liver disease are chronically fatigued. Consequently, they may rarely exercise and tend to lead relatively sedentary lifestyles. This creates a cycle that perpetuates further weight gain.

Finally, it is common for a person to experience considerable weight gain after receiving a liver transplant. This occurs because medications used in the prevention of liver graft rejection, such as cyclosporine and prednisone, can cause an increase in body fat and fluid retention. This problem can be remedied in many instances by slowly decreasing the dosage of prednisone until it is discontinued and changing from cyclosporine to tacrolimus. Liver transplant recipients are prone to adopt a diet high in fatty foods. This most likely occurs because their diets may have been severely restricted prior to the transplantation or their appetites may have been suppressed due to their illness and associated depression. After transplantation, a new sense of well-being, accompanied by an improved outlook on life, often leads to an increased appetite.

A Warning About Crash Diets and Diet Pills

The recommended way to lose weight is to adopt a healthy, balanced diet and to exercise regularly. It is easy to be tempted to take a shortcut through this approach via the use of crash diets or diet pills. This is definitely not recommended. These mass-market solutions may produce serious adverse, or perhaps even fatal, consequences in a person with liver disease. Many fad diets emphasize one particular category of nutrient, say protein, or even just one specific type of food, like grapefruit, to the exclusion of everything else. A healthy person's liver might be able to tolerate this approach, but a damaged liver often cannot. The nutritional imbalance that an ill-advised fad diet can create can easily throw a weakened liver into failure and land a person in the hospital. The same applies to some diet pills. Remember, everything that is ingested eventually has to be processed by the liver. Diet pills may add to the stress of an already burdened liver, thereby increasing the likelihood that a person's condition will worsen rather than improve.

EXERCISE FOR THOSE WITH LIVER DISEASE

Regular exercise is an important component necessary to combat liver disease. This isn't something that can be read in any medical textbook or taught in medical school classrooms. This may explain why most liver doctors don't realize how important exercise can be to maintaining their patients' health. But I've seen the benefits over and over again in my practice. People who are in good shape and who exercise on a regular basis not only feel better, but often respond more positively to medical treatment. People do not have to do a lot of exercise in order to reap the benefits. Nor does it pay to overdo it. The main thing is simply to get going. Regular exercise will increase energy levels, decrease stress on the liver, and, in many cases, even delay the onset of certain complications associated with liver disease. For people with liver disease, it is crucial to consult with a doctor before beginning any type of exercise program.

Some of the Benefits of Exercise

The benefits of exercising are numerous. First, exercise gives people a general sense of well-being and improved self-image. It is a known fact that if a person feels well mentally, her immune system will be stronger and give her that extra edge needed to fight disease.

Second, as previously discussed, exercising gives a person a boost of energy. Fatigue is probably the most common and one of the most bothersome symptoms that plagues people with liver disease. Many people with liver disease frequently feel like they don't have enough energy to make it across the room, let alone around the block. However, the best way to fight this seemingly relentless exhaustion is to exercise. Yes, this may seem like a vicious cycle, but most people find that it actually works. In part, fatigue may have to do with the fact that both the heart and the liver are working overtime to keep a good supply of filtered blood circulating throughout the body. Adding a regular exercise routine enables both organs to work more efficiently. Eventually, this will boost energy levels. While most people find it tough going at first, they eventually realize that the benefits are worth it.

Third, exercise improves cardiovascular function. As the body gets stronger and more aerobically fit, the cardiovascular system will be able to work more efficiently. Less effort will be required of the heart to pump blood to the liver and other body organs. Less effort on the heart equals stronger cardiovascular function and an increased overall energy level for a person with liver disease. It is extremely important to attempt to do some exercise while on interferon treatment, as this will decrease the fatigue, irritability, and depression often associated with this medication.

Fourth, exercise results in a reduction of total body fat. While nearly everyone knows that being overweight places a great deal of stress on the heart, most people don't realize that it also makes it harder for the liver to do its job. When total body fat is reduced, fat content in the liver is simultaneously reduced. This often results in a significant reduction of elevated liver enzymes, no matter what the underlying liver disorder may be. Eating right and getting plenty of exercise is probably the slowest way to lose weight known to humanity, but it's also the safest. That's especially true for people with liver disease. Combining a healthy diet with regular exercise is also the best way to keep from regaining the weight.

The Benefits of Exercise for Osteoporosis

Exercise is essential in order to decrease the incidence of potentially detrimental bone disorders. Osteoporosis is a bone disorder frequently associated with liver disease. It results in decreased bone density, leading to fragile, easily fractured bones. While osteoporosis is a disease that most frequently affects postmenopausal women, it can also affect premenopausal women and men with liver disease. Postmenopausal women are particularly susceptible to osteoporosis because as estrogen production stops, bone loss accelerates. Furthermore, women naturally have a lower percentage of muscle and bone mass than men. This further increases their risk of developing osteoporosis. Other risks for osteoporosis in people with liver disease include excessive alcohol use, primary biliary cirrhosis, advanced cirrhosis from any liver disease typically resulting in muscle wasting, and the use of prednisone. Fortunately, people can reduce the likelihood of developing osteoporosis by making exercise and a healthy diet part of their lifestyle.

Just as muscles grow in response to muscle contractions, bone strength and density increase when the muscles attached are contracting. Studies have shown that muscle and bone growth promoted by frequent weight-bearing exercise is vital to the prevention of osteoporosis. Supplementing the diet with at least 1,000 to 1,500 milligrams per day of calcium with vitamin D is also important. If a person already has osteoporosis, it needn't keep her from exercising, but she will have to use more caution to keep from breaking any bones. High impact aerobic exercises, which involve jumping and twisting, can increase the risk of injury and should be avoided. Low impact exercises, such as swimming and walking, are the safest choices for aerobic exercise. Weight-bearing exercises with light weights can generally be safely performed. Close attention should always be paid to proper form. Running on a hard surface, such as concrete pavement, should be avoided. Soft surfaces, such as specially designed running tracks or a sandy beach, are preferable.

The Types of Exercise for Liver Disease

People with liver disease should take up both aerobic and weight-bearing exercises, as they each play a different role in fighting liver disease. It is fortunate that there are an abundance of books, videotapes, and television programs that help teach, step by step, both types of exercises. It is important to use these self-help materials prior to starting any exercise regimen. Other helpful ideas include scheduling a few appointments with a personal trainer to design a fitness routine that personally meets the needs of a person with liver disease. Many fitness trainers will even work in their clients' homes. This is important, as many people are too self-conscious or too shy to exercise in a crowded gym, and/or lose self-motivation after the first few sessions at a gym. The chance of success is increased if a person chooses an exercise that she already enjoys and that can easily be done at least three times a week.

Timing is also important. It is fine to exercise at any time of the day that is personally convenient. However, by the end of the day, most people are usually too mentally and physically tired to do anything, least of all, run on a treadmill. That is why most people with liver disease find that they need to do their exercises first thing in the morning. While some people may find it difficult to get up in the morning in the first place, once they get started with an exercise regimen, it will become easier and easier. And people usually find that exercising in the morning helps give them an extra boost of energy to make it through the day. Finally, don't overdo it. It's more important to maintain a regular routine than to set any records.

Aerobic Exercises

Aerobic exercise trains the heart, lungs, and entire cardiovascular system to process and deliver oxygen more quickly and efficiently to every part of the body. It's the kind of exercise that gets the heart pumping. As one becomes more aerobically fit, the heart won't have to work as hard to pump blood to the rest of the body, including the liver. The pulse will begin to slow down, making it easier for the liver to send the blood it has just filtered back to the rest of the body. The benefits of being an aerobically fit person include an overall improved energy level, which translates into decreased fatigue. Fortunately, a person does not have to wear high-fashion workout clothes or go to a fancy gym to get aerobic exercise. Walking briskly, bicycling (either stationary or regular), swimming, or using a treadmill all provide solid aerobic benefits. Many people start off with something easy, such as walking around the block. A helpful hint is to start by walking up and down the street close to home. In that way, if a bout of fatigue suddenly occurs, it won't take long to get home.

Weight-Bearing Exercises

Weight-bearing exercises build up both bones and muscles. For many reasons, it is important for all people with liver disease to incorporate weight-bearing exercises into their daily exercise routines. First, people with liver disease need good strong bones because they are prone to osteoporosis. Weight training is the best way to fight against this, as stronger muscles equal stronger bones. Second, in advanced stages of liver disease, the body is forced to recruit muscle as a source of energy, and people are at risk of developing severe muscle wasting and greatly diminished strength. However, if a person has a reserve of muscle built up on her body, it will take a much longer time for this complication of liver disease to develop. Third, people who have too much fat on their bodies are prone to worsen their underlying liver condition by developing fatty liver and possibly NASH. Weight training reduces the amount of fat on the body and increases muscle mass. Therefore, the chance of developing fatty liver will be reduced. Finally, since muscle weighs more than fat, weight training is the perfect means of gaining lean healthy weight for those people who are underweight.

Once again, there are lots of self-help books and videotapes that describe how to create a personalized weight-bearing exercise routine. It's a good idea to hire a personal fitness trainer, who can design a personalized routine specific to an individual's needs. It is important that the trainer be aware of the client's liver disorder, and that sometimes she will not be able to exercise to her fullest capacity. A person with liver disease should never push herself or allow herself to be pushed by a trainer. If she feels too tired or if a body part feels strained, she should stop exercising until she feels better. Fitness training has become a field that requires certification, so make sure that the trainer is certified.

It is important to remember to work out every part of the body evenly. (There are eleven distinct body parts to work out.) In that way, the chances of injury are decreased. A few stretching exercises should always be performed to warm up the muscles before doing weight-bearing exercises. The amount of weight being lifted should allow for eight to twelve repetitions. Each *repetition* (rep) is defined as one full and individual execution of a particular lifting exercise. A *set* is a distinct grouping of repetitions, followed by a brief rest interval. Three sets of a given type of exercise should be performed. Aim to work out each body part at least once a week. Twice a week is ideal.

Putting Together an Exercise Program

Nobody expects a person beginning an exercise regimen to run a marathon or enter a bodybuilding contest. Setting impossibly high standards only guarantees failure. But if a person starts with easy goals and works her way up, she is much more likely to make exercise part of her daily routine. A good beginning regimen might include ten to twenty minutes of aerobic exercise, followed by a few weight-bearing exercises, three times a week. Everyone should work at her own pace until she is working out daily or at least five times per week. But even if a person can exercise only for a few minutes at a time, there is no need to despair. Doing a little exercise is better than doing none at all. It will get easier as time goes on.

When a person is in an acute phase of hepatitis or is experiencing a severe exacerbation or relapse of disease, any form of intense exertion should be avoided. There's no need for enforced bed rest, however. A person should listen to her body. If she is exhausted, then it's time to rest. If she's up to physical activity, then by all means she should be active. But, she must be aware of her personal limitations and know when it's time to call it quits. The liver has only so much energy to distribute to the rest of the body, so it's never wise to overdo it. Again, it is crucial to consult with the doctor prior to commencing any exercise program.

CONCLUSION

While a healthy diet and suitable exercise regimen should not be a substitute for conventional medical treatment, it should be considered an essential addition to therapy. In fact, following the appropriate regimen could actually improve the long-term outcome of some people with liver disease and can help prevent or delay the onset of some complications associated with liver disease. Furthermore, proper nutrition and exercise can also minimize the need for the use of excessive medications in many cases. Since everyone has individual needs and requirements related to diet and exercise, it is important to seek out a liver specialist, nutritionist, and/or fitness trainer with the expertise for guidance in the right direction. This chapter provided a general guideline upon which to form a basis for a personalized nutrition and exercise program.

The next and last chapter of this book provides the answers to lifestyle-related questions commonly asked by people living with liver disease, their friends, and their loved ones.

24

Pregnancy, Sex, Medications, and Prevention

In most cases, a person who has been diagnosed with liver disease can continue to live a normal, active life. However, there is some information that people with liver disease should know in order to keep themselves healthy, to protect themselves from additional liver damage, and to help keep their loved ones and close contacts free of liver disease. This chapter discusses four topics that commonly concern people living with liver disease—pregnancy, sex, medications, and prevention.

First, people with liver disease and their spouses invariably want to know to what extent the liver disease will impact pregnancy and the health of their offspring, and if pregnancy will have an effect on the course of the disease. Typically, they are surprised to learn that most women with liver disease have had successful, uncomplicated pregnancies and healthy children, without further damage to their livers. The first section of this chapter discusses these issues and also covers what the consequences may be if a woman develops liver disease during pregnancy.

The second topic discussed in this chapter concerns sex-related issues. Although most people with liver disease experience normal sexual functioning and interest, some people do suffer from sexual dysfunction, ranging from a decreased interest in sex to an inability to achieve an erection. In addition, the forms of contraception that are safest for people with liver disease and which types of hepatitis and liver disease can be sexually transmitted are covered under this topic as well.

The third topic discussed in this chapter relates to the impact that certain medications unrelated to the treatment of liver disease may have on the liver. Which medications are safe and which medications are potentially dangerous for people with liver disease are discussed. Some people are more susceptible than others to drug-induced (medication-induced) liver problems. While many of these factors are alterable (such as reducing the amount of alcohol consumed), other factors (such as age) cannot be changed. Also covered under this topic are the effects of acetaminophen (Tylenol) and aspirin and other nonsteroidal anti-inflammatories (NSAIDs) on the liver. Also, since many people do not realize that recreational drugs can be harmful to the liver and that they can sometimes cause hepatitis or decrease the effectiveness of medications used to treat liver disease, this subtopic is also addressed.

The last section of this chapter discusses a topic of special importance—the prevention of liver disease. Two separate issues will be covered: how to prevent the spread of liver disease to others and how to prevent the occurrence of additional liver diseases in a person who already has liver disease. This section focuses on the importance of obtaining the hepatitis A and B vaccinations and also discusses some general preventative strategies that are recommended for those living with liver disease and for the people in their lives.

PREGNANCY AND THE LIVER

The issues surrounding pregnancy and the liver are many. This section will address several of these issues, including how pregnancy may affect the liver and the general health of a woman with preexistent chronic liver disease. Another issue covered is what impact chronic liver disease may have on the fetus. This section will also discuss some liver diseases that may occur in pregnant women with no prior history of liver disease.

Pregnancy in Women With Preexistent Chronic Liver Disease

Most women with liver disease can become pregnant, have uncomplicated pregnancies, and go on to give birth to healthy babies. However, in some circumstances, liver disease may adversely affect pregnancy and childbirth. The following pages discuss pregnancy in women with preexistent chronic liver diseases, including decompensated cirrhosis, chronic hepatitis B and C, autoimmune hepatitis, and others.

Decompensated Cirrhosis and Pregnancy

Cirrhosis (see Chapter 6) is often associated with *amenorrhea* (lack of menses) and infertility. Consequently, women with cirrhosis—especially decompensated cirrhosis—may have difficulty conceiving. As a result of their advanced liver disease, women with decompensated cirrhosis who do conceive have an increased risk of serious complications during pregnancy. Approximately 15 to 20 percent of these women suffer spontaneous abortion (miscarriage). Also, there is an increased risk for premature childbirth or stillbirth. Furthermore, women with decompensated cirrhosis are at an increased risk for the development of liver failure during pregnancy, although it is unknown how often this occurs.

Bleeding from esophageal varices is probably the biggest pregnancy-related health risk for women with decompensated cirrhosis. Variceal bleeding is most common during the second trimester, occurring in approximately 20 to 45 percent of women with portal hypertension. Ten percent of the time, women with decompensated cirrhosis experience variceal bleeding during labor and immediately after childbirth. Death of the mother from uncontrollable variceal hemorrhage occurs approximately 10 to 18 percent of the time during the course of pregnancy—depending on the trimester, the baby sometimes has a chance for survival. It has been noted that pregnant women with alcoholic cirrhosis appear to have the worst prognosis. Those with primary biliary cirrhosis appear to have the best prognosis.

Despite the increased risk of complications, many women with decompensated cirrhosis successfully proceed through pregnancy and childbirth without any complications. It is important for these women to be monitored regularly by a liver specialist and to choose an obstetrician who has experience with high-risk pregnancies. Women with decompensated cirrhosis who are thinking about becoming pregnant should undergo an upper endoscopy, which can assess the presence and degree of esophageal varices. If a woman has esophageal varices, she should be placed on a beta-blocker, such as propanolol (Inderal). It should be kept in mind that beta-blockers may pose risks to a fetus, including a slow heart rate and potential growth retardation. Such risks must be weighed against the potential benefit to be gained by preventing bleeding from esophageal varices. Women who have previously bled from esophageal varices are advised to refrain from becoming pregnant. For these women, if pregnancy is still desired despite the high risks, it is strongly recommended that a transjugular intrahepatic portosystemic shunt (TIPS) or other shunt procedure be performed before pregnancy occurs—as this may decrease the risk of bleeding from esophageal varices.

Chronic Hepatitis B and Pregnancy

Women with chronic hepatitis B (see Chapter 9) generally do quite well during pregnancy, providing that they have not progressed to decompensated cirrhosis. Although it has been reported, a flare-up of hepatitis B during pregnancy is very uncommon. Transmission of the hepatitis B virus (HBV) to the fetus during pregnancy (known as vertical transmission) is rare, but can occur if the placenta leaks blood into the fetus (for example, during a threatened miscarriage). However, perinatal transmission (transmission from mother to infant during childbirth) is very common, occurring in more than 90 percent of the cases where the mother is HBeAg and/or HBV DNA positive. Newborn infants are usually asymptomatic (without symptoms). Some will eventually develop symptoms, other will not (see Chapter 9).

Universal vaccination of all newborns (whose mothers are HBeAg and/or HBV DNA positive) with both the hepatitis B immune globulin (HBIG) shot and the hepatitis B vaccine is now mandatory (see page 385 for a discussion of vaccinations). This prevents transmission of HBV from the infected mother to the infant more than 90 percent of the time.

Treatment of pregnant women who have actively infectious chronic hepatitis B should be delayed until after childbirth because the medications used to treat this disease are *teratogenic*—capable of causing birth defects.

Chronic Hepatitis C and Pregnancy

Women with chronic hepatitis C (see Chapter 10) usually have uneventful pregnancies, provided that the liver disease is stable and she has not progressed to decompensated cirrhosis. As a general rule, a stable liver equals a safe pregnancy. Transmission of the hepatitis C virus (HCV) to the newborn is very uncommon. The likelihood of transmission is increased by the presence of the human immunodeficiency virus (HIV)—the virus that causes AIDS. The risk of transmitting HCV may also be increased by the presence of very high HCV viral loads (for example, five million) at the time of childbirth. However, some studies have shown that transmission of HCV to the newborn does not occur regardless of the mother's HCV viral load.

It is not necessary to test infants for the presence of the HCV Ab during their first six months of life. Due to passive transfer of this antibody from the mother during childbirth, HCV antibodies will usually be present in the newborn. However, this in no way indicates that the infant has hepatitis C. In fact, in most cases, HCVAb disappears in infants after six months. Breast-feeding has not been associated with the transmission of HCV and is considered safe.

Treatment of pregnant women with hepatitis C should be delayed until after they have given birth. This is because ribavirin, a common medication used in the treatment of hepatitis C, has been shown to be teratogenic (capable of causing birth defects). Interferon, another common medication for hepatitis C, may also be teratogenic.

Autoimmune Hepatitis and Pregnancy

In many cases, severe, active autoimmune hepatitis (AIH; discussed in Chapter 14) causes women to stop menstruating, and as a result, these women cannot become pregnant. However, when treated with corticosteroids and azathioprine, their menstrual cycles usually return to normal and pregnancy can be achieved. Women with AIH generally have successful pregnancies and deliveries.

Flare-ups of AIH may occur during pregnancy, although such occurrences are usually rare due to the immunosuppressive effects of pregnancy. In fact, some women have even experienced a remission of AIH during pregnancy. To further minimize the chance of an AIH flare-up, a pregnant woman should remain on therapy during pregnancy. At low dosages, both prednisone and azathioprine have been demonstrated to be safe for use during pregnancy. However, as a precaution, it is recommended to discontinue using azathioprine as soon as pregnancy is discovered as some studies have found this medication to be teratogenic. Furthermore, if contemplating pregnancy, it is advised to discontinue azathioprine approximately six months before conceiving. Urodeoxycholic acid and cholestyramine, two other medications often used in the treatment of AIH are considered safe during pregnancy. There are also a few instances in which pregnancy should be delayed at least one year because a poor outcome is likely. These situations include an AIH flare-up, any liver-related complication, such as variceal bleeding, or the withdrawal of prednisone.

Although rare, stillbirths and premature labor have been reported among women with AIH. Conservative management during pregnancy, which includes fluid and sodium restriction and the elimination of all unnecessary medications, enhances the likelihood of a successful outcome for both the mother and her unborn baby.

Alcoholic Liver Disease and Pregnancy

Women with alcoholic liver disease (ALD; see Chapter 17) are often infertile. Women with ALD who do become pregnant and continue to drink alcohol during pregnancy put their infants at high risk for a number of abnormalities. These abnormalities are collectively referred to as the *fetal-alcohol syndrome.* Infants suffering from fetal-alcohol syndrome may be born with enlarged, scarred livers and elevated transaminase levels. Other abnormalities often found in these newborns include mental retardation, delayed maturity and growth, and defects in the skull, face, and brain. It is extremely important for all women, especially those with ALD, to avoid alcohol during pregnancy.

Primary Biliary Cirrhosis and Pregnancy

Women with primary biliary cirrhosis (PBC; see Chapter 15) generally have uneventful pregnancies and deliveries. However, some studies have noted a greater-than-average incidence of stillbirths, spontaneous abortions (miscarriage), and declining liver function among these women. Pruritus can worsen during pregnancy and may be successfully and safely treated with cholestyramine. Ursodeoxycholic acid, which is used to treat PBC, is generally considered to be safe during pregnancy.

Liver Tumors and Pregnancy

Most liver tumors (see Chapter 19) found in women who are of child-bearing age are benign (noncancerous). These tumors include hepatic adenomas, focal nodular hyperplasia, and hemangiomas. They may enlarge and rupture when exposed to high levels of estrogen, as occurs during pregnancy. Fortunately, such complications during pregnancy are very rare. If rupture does occur, immediate surgery is required, which may put the fetus at risk.

Liver Transplantation and Pregnancy

Despite having undergone a liver transplant (see Chapter 22), women may become pregnant and can successfully complete their pregnancies. However, it is advisable that they wait at least one year and preferably at least two years from the time of transplantation before becoming pregnant. Immunosuppressive medications may be continued during pregnancy as there is little risk that they will adversely affect the fetus. In general, there is an increased incidence of premature deliveries and low birth-weight among women who have undergone liver transplantation. Women who become pregnant after liver transplantation must be carefully observed by a liver specialist, as well as by an obstetrician who specializes in high-risk pregnancies.

Liver Diseases That May Develop During Pregnancy

During pregnancy, liver disease can develop in a person who did not have anything wrong with her liver before becoming pregnant The following pages discuss the liver diseases that most commonly occur during pregnancy—viral hepatitis and drug-induced hepatitis—in otherwise healthy women. Gallstones commonly occur during pregnancy, and women with certain liver diseases (such as PBC) have an increased risk for the development of gallstones. Furthermore, due to the gallbladder's close proximity to the liver (see Figure 1.1 on page 9), the presence of gallstones often mimics liver disease by virtue of causing elevations in LFTs. Therefore, gallstones will also be discussed in this section.

Viral Hepatitis and Pregnancy

When viral hepatitis occurs during pregnancy, it is no different from viral hepatitis as it occurs in nonpregnant women—with the exception of pregnant women infected with the hepatitis E virus (HEV). Viral hepatitis is the most common cause of jaundice occurring during pregnancy. Other causes of jaundice can include medications and gallstones. Read on to learn more about how the different types of viral hepatitis affect pregnancy.

Hepatitis A. Hepatitis A has been reported to occur in approximately 1 out of 1,000 pregnancies. The course of the infection is not affected by pregnancy. Therefore, pregnant women infected with the hepatitis A virus (HAV) do not become any sicker than HAV-infected nonpregnant women. However, if HAV is contracted during the third trimester, there may be an increased risk of premature labor, although this is uncommon. Transmission of HAV to the newborn may occur, but is rare. HAV, when transmitted from mother to newborn, has not been shown to increase the risk of miscarriage or fetal abnormalities. It is safe for newborns and pregnant women to receive immune globulin injections for hepatitis A and the hepatitis A vaccine (see page 383), if exposed to hepatitis A.

Hepatitis B. Acute hepatitis B has been reported to occur in approximately 2 out of every 1,000 pregnancies. The course of the infection is not affected by pregnancy. Transmission of the hepatitis B virus (HBV) to the newborn commonly occurs during childbirth when the baby passes through the birth canal. This happens approximately 10 to 20 percent of the time, if the mother is only HBsAg positive during the third trimester. However, if the mother is both HBeAg and HBV DNA positive during the third trimester, the incidence of transmission increases to over 90 percent.

Newborns infected with HBV usually have no symptoms, although they usually develop either chronic hepatitis B or become chronic carriers of the virus. Therefore, any newborn whose mother is HBsAg positive should receive the hepatitis B immune globulin shot (HBIG) and the hepatitis B vaccination (see page 385). For women exposed to HBV during pregnancy, the immune globulin shot and the hepatitis B vaccination—both of which have been shown to be safe and effective for pregnant women—should be obtained.

Hepatitis C. It is unknown how often pregnant women contract acute hepatitis C. However, it is believed that the course of infection of hepatitis C is not affected by pregnancy, and that hepatitis C does not adversely affect the outcome of pregnancy. Therefore, pregnant women who become infected with the hepatitis C virus (HCV), do not become any sicker than nonpregnant women. The risk of transmission of HCV to the newborn is extremely low. This risk increases when there is coinfection with HIV. The risk may also increase when there are high viral loads of HCV, although this has been disputed. However, even in these people, the risk of transmission of HCV to the newborn is estimated to be less than 10 percent. Unfortunately, there is no protective vaccination available.

Hepatitis D. Acute hepatitis D infects only people who have hepatitis B. Transmission of the hepatitis delta virus (HDV) to the newborn during pregnancy and/or childbirth is exceedingly uncommon.

Hepatitis E. Hepatitis E occurs most commonly in Third World countries and is very rare in the United States. This virus has a very severe course in pregnant women. Therefore, pregnant women are advised not to travel to Third World countries. Hepatitis E results in fulminant hepatitis in approximately 20 percent of pregnant women. In fact, when the virus is acquired during the third trimester of pregnancy, approximately 20 percent of women die. Hepatitis E also increases the incidence of fetal complications and fetal death. Currently, there is no vaccine available to prevent hepatitis E, but one is undergoing testing.

Drug-Induced (Medication-Induced) Liver Disease

If a woman with normal liver function before pregnancy develops liver-related abnormalities during pregnancy, drug-induced liver disease should be suspected. However, drug-induced liver disease is no more common in pregnant women than it is in nonpregnant women. Some medications that are commonly associated with liver abnormalities during pregnancy include the following: the antibiotic erythromycin estolate, the thyroid medication propylthiouracil, the anesthetic halothane, and the antipsychotic medication chlorpromazine. Pregnant women are advised to use alternatives to these medications whenever possible. (The topic of drug-induced liver disease is discussed in more detail on page 377).

Gallstones

Being of the female gender and pregnancy are both risk factors for the development of gallstones. Thus, gallbladder disease is common during pregnancy. Furthermore, women with certain liver diseases, such as PBC, have an increased risk for the development of gallstones. The incidence of gallstones ranges from approximately 3 to 12 percent in pregnant women, and rises during the second and third trimesters and also with the number of pregnancies. Approximately 65 percent of women with gallstones have no symptoms. In fact, the presence of gallstones is usually discovered during a pelvic sonogram done during the routine evaluation of the pregnancy. In cases where gallstones are asymptomatic, no treatment is necessary. In fact, in 13 to 28 percent of women, gallstones disappear within a year of childbirth.

People who suffer from pain due to gallstones, a condition known as *biliary colic,* typically have abdominal or right upper quadrant pain radiating to their right shoulders or backs. The pain usually lasts about three hours per episode. The pain often occurs after a meal has been consumed and is sometimes associated with nausea and vomiting. During pregnancy, symptoms typically worsen as childbirth nears. LFTs are often elevated and may mimic LFT elevations that can occur with hepatitis or with other liver diseases. Therefore, it is important to be aware of the frequency with which gallstones can occur during pregnancy.

If gallbladder disease becomes complicated by infection or inflammation of the pancreas (*gallstone pancreatitis*), surgery becomes necessary. The surgery will involve removing the entire gallbladder containing the gallstones. It is safest to perform this surgery either during the second trimester or after childbirth. Gallbladder surgery during the first trimester is associated with spontaneous abortions (miscarriage), whereas gallbladder surgery during the third trimester is associated with premature labor. Removal of the gallbladder and gallstones can be safely performed during pregnancy with a technique known as laparoscopic gallbladder surgery. This involves the insertion of a laparoscope into the umbilicus to remove the gallbladder. With this technique, the large incision and long hospital stay required of open gallbladder surgery is avoided.

SEX AND LIVER DISEASE

Two sex-related issues that commonly concern people with liver disease are sexual function/dysfunction and methods of contraception. This section discusses these issue in detail. The medical treatment of sexual dysfunction in men, and which types of hepatitis can be transmitted sexually are also addressed.

Sexual Function and Dysfunction

Most people with chronic liver disease have normal sexual function and normal interest in sex. However, some people do complain of decreased libido, decreased ability to achieve and maintain an erection (a condition known as *erectile dysfunction*), and decreased satisfaction with sex.

Decreased sexual interest and erectile dysfunction occur in approximately 2 percent of healthy, middle-aged males without liver disease. This is about the same incidence noted in males in the early stages of liver disease. Men with advanced liver disease, however, are more likely to experience testicular dysfunction, loss of body hair, gynecomastia (enlarged breasts), redistribution of body fat, a female configuration of pubic hair, decreased muscle mass, decreased sexual desire, and erectile dysfunction. These characteristics are due to the changes in hormone levels that can occur in such men with advanced liver disease. The male hormone, *testosterone,* is typically low and the female hormone, *estrogen,* is typically high in such men. These findings are particularly applicable to men with alcoholic liver disease, as alcohol abuse (even in the absence of liver disease) may cause decreased testosterone levels, and thereby lead to sexual dysfunction.

Women with liver disease appear to have normal sexual function, with the exception of women whose liver disease is due to excessive alcohol consumption. Women who have undergone a liver transplant generally experience improvements in sexual interest, body image, and sexual intimacy.

Any chronic illness may be associated with sexual dysfunction. This is particularly true for liver disease, since it is so often associated with fatigue and depression, each of which can contribute to a decreased interest in sex. In addition, medications used in the treatment of liver disease, particularly interferon, may cause sexual dysfunction and decreased libido—especially in men. When medication is discontinued, the medication-induced sexual dysfunction abates. Other medical conditions unrelated to liver disease may also cause or contribute to sexual dysfunction. Therefore, people need to openly discuss sexual problems with their doctors to determine if some other medical condition, such as a prostate disorder or a psychiatric disorder, exists.

Treatment for Sexual Dysfunction in Men

Viagra (silenafil citrate) is the first oral medication for the treatment of erectile dysfunction to be approved by the FDA. The effects of Viagra on people with liver disease or in people who have undergone liver transplants have not been specifically studied. Moreover, Viagra's interaction with medications used to treat liver disease or medications used after transplantation has not been evaluated. Therefore, the adverse effects of Viagra, if any, in people with liver disease (whether pre- or post-transplant) are not conclusively known. It has been noted, however, that about 2 percent of men experience abnormal liver function tests as a result of taking Viagra.

For people without liver disease, the recommended dose of Viagra is 50 milligrams taken one hour prior to sexual activity. As this drug is metabolized through the liver, people with liver disease are advised to decrease this dose to 25 milligrams. Careful monitoring by a doctor, preferably a liver specialist, of a patient's liver function is essential for anyone with liver disease who uses this drug. People post-liver transplant using Viagra are advised to additionally have the levels of their antirejection medications checked with increased frequency. However, it is perhaps more advisable to refrain from using Viagra until studies documenting its effects on people with liver disease and on those who have received liver transplants have been published.

There is no evidence that conclusively establishes whether testosterone replacement treatment improves sexual function in men with chronic liver disease. Furthermore, testosterone may even be dangerous for those with liver disease. Therefore, this type of treatment cannot be recommended until further research has confirmed its effectiveness.

Contraception

People often assume that most forms of hepatitis and liver disease are easily transmitted through sexual contact. Such an assumption is incorrect. In fact, the only liver disease with a high rate of sexual transmission is hepatitis B. Men with infectious hepatitis B should use a condom until such time as their partners have completed the hepatitis B vaccination series (see page 385) and have demonstrated immunity—as evidenced by the presence of HBsAb in their blood. Likewise, any woman with infectious hepatitis B should have their partners use condoms until such time as their partners have completed the hepatitis B vaccination series and have demonstrated immunity.

The incidence of sexual transmission of hepatitis C is very low, and most such cases likely stem from a mingling of blood during sexual contact. Since there is no vaccination available for hepatitis C, men with chronic hepatitis C who are not in long-term monogamous relationships should wear condoms. This is especially important for those men who have multiple sex partners, who engage in anal sex (where the incidence of bleeding is higher than with genital sex), who have breaks or sores on their genitals (such as herpes sores, which may bleed), or who have frequent prostate infections. Similarly, women with chronic hepatitis C who are not in long-term monogamous relationships should have their partners wear condoms if any of the above-mentioned circumstances apply. Extra precautions should be taken in situations where a woman with chronic hepatitis C is menstruating. However, it should be emphasized that for people in stable, monogamous relationships, the incidence of sexual transmission of the hepatitis C virus (HCV) to the partner is extremely low. In fact, only about 3 to 6 percent of sexual partners of HCV-infected people are also positive for HCV. And since this statistic is based on indirect evidence, it is unclear whether the sexual partners of the HCV-infected people quoted in these studies became infected through sexual acts or by some other route.

People with liver diseases other than hepatitis B or hepatitis C (as well as the sexual partners of these people) need not take any special sexual precautions. Autoimmune hepatitis, primary biliary cirrhosis, fatty liver, NASH, alcoholic liver disease, and hemochromatosis are not liver diseases that can be transmitted sexually. As these diseases probably, to some degree, have a genetic basis, people (male and female) with one of these diseases may pass the susceptibility for the disease on to their offspring.

Although birth control pills are an effective form of contraception, they will not prevent the spread of a sexually transmitted disease nor do they lessen the likelihood of such a disease being transmitted. People with a benign liver tumor (hemangioma, focal nodular hyperplasia, or hepatic adenoma) are advised to avoid birth control pills containing estrogen, as estrogen may cause enlargement or rupture of these tumors. Furthermore, estrogen has been shown to cause and also worsen jaundice and cholestasis. Therefore, it is advisable for all women with liver disease to avoid taking estrogen-containing birth control pills. As an alternative, women may wish to consider the long-acting contraceptive *medroxyprogesterone* (Depo-Provera), which is preferable because it does not contain estrogen. Instead, it contains progesterone, another hormone. However, women should be aware that progesterone-containing birth control pills may cause sodium retention, thereby making these contraceptives unsuitable for women with ascites. Intrauterine devices (IUDs) are associated with an increased tendency to bleed when used by a woman with cirrhosis who has a decreased platelet count. Such women are advised to avoid the use of IUDs.

MEDICATIONS AND THE LIVER

There are over 1,000 drugs and chemicals that are capable of causing injury to the liver, some of which appear in Table 24.1 on page 381. The terms *drug-induced liver disease, drug hepatotoxicity,* and *drug-induced hepatitis* are used to describe those instances in which a medication or chemical substance has caused injury to the liver. In fact, drug-induced liver injury may account for as many as 10 percent of hepatitis cases in all adults, 40 percent of hepatitis cases in adults over fifty years old, and 25 percent of the cases of fulminant liver failure.

Since all medications are processed through the liver at least to some degree, people with liver disease must become aware of which medications can cause liver damage, which medications can worsen preexisting liver disease, and which medications are safe to take. It is the liver's job to detoxify any substances that are potentially harmful to the body. An already damaged and weakened liver must work much harder than a healthy liver in order to accomplish this task. When a person with liver disease ingests a potentially hepatotoxic drug, this puts additional stress on the liver and can result in further liver injury or possibly even liver failure. Even people with a healthy liver can develop liver disease as a consequence of ingesting a toxic medication or drug.

In general, people with liver disease should avoid medications known to be hepatotoxic. People who must be treated with a medication that is potentially hepatotoxic should have their LFTs closely monitored by their doctors. If a person's LFTs become greater than three times baseline values, the medication causing these elevations should be discontinued. Also, it is essential that people with liver disease inform their liver specialists of every medication or drug that they are taking— including holistic remedies or recreational drugs. There is no reason for the patient to expect the doctor to be judgmental. Her goal is the same as the patient's goal. Therefore, complete information should be provided to the doctor concerning prescription medications, over-the-counter medications, and alternative therapies. Remember, a doctor's objective is to help her patient get better and to help protect her patient from unintentional or additional liver damage.

How Drugs Cause Liver Disease

A particular drug may cause liver damage for many reasons. First, there are some drugs that are intrinsically toxic to the liver. These drugs can cause liver injury when the drug is taken in a dosage that exceeds the recommended dosage. This form of drug hepatotoxicity is what is known as "dose-dependent." The greater the amount by which the dosage taken exceeds the recommended dose, the more likely it is that the drug will cause liver injury. Drugs in this category are usually broken down by the cytochrome P450 enzyme system, discussed in Chapter 1. Under normal circumstances, the cytochrome P450 enzyme system usually converts toxic substances into nontoxic ones. However, in situations of drug hepatotoxicity, the reverse happens. A nonhepatotoxic drug is broken down into hepatotoxic byproducts. These byproducts cause liver damage as they begin to accumulate. An example of a drug in this category is the headache and minor pain reliever acetaminophen (Tylenol), which is discussed on page 381. The drugs in this category may also cause liver injury if taken in excess in combination with another hepatotoxic substance, such as alcohol.

Second, there are some drugs that can trigger an idiosyncratic reaction (an abnormal, unexpected hypersensitivity) to a normal dose of the drug similar to an allergic reaction, even though a normal dose may have been taken. Such a reaction is not related to the quantity of the drug ingested, and, furthermore, the ensuing liver injury is unpredictable. The type of drug hepatotoxicity is often accompanied by fatigue, fever, and rash. It usually develops after a person has already been taking the drug for a few weeks. An example of a drug in this category is the anticonvulsant phenytoin (Dilantin).

Finally, a person's susceptibility to a potentially hepatotoxic drug is enhanced by many factors. Some of these factors are within the person's control, such as quitting cigarette smoking and abstaining from excessive alcohol intake. But other factors cannot be altered. These include advancing age and being of the female gender. Some of the factors, both alterable and permanent, are listed below. (See Table 24.1 on page 380 for more information concerning most of the medications mentioned in this list.)

- **Age.** Adults are more prone to liver injury from certain hepatotoxic drugs. such as isoniazide (INH), a drug used to treat tuberculosis.

- **Gender.** Females are more susceptible than males are to most forms of drug-induced liver disease—especially drugs that can cause chronic hepatitis, such as methyldopa (Aldomet), which is a drug used to treat hypertension (high blood pressure).

- **Genetics.** Some people have a genetically based impaired ability to break down potentially hepatotoxic drugs, such as phenytoin (Dilantin)—a drug used to treat seizures—into safe byproducts.

- **Dose.** The higher the dose the more likely the chance for liver toxicity. This applies to drugs, such as acetominophen (Tylenol), which is intrinsically toxic to the liver.

- **Duration.** For some drugs, such as methotrexate (a type of chemotherapy), the longer it is used, the greater the likelihood of liver damage or even cirrhosis.

- **Kidney damage.** People with poorly functioning kidneys are more prone to the hepatotoxicity of some drugs, such as tetracycline, an antibiotic.

- **Alcohol.** Alcohol consumption enhances the hepatotoxicity of certain drugs, such as acetaminophen.

- **Cigarettes.** Cigarette smoking enhances the hepatotoxicity of certain drugs, such as acetaminophen.

- **Drug interactions.** Taking two hepatotoxic drugs in combination can greatly increase the likelihood of liver damage compared with when one hepatotoxic drug is taken alone.

- **AIDS.** The presence of AIDS increases the likelihood of hepatotoxicity from certain drugs, such as sulfamethoxazole-trimethoprim (Septra).

- **Rheumatoid arthritis (RA) and systemic lupus erythematosus (SLE).** People with these autoimmune disorders are more prone to the hepatotoxic effects of aspirin than people without these disorders.

- **Obesity.** Obesity increases the susceptibility of halothane-induced liver injury. (Halothane is a type of anesthesia.)

- **Nutritional status.** Fasting increases a person's susceptibility to acetaminophen-induced liver injury.

Characteristics of Drug-Induced Liver Disease

Many drugs have the ability to cause any form of liver disease, including acute and chronic hepatitis, fatty liver, cirrhosis, liver failure, and even some liver tumors. People with drug-induced liver disease may be asymptomatic with only mildly elevated LFTs, or they may be severely ill with liver failure and consequently in need of a liver transplant. Or they may be somewhere in between. Drug-induced liver disease can result in exactly the same symptoms and signs as those that characterize the same disease when not induced by drugs. It is essential for both the patient and the doctor to consider the potential hepatotoxicity of all drugs that the patient is taking and to promptly discontinue the use of such medications whenever an adverse effect on the liver is suspected. Continuing to use a drug after liver-related symptoms and signs have appeared greatly increases the chances of serious liver damage.

Drug-induced liver injury may be diagnosed through blood work. Some medications may cause hepatocellular liver injury. This is manifested by elevations in the transaminases AST and ALT. Other medications may cause cholestatic liver injury. This is manifested by elevations in AP and GGTP. And some medications may cause both types of liver injury. Still other medications may cause elevated bilirubin levels. Patients with elevated bilirubin levels exhibit signs of jaundice, with yellowing of the skin and eyes, and a darkening of the urine.

Drug-induced liver disease can be expected to occur in most, but not all cases, between five and ninety days from initial exposure to the hepatotoxic drug. Thus, people taking potentially hepatotoxic drugs should be monitored with blood tests during this time period. If a greater than threefold increase from baseline LFT levels occur, the medication should be discontinued. LFTs should improve within two to four weeks from when the medication was discontinued.

Since more than 1,000 drugs are potentially hepatotoxic, a comprehensive list detailing every hepatotoxic drug is beyond the scope of this book. However, Table 24.1 on page 381 lists some commonly used medications that may cause liver injury in some people. It is important to remember that not everyone will sustain liver injury as a result of using one of these drugs. And it is important to keep in mind that, as discussed on page 378, there are numerous variables that increase a person's susceptibility to the hepatotoxicity of these medications. Still, any person with liver disease who is using one or more of these medications needs to be carefully monitored. Careful monitoring is particularly crucial when such a person is using two or more hepatotoxic drugs in combination with alcohol. People with liver disease are best advised to use an alternative to one of these potentially hepatotoxic medications whenever possible.

Painkillers and Liver Disease

Acetaminophen (Tylenol) is a medication used to control pain (known as an *analgesic*) and fever (known as *antipyretic*). It does this without producing the stomach discomfort often experienced with aspirin and other nonsteroidal anti-inflammatories (NSAIDs). This characteristic has resulted in acetaminophen becoming a very popular alternative to NSAIDs. In small doses (less than 4 grams per day, or eight pills taken over a twenty-four hour period of time) acetaminophen is quite safe for the liver—unless combined with alcoholic beverages (see below). (Note: each acetaminophen tablet or pill typically contains 500 milligrams of acetaminophen.) In fact, acetaminophen is the recommended medication for relieving minor aches, pains, and headaches in people with liver disease.

However, when taken in excessive quantities or when combined with alcohol, acetaminophen may cause death due to liver failure. In fact, an overdose of acetaminophen is the most common cause of fulminant hepatic failure as well as the most common cause of drug-induced liver disease in the United States. And, after acetaminophen became readily available in 1960 as an over-the-counter medication, it became one of the most popular means of attempting suicide. For liver injury to occur, acetaminophen must generally be consumed in quantities exceeding 15 grams within a short period of time, such as in a single dose. Although uncommon, ingestion of 7 to 10 grams at one time may also cause liver damage.

The consumption of alcohol in conjunction with acetaminophen significantly

Table 24.1. Some Medications With Potential Hepatotoxicity

Medication	Use	Possible Liver Disorder
Anabolic steroids	For muscle growth	Liver tumor
Chlorpromazine (Thorazine)	Antipsychotic	Pseudo-PBC
Cimetidine (Tagamet)	Treats ulcers	Acute hepatitis and Cholestasis
Ciprofloxin	Antibiotic	Cholestatic hepatitis
Clindamycin (Cleocin)	Antibiotic	Acute hepatitis
Cocaine	Psychotropic	Acute hepatitis
Corticosteroids (prednisone)	Anti-inflammatory	Fatty liver
Coumadin	Blood thinner	Acute hepatitis and Cholestasis
Cyclosporine A	For immunosuppression	Cholestasis
Diazepam (Valium)	Psychotropic	Acute hepatitis and Cholestasis
Erythromycin estolate	Antibiotic	Cholestasis
Halothane	Anesthesia	Acute/chronic hepatitis
Ibuprofen (Motrin)	Analgesic	Acute hepatitis
Methotrexate	Treats rheumatoid arthritis	Cirrhosis
Methyldopa (Aldomet)	Treats hypertension	AIH
Metronidazole (Flagyl)	Antibiotic	Acute hepatitis
Naproxen (Anaprox)	Analgesic	Acute hepatitis and Cholestasis
Omeprazole	Treats ulcers	Hepatitis
Oral contraceptives	Birth control	Liver tumor
Phenytoin (Dilantin)	Anticonvulsant	Acute hepatitis
Salicylates (aspirin)	Analgesic	Acute/chronic hepatitis
Tamoxifen	Treats breast cancer	Acute hepatitis
Tetracycline	Antibiotic	Fatty liver

increases the likelihood that a person will incur severe liver damage. Therefore, people who consume alcohol on a regular basis should probably limit acetaminophen intake to a maximum of 1 to 2 grams per day (that is, two to four pills within a twenty-four hour period). Still, the best advice for people with liver disease is to totally abstain from alcohol.

People should take special note that acetaminophen is also an active ingredient in more than 200 other medications, including Nyquil and Anacin 3. Therefore, it is essential to read the labels of all over-the-counter medications carefully. Other commonly used medications, such as omeprazole (Prilosec), phenytoin (Dilantin), and isoniazid (INH), may increase the risk of liver injury caused by acetaminophen. It is always in the liver patient's best interest to consult with a liver specialists prior to taking any medication.

Acetylsalicylic acid (aspirin) and other NSAIDs are drugs that are widely used for their anti-inflammatory and analgesic effects. They also have the potential to cause drug-induced liver disease. In fact, many NSAIDs have been withdrawn from the market due to hepatotoxicity. All NSAIDs have the potential to cause liver injury. However, some NSAIDs are more hepatotoxic than others. The NSAIDs that are presently on the market that have been frequently associated with liver injury are aspirin (ASA), diclofenac (Voltaren), and sulindac (Clinoril). Therefore, people with liver disease should avoid using these NSAIDs. Older women seem to be particularly susceptible to the hepatotoxicity of NSAIDs and are best advised to avoid NSAIDs altogether. People with decompensated cirrhosis are at increased risk for the kidney toxicity of NSAIDs. Since this may lead to hepatorenal syndrome (see Chapter 6), people with advanced liver disease are best advised to totally avoid all NSAIDs.

Recreational Drugs and Liver Disease

It is important for people with liver disease to refrain from using any form of recreational drugs. In fact, it has been shown that both cocaine and Ecstasy (an amphetamine) can potentially cause hepatitis. Furthermore, cannabis (marijuana) may decrease the effectiveness of interferon therapy and may diminish or nullify a person's response to this medication. As discussed in previous chapters, intravenous and intranasal drug use have been associated with the transmission of hepatitis B and C.

Tobacco and Liver Disease

Cigarette smoking may induce certain cytochrome P450 enzymes in the liver, thereby increasing the susceptibility of these people to the potentially hepatotoxic effects of some drugs, including acetaminophen. Smoking may also diminish the liver's ability to detoxify dangerous substances, and it may affect the dose of medication required to treat a particular liver disease. Furthermore, cigarettes may worsen the course of alcoholic liver disease. Also, cigarettes have been associated with a possible increased incidence of liver cancer. Therefore, people with liver disease should refrain from cigarette smoking.

There is no conclusive evidence that other forms of tobacco use, such as pipe and cigar smoking or the use of chewing tobacco, have an adverse effect on the liver. However, it is likely that these forms of tobacco have similar effects on the liver as cigarette smoking. Therefore, it is recommended that people with liver disease refrain from these forms of tobacco use, as well.

PREVENTION OF LIVER DISEASE

People living with liver disease must address two separate issues regarding prevention. The first concerns preventing the spread of a potentially infectious liver disease—namely viral hepatitis—to others. Fortunately, the hepatitis A and B vaccinations are available and are effective means of preventing these forms of viral hepatitis. The second issue concerns the importance of preventing additional liver diseases in people already living with liver disease. People with chronic liver disease often experience a severe if not life-threatening course of disease when infected with acute hepatitis A. And some people who have had a liver transplant are at risk for developing hepatitis B, which could lead to dysfunction of the transplanted liver, fulminant hepatitis, and/or cirrhosis. It is of utmost importance that all people with chronic liver disease receive the immunizations for hepatitis A and B. The following discusses the importance of vaccination, both for people living with or in close contact with someone who has viral hepatitis and for all people with chronic liver disease of any type. Also discussed are some general preventative strategies of which all people with liver disease, their loved ones, and their friends should be aware.

Hepatitis A Vaccination

The hepatitis A vaccination was first approved by the FDA in 1995. Manufactured by SmithKline Beecham Biologicals, this vaccination is called HAVRIX. In 1996, the FDA approved VAQTA, a hepatitis A vaccination manufactured by Merck and Company, Inc. As such, there are currently two hepatitis A vaccinations available, which are equally effective. The hepatitis A vaccination is made by growing the hepatitis A virus (HAV) in a cell culture, after which the virus is killed with a toxic substance known as *formalin*. A vaccine manufactured in this method is known as a formalin-inactivated vaccine.

The hepatitis A vaccination is given via an injection into the shoulder muscle. This is known as an intramuscular (IM) deltoid injection. Side effects from the vaccination are rare. If experienced, they may include mild soreness at the site of the injection, a headache, and a low-grade fever. When a person receives the vaccination, her body's immune system will manufacture protective antibodies that guard her against a future hepatitis A infection. Because the HAV in the vaccination is dead and, therefore, is incapable of multiplying or causing disease, inoculation with the hepatitis A vaccination cannot possibly cause a person to become infected with HAV or make her capable of transmitting HAV to others.

Within two weeks of receiving the hepatitis A vaccination, 80 percent of people develop the hepatitis A antibody (HAV Ab). And within one month of receiving the vaccination, 95 to 99 percent of people develop immunity to hepatitis A. Another dose of the hepatitis A vaccination is given six to twelve months after the initial injection. This second injection has the effect of extending the duration of protection. After receiving both doses of the hepatitis A vaccination, a person is totally protected against future hepatitis A infections. This protection lasts at least ten years, if not longer.

Although HAV does not cause chronic liver disease, infection with this virus can make a person quite ill (see Chapter 8). In fact, some people are ill for as long as six months. Moreover, approximately 100 to 150 people die each year from fulminant liver failure caused by hepatitis A. It has been recognized that older people and those with chronic liver disease are especially likely to suffer a poor outcome when infected with HAV. Therefore, it is essential that all people with chronic liver disease (especially those over thirty years old) receive the hepatitis A vaccination. It is further recommended that all people who are awaiting a liver transplant or who have received a transplant be vaccinated. The vaccination of food handlers and day-care-center workers should also be considered.

Other groups of people who are at increased risk for hepatitis A and who should, therefore, receive the hepatitis A vaccination include:

- People traveling to, or working in, areas of the world where hepatitis A infection is common.

- Men who have sex with men.

- People who use intravenous or other illegal injection drugs.

- People with blood clotting factor disorders.

- People who work with nonhuman primates.

- Laboratory workers handling hepatitis A-contaminated blood or stools.

Routine inoculation in children older than two years old with the hepatitis A vaccination was approved in 1999 for states with a consistently high incidence of hepatitis A (20 people per 100,000 population). Known as "high rate communities," they include Arizona, Alaska, Oregon, New Mexico, Utah, Washington, Oklahoma, South Dakota, Nevada, California, and Idaho. "Intermediate rate communities," including Missouri, Texas, Colorado, Arkansas, Montana, and Wyoming, where the incidence of hepatitis A falls between 10 people per 100,000 population (the national average), and 20 people per 100,000 do not mandate childhood hepatitis A vaccination, but would be wise to enact such a mandate. In fact, mandatory childhood hepatitis A vaccination for all children could make hepatitis A a disease of the past, or at least it would significantly decrease the incidence of hepatitis A in the United States. Hopefully, future policy changes will be directed toward accomplishing this goal.

If a person has had hepatitis A already or has been exposed to HAV at any time in the past, she is protected from reinfection lifelong. Past exposure can be detected by obtaining a blood test for the hepatitis A antibody (HAV Ab). If a person tests positive for HAV Ab, there is no reason to get the vaccination because it will not provide any additional benefit. The hepatitis A vaccination will not protect a person from hepatitis B or C or from any form of hepatitis or liver disease other than hepatitis A.

Immune Globulin (IG) for Hepatitis A

Prior to 1995, when the hepatitis A vaccination first became available in the United States, an injection of immune globulin (IG) was the only way to protect a person who had been exposed to someone with acute hepatitis A. IG is a preparation composed of multiple antibodies (immunoglobulins). It is made from human plasma that has been pooled from many people. This plasma is sterilized and must test negative for other infectious diseases. (All IG in the United States has tested negative for hepatitis B, hepatitis C, and HIV.)

Since the hepatitis A vaccine does not provide immediate protection against acute hepatitis A, IG continues to be an important form of protection for people who have been recently exposed to HAV. IG is typically given as a single intramuscular injection and is effective only if it is administered within two weeks of exposure to HAV. While IG provides immediate protection against hepatitis A, its beneficial effects are strictly short-term. The protection from HAV that IG provides usually lasts no more than three to five months. Therefore, if a person who received IG is exposed to someone with acute hepatitis A five months or more after receiving the injection, they will be at risk for infection once again. Although IG cannot prevent infection in a person who already has acute hepatitis A, it may reduce the severity of the disease.

Hepatitis B Vaccination

The development of the hepatitis B vaccine represents one of the most important advances in the medical field. This is the first and only vaccine in history that can simultaneously prevent liver cancer, cirrhosis, and a sexually transmitted disease—hepatitis B. The FDA approved the hepatitis B vaccine in 1981, and it became commercially available in 1982. The original hepatitis B vaccine was made from the plasma of people chronically infected with hepatitis B. While this version of the vaccine is still available, it has been phased out of use in the United States since 1986, when the FDA approved Recombivax, an improved version of the vaccine. Recombivax, which is manufactured by Merck, Sharp and Dohme, is made from common baker's yeast.

There are currently two separate hepatitis B vaccines in use, Recombivax and Engerix-B. Engerix-B, which is manufactured by SmithKline Biologicals, was approved by the FDA in 1989. As with the hepatitis A vaccine, a person cannot develop hepatitis B infection as a result of receiving the injection, nor can they transmit the virus to others by receiving the vaccine. The vaccination is administered via an intramuscular injection in the shoulder muscle, and it rarely produces side effects. If experienced, side effects can include mild soreness at the site of injection, headache, and low-grade fever.

Adults are given three injections. The initial injection, a second injection one month after the initial one, and a third one, six months after the initial one. Approximately 95 to 99 percent of adults are protected against hepatitis B as a result of receiving the three injections. Protection is manifested on blood work by a hepatitis B surface antibody (HBsAb) titer of greater than 10 IU/ml (international units per milliliter). When such a lab value appears on blood work, this signifies that a person is completely protected against a future hepatitis B infection for at least ten years and possibly lifelong. An additional hepatitis B injection is normally not necessary. It is currently only recommended for people with poor immune systems, such as those people with AIDS, or people whose HBsAb levels are lower than 10 IU/ml.

Hepatitis B can lead to cirrhosis, liver failure, and liver cancer. Since the hepatitis B vaccine prevents hepatitis B infection from occurring, it is crucial for all people at risk for hepatitis B to obtain the vaccination. In fact, the hepatitis B vaccine has now been incorporated into the immunization programs in more than eighty countries. And, in 1991, the Advisory Committee on Immunization Practices (ACIP) mandated the routine universal vaccination of all newborns in the United States. Routine prenatal screening of all pregnant women for HBsAg is now the standard of care. Infants born to HBsAg positive mothers should receive both the hepatitis B vaccination and the hepatitis B immune globulin (HBIG; see below) within twelve hours of birth.

It is currently recommended that children receive the vaccination at age eleven or twelve if they did not receive it at birth. Many states have laws or regulations requiring the administration of the hepatitis B vaccination to children prior to beginning daycare or school.

Other groups of people who are at increased risk for hepatitis B, and who therefore should receive the hepatitis B vaccination include:

- People of any age who have multiple sexual partners.

- Men who have sex with other men.

- People who use intravenous or other illegal injection drugs.

- People with blood clotting factor disorders.

- Those who have intimate or household contact with a person who is a hepatitis B carrier (HBsAg positive).

- People who work in health care.

- Public safety workers who may come into contact with blood.

- People receiving hemodialysis.

- People who live or work in an institution for the developmentally disadvantaged.

- Prison inmates.

- Alaskan Natives and Pacific Islanders.

It is also advisable for any person with chronic liver disease to obtain the hepatitis B vaccination. The hepatitis B vaccination will eliminate the risk of acquiring hepatitis B through a liver transplant. It will also increase the number of potential donor livers available to a person awaiting transplant, because it will enable the use of a HBcAb positive donor organ. Finally, since it appears that coinfection with both HBV and HCV greatly increases a person's chance of developing liver cancer, obtaining the hepatitis B vaccination is crucial for people with chronic hepatitis C.

If a person has been exposed to hepatitis B at some time in the past, the vaccination will not afford them any benefit. Therefore, there is no reason for a person who is HBcAb or HBsAb positive to receive the hepatitis B vaccination. The hepatitis B vaccine will not protect a person against hepatitis A or C, and it will not protect a person against any form of hepatitis or liver disease other than hepatitis B.

Hepatitis B Immune Globulin (HBIG)

Hepatitis B immune globulin (HBIG) is made from plasma that has been pooled from many people who have high levels of the hepatitis B surface antibody (HBsAb). HBIG provides immediate but temporary protection to people who have been exposed to someone with infectious hepatitis B and to those who have accidentally been exposed to the blood or body fluids (for example, in a needle stick injury or blood splashing accident) of someone with infectious hepatitis B. Therefore, within two weeks of contact, HBIG should be administered to any person who has had exposure to hepatitis B-infected blood or who has had close or intimate contact with someone with infectious hepatitis B. As previously noted, infants born to mothers who are HBsAg positive should receive HBIG within twelve hours of birth. These infants must also obtain the hepatitis B vaccination series of shots. The hepatitis B vaccination may be obtained at the same time as HBIG. However, when the two are administered at the same time, they should not be injected into the same shoulder.

Combination Hepatitis A and B Vaccination

A combined hepatitis A and B vaccination is currently awaiting FDA approval in the United States. Once available, this vaccination should simplify immunization schedules and promote the important goal of routinely immunizing the population against hepatitis A and B. Since, with a combined vaccination, fewer injections would be required to achieve protection against these two viruses, it seems certain that members of the public would be more likely to avail themselves of the vaccination.

Hepatitis C Vaccination

The development of a vaccination against HCV is being doggedly researched. Yet this challenging quest faces some considerable obstacles. One of the major barriers to the development of a vaccine involves the complex population of mutant strains of the hepatitis C virus, known as quasispecies, that can exist in a person infected with hepatitis C. The existence of quasispecies is also one factor responsible for the failure of so many people to respond to antiviral therapy. It is also one of the reasons why so many people relapse after initially responding to antiviral therapy. During treatment, mutant strains that are resistant to further therapy often emerge. Thus, to be effective, a vaccine would need to protect a person against many different HCV variants. Indeed, if and when an effective, safe vaccination against HCV is produced, it would surely rank as a major advance in the annals of medicine.

Immune Globulin for Hepatitis C

It has not been convincingly demonstrated that immune globulin would protect a person who has been exposed to hepatitis C from getting infected with the virus. Therefore, it is not recommended that a person in this situation obtain an immune globulin injection.

Hepatitis D Vaccination

There is presently no vaccine available against the hepatitis delta virus (HDV), nor is there an immune globulin available that can combat this virus. However, the hepatitis B vaccination will effectively prevent the occurrence of hepatitis D in a person who did not have hepatitis B at the time she was vaccinated. For people who already have chronic hepatitis B, obtaining the hepatitis B vaccination will not provide any protection against becoming additionally infected with HDV. Animal research, however, appears promising. In those animals experimentally vaccinated, while infection with HDV was not prevented, the resultant liver disease was not as severe. Clearly, further investigation needs to be conducted in this area.

General Preventative Strategies

While it is impossible to prevent some liver diseases, there are many strategies that people can adopt to protect their livers and to maximize their health. All people—especially women—should consume alcohol only in moderation. People with liver disease should eliminate alcohol from their lives altogether. People with a family history of hemochromatosis or primary biliary cirrhosis should have blood work performed to test for these liver diseases. If either disease is found to be present, treatment should be started as soon as possible. For the best results to be achieved, treatment should begin during the earliest stages of the disease before any symptoms develop. As a general rule, all people should attempt to maintain a normal weight and to keep their diets low in saturated fats. This may minimize the likelihood of developing fatty liver and nonalcoholic steatohepatitis (although other factors may have a role in the development of these diseases). As much as possible, all hepatotoxic medications should be avoided. Cigarette smoking should be terminated, as it has been linked to the development of liver cancer and may enhance the hepatotoxicity of some medications.

The hepatitis A virus can be killed by boiling infected foods for three minutes and by disinfecting surfaces infected with the virus with bleach. It is best to avoid eating raw or partially cooked mollusks (clams, oysters, mussels, and scallops), as these fish often live in HAV-contaminated rivers and seas. When traveling to areas of the world known to have a high incidence of hepatitis A, it is especially important to eat well-cooked foods and to drink only bottled water. Sanitizing diaper-changing tables is also important, as hepatitis A-infected infants are typically a silent source for the spread of hepatitis A infection. Meticulous hand washing is of a great importance after using the bathroom, before eating a meal, and when preparing food for others.

Not engaging in unprotected sex will greatly reduce the likelihood of infection with HBV. While the risk of sexual transmission of HCV is rare, protected sex is recommended if a person engages in anal sex, has multiple sexual partners, has frequent prostate infections, or has open cuts or sores on the genitalia. People with hepatitis B or C should avoid sharing anything that may contain even the tiniest amount of their blood, including toothbrushes, razors, and nail clippers.

In order to further reduce the likelihood of spreading hepatitis B and C, people who are using injection drugs should never share needles with others or inject themselves with a used needle. A drop of blood so minuscule that it cannot be detected by the human eye may contain hundreds or even thousands of hepatitis B and/or C particles. Even meticulous cleaning may not totally eradicate the virus from a needle. If a person needs unused needles but cannot obtain them, she should seek out a needle exchange program. Or needle use can be limited to auto-destruct syringes. These needles are nonreusable because they are designed to self-destruct after one use so that they cannot be reused or shared with others. Of course, the best advice for a person who continues to actively use illicit drugs is to discontinue this activity immediately and seek help at a drug rehabilitation center. Also, anyone who intends to get a tattoo or have a body part pierced should make sure that they deal only with establishments that are clean and adhere to meticulous sterilization practices.

Finally, while the risk of transmission of hepatitis B and C through a blood transfusion is extraordinarily low, if a person will be undergoing surgery and may need a blood transfusion, she may wish to donate her own blood or to select a specific person (usually a relative) to donate blood to her. This is known, respectively, as autologous blood and directed blood donations. If this route of blood donation is desired, it should, if possible, be planned out well in advance of surgery.

CONCLUSION

Hopefully, this chapter has shed some light on many significant issues that involve the daily lives of all people with liver disease. Issues regarding pregnancy and sex, medications and their effects on the liver, the importance of obtaining the hepatitis

A and B vaccinations, and how to prevent the spread of liver disease, were all discussed. However, the key point of this chapter is that most people with liver disease can enjoy a good quality of life, but they must make certain modifications in their lifestyles in order to help make such a goal possible.

Conclusion

With the knowledge you have acquired from this book, you now know how integral the liver is to every aspect of your health and daily functioning. You know how to choose a qualified doctor and which questions are most important to ask. If you are a person with liver disease, you have the information you need to actively participate with your doctor in your treatment. You know what therapies are available to treat your liver disorder, and what new therapies are on the horizon. You're aware that certain changes in your lifestyle can improve your health and help you win the battle against liver disease. In addition, you know how to protect yourself from getting certain types of liver diseases, and how to protect your loved ones from becoming infected. You learned that liver transplantation can transform a debilitated person into someone who is active and productive. And, most important, you have also learned that being diagnosed with liver disease does not necessarily mean that you cannot lead a full and active life.

This book has also sought to emphasize a more subtle point, one that is quite important yet often overlooked. Namely, that the treatment of liver disease is a shared responsibility between the patient and the doctor. This is a key issue that I stress in running my medical practice. I believe that it is crucial for a patient to have a clear understanding of his or her liver disease and what can be done to control it. Moreover, I believe that it is important to keep patients abreast of the latest information concerning liver disease and its treatment. By adhering to this strategy, I believe that patients will be best equipped to take control of their health and to work in tandem with their doctor towards the ultimate goal of fighting their disease. As I stated at the outset of this book, congratulations are in order—because by reading this book you have already taken a huge step towards achieving this objective. There are many challenges that you face when diagnosed with liver disease. Hopefully, this book has enabled you to face these challenges with confidence and a positive outlook, thereby enhancing the likelihood that the best possible outcome will be achieved. You now have the power of knowledge, please use it in the best of health to conquer your liver disease.

APPENDIX

Resource Groups and Internet Websites

The following are some useful resource groups and Internet websites for the person seeking further information on hepatitis and liver disease. Please keep in mind that the author does not vouch for the accuracy of the information contained in these sites.

PART ONE

American Association for the Study of Liver Disease (AASLD)
1729 King Street, Suite 100
Alexandria, VA 22314-2720
703–299–9766
www.hepar-sfgh.ucsf.edu

American Board of Internal Medicine (ABIM)
800–441–2246

American Board of Medical Specialties (ABMS)
1007 Church Street Suite 404
Evanston, IL 60201-5913
847–491–9091
www.abms.org

American Gastroenterological Association (AGA)
7910 Woodmont Avenue, Suite 700
Bethesda, MD 20814
www.gastro.org

American Digestive Health Foundation (ADHF)
301–654–2635
www.adhf.org

American Liver Foundation (ALF)

National Chapter
75 Maiden Lane, Suite 603
New York, NY 10038

New York Chapter
80 Wall Street, Suite 1015
New York, NY 10005

800–GO LIVER (800–465–4837)
www.liverfoundation.org

American Medical Association (AMA)
800–AMA-3211
www.ama-assn.org

Canadian Liver Foundation
800–563–5483
www.liver.ca/docs.org

Dr. C. Everett Koop's website
www.dr.koop.com

Dr. Melissa Palmer
1097 Old Country Road
Plainview, NY 11803

444 Lakeville Road
New Hyde Park, NY 11040

500 Portion Road
Lake Ronkonkoma, NY 11779

516–939–2626
www.liverdisease.com

Latino Organization for Liver Awareness (LOLA)
P.O. Box 842 Throggs Neck Station
Bronx, NY 10465
888–367–LOLA

National Institutes of Diabetes and Digestive and Kidney Diseases (NIDDK)
www.niddk.nih.gov

National Center for Biotechnicology Information PubMed
www.ncbi.nlm.nih.gov/PubMed

PART TWO

Amgen, Inc.
1 Amgen Center Drive
Thousand Oaks, CA 91320-1789
888–508–8088
800–282–6436
805–447–1000
www.AMGEN.com

Hepatitis Foundation International
800–891–0707
www.HepFi.org

Hepatitis B Foundation
215–489–4900
www.hepb.org

Hepatitis B Coalition
651–647–9009
www.immunize.org

Hepatitis C Home Access Kit
888–888–HEPC

Centers For Disease Control— Hepatitis Branch
888–4HEPCDC (443–7232)
www.cdc.gov.ncidod/diseases/hepatitis/
   index.htm

CenterWatch—Clinical Trials Listing Service
www.centerwatch.com/

Hepatitis Information Network
www.hepnet.com

Roche Pharmaceuticals
340 Kingslands Street
Nutley, NJ 07110-1199
800–526–0625
800–433–6676
www.roche.com

Schering-Plough Corp.
2000 Galloping Hill Road
Kenilworth, NJ 07033-0530
www.schering-plough.com
888–HEP-2608 (888–437–2608)
800–521–7157
www.beincharge.com
www.schering-plough.com

PART THREE

Chronic Autoimmune Liver Disease Support Group
www.members.aol.com

Primary Biliary Cirrhosis Support Group
www.hometown.aol.com

Axcan Pharma
www.axcan.com

Al-Anon and Alateen
www.Al-Anon-Alateen.org

Alcoholics Anonymous
www.alcoholics-anonymous.org

Alcohol and Health
www.glness.com

National Institute on Alcohol Abuse and Alcoholism
www.etoh.niaaa.nih.gov

Iron Overload Disease Association
www.ironoverload.org
561–840–8512

The Hemochromatosis Foundation
518–489–0972
www.hemochromatosis.org

American Hemochromatosis Society
www.americanhs.org

Liver Cancer Network
www.livercancer.com

Living with Liver Cancer
www/rattler.cameron.edu/liver.com

PART FOUR

Office of Dietary Supplements
National Institutes of Health
Building 31 Room 1B
31 Center Drive
Bethesda, MD 20892
301–435–2920
www.odp.od.noh.gov

Herbs and Dietary Supplements
www.dietary-supplements.info.nih.gov

American Association of Naturopathic Physicians (AANP)
601 Valley Street, Suite 105
Seattle WA 98109
206–328–8510
www.infinite.org

Herbnet
www.herbnet.com

Herb Research Foundation
1007 Pearl Street, Suite 200
Boulder,CO 80302
303–449–2265
www.herbs.org

Food and Drug Administration (FDA)
www.fda.org

United States Department of Agriculture National Agricultural Library
Food and Nutrition Information Center
301–504–5719
www.nal.usda.gov

United Network For Organ Sharing (UNOS)
804–330–8500
www.unos.org

Transplant Recipients International Organization, Inc. (TRIO)
202–293–0980
www.primenet.com

American Share Foundation
www.asf.org

Centers for Disease Control and Prevention (CDC)
www.cdc.gov

Immunization Acion Coalition
www.immunix.org

SmithKline Beecham
P.O. Box 7929 FP 2005
Phila, PA 19101
800–366– 8900
www.sb.com

Glossary

This glossary should be used as a guide to assist you in defining words used throughout this book and words commonly used by doctors when they refer to hepatitis and liver disease. Not included in this glossary are the definitions of various liver diseases, different types of doctors, or medications used for liver disease. Refer to the appropriate chapters for detailed discussions on each of these topics.

Abdomen. The part of the body below the ribcage and above the pelvis; does not include the back of the body.

Acute hepatitis. Hepatitis with a course of six months or less.

Acute liver failure. The rapid development of liver failure associated with coagulopathy.

Adhesions. Scar tissue commonly resulting from prior abdominal surgery (but also has many other causes).

Adipose tissue. Fatty body tissue.

Alanine aminotransferase (ALT or SGPT). One of the transaminases (only found in the liver); high levels may indicate inflammation and/or injury to liver cells.

Albumin. A protein produced by the liver. A low level is an indicator of poor health and nutrition, and/or a poorly functioning liver.

Aldosterone. A steroid hormone that regulates salt and water balance in the body.

Alkaline phosphate (AP). One of the cholestatic liver enzymes found primarily in the liver and the bones but may also be found in the intestines, kidneys, and placenta.

Alpha-fetoprotein. A tumor marker often indicative of liver cancer when levels are very elevated.

ALT. *See* Alanine aminotransferase.

Alternative medicine. Any therapy used to treat an illness that is not within the realm of conventional and/or accepted medical therapies.

Amenorrhea. A lack of menstruation.

Amino acids. The building blocks of protein.

Ampulla (of vater). A tiny opening in the duodenum that leads to the common bile ducts.

Analgesic. A medication or substance used to control pain.

Analogue. A compound that resembles another compound in structure and function.

Androgen. A steroid hormone responsible for masculine traits.

Anemia. A condition in which the blood is low in red blood cells.

Angiogenesis. The development of new blood vessels.

Anicteric. Not icteric or not jaundiced; bilirubin level normal.

Antibody (Ab). A protein of the immune system that fights against foreign substances (antigens) with the goal of destroying and eliminating them from the body.

Antifibrotic. The ability to reduce scarring (fibrosis, not cirrhosis).

Antigen (Ag). A substance foreign to the body, capable of stimulating an immune response, noted by the formation of antibodies.

Anti-inflammatory. Capable of reducing inflammation.

Antimitochondrial antibody. An autoantibody occurring in most people with primary biliary cirrhosis.

Antinuclear antibody (ANA). An autoantibody produced in most people with autoimmune hepatitis.

Antioxidants. A group of enzymes and/or other substances, some of which are produced by the body as a defense against free radicals, specifically oxygen free radicals.

Antipyretic. A medication or substance used to control fever.

Antitumor. Able to fight cancer.

Antiviral. Able to fight viruses.

AP. *See* Alkaline phosphate.

Arrhythmia. Irregular heartbeat.

Arteriogram. An x-ray of an artery after the injection of dye.

Arthralgias. Joint aches.

Ascites. The accumulation of fluid in the peritoneal cavity; the most common complication of portal hypertension.

Aspartate aminotransferase (AST or SGOT). One of the transaminases; high levels may indicate inflammation and/or injury to liver cells; also found in other organs, such as the kidneys and heart.

AST. *See* Aspartate aminotransferase.

Asterixis. An uncontrollable flapping of the hands that often occurs with encephalopathy.

Asymptomatic. Having no symptoms of disease.

Autoantibody. Antibodies produced by the immune system targeted against a person's own organs or tissues.

Autoimmune reaction. A condition in which the body's immune system attacks its own organs and tissues as it identified them as being foreign or intruders.

Barbiturate. A central nervous system depressant medication.

Benign. Not cancerous.

Bile. A bitter, greenish mixture of acids, salts, pigments, cholesterol, proteins, and electrolytes produced by liver cells and stored in the gallbladder, which aids in the digestion of fats and is a neutralizer of poisons.

Bile acid. A major component of bile closely involved in both the production and the elimination of cholesterol.

Bile ducts. Ducts that carry bile into the intestines and the gallbladder from the liver.

Bile ductules. Small bile ducts.

Biliary Colic. Pain typically associated with an attack of gallstones characterized by right upper quadrant pain radiating to the right shoulder or back.

Bilirubin. A yellow-colored pigment produced by the liver when it recycles old red-blood cells; a component of bile, responsible for its yellow color.

Biopsy. *See* Liver biopsy.

Blanch. To turn white with the application of light pressure.

Board Certified. A designation that indicates that a doctor has completed rigorous training in the specialty and has passed an intensive set of boards (exams) in that specialty.

Board Eligible. A designation indicating that a doctor has completed training in the specialty but either has not taken or has not passed the boards in that specialty.

Bruit. *See* Hepatic bruit.

Calcinosis. Abnormal deposits of excess calcium in parts of the body.

Caput medusa. Dilated blood vessels that snake out from the umbilicus in people with massive ascites.

Carbohydrate-deficient transferrin (CDT). A blood test that may be an indicator of excessive alcohol use.

Cardiomegaly. Enlargement of the heart.

Cardiomyopathy. Enlargement of the heart due to a chronic disorder of heart muscle.

CAT scan. *See* Computerized axial tomography.

CBC. *See* Complete blood count.

CDT. *See* Carbohydrate-deficient transferrin.

Celiac sprue. An autoimmune disorder characterized by gluten intolerance.

Chelation therapy. A form of iron reduction therapy involving infusion of an iron-binding drug either into a vein or beneath the skin, which promotes the elimination of iron from the body.

Chelator. A binding agent.

Cholangitis. An infection in the bile ducts that can occur in a person with gallstones or with primary sclerosing cholangitis, for example.

Cholecystectomy. Surgical removal of the gallbladder.

Choledocholithiasis. Gallstones in the bile duct.

Cholestasis. Impairment or failure of bile flow, manifested by elevated levels of GGTP and AP.

Cholestatic liver enzymes. *See* Alkaline phosphate (AP); Gamma-glutamyl transpeptidase (GGTP).

Cholestatic liver injury. Liver injury in which there is an impairment or failure of bile flow within the bile ducts.

Chromosome. A substance containing most or all of the deoxyribonucleic acid (DNA) or ribonucleic acid (RNA) composing the genes of an individual.

Chronic hepatitis. Hepatitis occurring for longer than six months.

Cirrhosis. Irreversible scarring of the liver.

Coagulopathy. A disorder of clotting, causing a tendency to bleed, manifested by a prolonged prothrombin time of greater than three seconds; indicative of severe liver damage or liver failure.

Cocarcinogen. A substance that when combined with another carcinogenic factor hastens the progression to cancer.

Cocktail therapy. Combining more than one drug with different modes of action to treat a virus.

Coenzyme. An enzyme helper.

Coinfection. Infection with two viruses (such as HBV and HDV) at the same time.

Collateral shunts. The formation of alternative passageways for blood flow due to portal hypertension.

Combination therapy. Therapy with more than one drug at the same time to treat a disease.

Compensated cirrhosis. Cirrhosis without the development of complications, such as internal bleeding, jaundice, ascites, and encephalopathy. Also known as stable cirrhosis.

Complete blood count (CBC). A blood test that includes the levels of the white blood cell count, the red blood cell count, and the platelet count.

Compound pharmacist. A pharmacist who prepares, mixes, assembles, packages, and labels medication from scratch.

Computerized axial tomography (CAT scan or CT scan). An imaging study that uses gamma-radiation to transmit an x-ray beam through an organ.

Congestive gastropathy. Buildup of pressure in the stomach due to cirrhosis, which can lead to inflammation and bleeding.

Contraindicated. Inadvisable to use.

CREST syndrome. An autoimmune syndrome, characterized by calcinosis, Raynaud's phenomenon, esophageal dysmotility, sclerodactyly, and telangiectasias.

Cytochrome P450 system. A complex group of specialized enzymes within the liver that are responsible for the conversion of fat-soluble drugs or substances to water-soluble drugs or substances.

Cytokines. Substances secreted by cells of the immune system involved in regulating the intensity and duration of the immune response.

Cytoprotective substances. Medications or other substances that can protect cells.

Decompensated cirrhosis. Cirrhosis accompanied by complications that include internal bleeding, jaundice, encephalopathy, and/or ascites. Also known as unstable cirrhosis.

Deoxyribonucleic acid (DNA). A component of chromosomes that caries genetic and hereditary information.

Diuretic. A water pill.

DNA. *See* Deoxyribonucleic acid.

Duodenum. The first part of the small intestine.

Dupuytren's contracture. A puckering of the palm that prevents a person from totally straightening his or her hand; common in people with alcoholic cirrhosis.

Dysphagia. Trouble swallowing.

Edema. Fluid accumulation commonly in the legs around the ankles. *See also* Pedal edema.

Electrolyte. Any compound that in solution conducts electricity and is decomposed (electrolyzed) by it. Sodium chloride (salt), calcium, and potassium are examples of electrolytes.

ELISA. *See* Enzyme-linked immunosorbent assay.

Encephalopathy. Altered or impaired mental status occurring in people with cirrhosis, which can lead to coma.

Endemic. A disease prevailing continually in a restricted region.

Endoscope. A tube with a light at the end of it that is used to visualize internal organs, including the esophagus, stomach, duodenum, and large intestine.

Endoscopic retrograde cholangiopancreatography (ERCP). A special endoscope used to visualize the bile ducts and pancreatic ducts.

Endoscopy. Examination of internal organs using an endoscope.

Endotoxin. A poisonous substance in the cell wall of certain bacteria.

Enteric. Introduced into the body by way of the digestive tract.

Enzyme. A protein that induces chemical changes in other substances, while remaining unchanged by the process.

Enzyme-linked immunosorbent assay (ELISA). A laboratory technique used to determine the presence of an antibody (such as the hepatitis C antibody) in the blood.

ERCP. *See* Endoscopic retrograde cholangiopancreatography.

Erectile dysfunction. The decreased ability to achieve and maintain an erection.

Erythropoietin. A protein made by the body that can stimulate the formation of new red blood cells.

Esophageal dysmotility. Abnormal movements of the esophagus.

Esophageal varices. Enlarged blood vessels or varicose veins in the esophagus.

Esophagitis. Inflammation of the esophagus.

Esophagus. Food pipe; the portion of the digestive tract located between the pharynx and the stomach.

Estrogen. A steroid hormone responsible for feminine traits.

Excoriations. Severe scratch marks associated with breaks in the skin that often bleed.

Extrahepatic. Outside the liver.

Extrahepatic cholestasis. Bile duct blockage or injury occurring outside the liver.

Fatigue. The most common symptom of liver disease, characterized by a diminished ability to exert oneself, usually associated with a feeling of being tired, sleepy, bored, weak, and/or irritable.

Fenestrations. Wide-open holes in the blood vessels of the liver.

Fermentation. An enzymatically controlled transformation of a complex compound into simple compounds.

Ferritin. The storage form of iron.

Fetal alcohol syndrome. A number of abnormalities that may occur in infants born to women who drink alcohol excessively during pregnancy.

Fetor hepaticus. A foul, sweetish, or feces-like smell on the breath; often can be a sign of either acute or chronic liver failure, and often precedes encephalopathy.

Fibrosis. The initial stage of the formation of scar tissue in the liver, which is sometimes reversible.

Finger clubbing. A sign of liver disease, occurring especially in people with primary biliary cirrhosis, manifested by the enlargement and rounding of the tips of the fingers.

Flatulence. Increased gas production.

Focal nodular hyperplasia. A benign liver tumor made of liver cells that have multiplied numerous times around an abnormally formed hepatic artery.

Free radicals. Toxic, highly reactive compounds that are naturally produced by the body.

Fulminant hepatitis. A particularly serious form of acute hepatitis associated with jaundice, coagulopathy, and encephalopathy.

Fulminant liver failure. Acute liver failure accompanied by the development of encephalopathy within eight weeks of onset of symptoms or within two weeks of the onset of jaundice.

Gallbladder. A pear-shaped organ located beneath the liver. Its main function is to store and concentrate bile.

Gallstones. Stones that form in the gallbladder.

Gamma-glutamyl transpeptidase (GGTP). One of the cholestatic liver enzymes, which is found predominantly in the liver and is, therefore, a sensitive marker for certain liver disorders.

Gastric varices. Enlarged blood vessels or varicose veins in the stomach.

Gastritis. Inflammation of the stomach.

Genotype. The genetic makeup of the different HCV mutants in the hepatitis C viral population of an individual.

GGTP. *See* Gamma-glutamyl transpeptidase.

Gilbert's disease. A benign familial disorder of bilirubin metabolism, manifested by an elevated level of bilirubin on blood tests.

Glucose. A carbohydrate molecule; sugar.

Glutathione peroxidase. An antioxidant enzyme produced by the liver that protects the liver from free-radical damage.

Gluten. A protein found in wheat, rye, oats, and barley.

Gluten intolerance. The inability to absorb gluten.

Glycogen. A form of carbohydrate stored in the liver.

Gout. A disease characterized by painful inflammation of joints and an elevated uric acid level in the blood.

Granulomas. Nodules filled with a variety of inflammatory cells.

Gynecomastia. Breast enlargement.

HCC. *See* Hepatocellular carcinoma.

Hemangioma. The most common benign tumor of the liver, often referred to as a blood tumor.

Hematemesis. Vomiting of bright red blood, often due to bursting of esophageal varices.

Heme. Blood.

Hemodialysis. A medical procedure used to treat people with kidney failure involving the removal of blood from an artery, cleaning the blood, and then replacing it in the person through a vein.

Hemoglobin. An iron-containing protein, which is part of a red blood cell, that carries oxygen to other organs and tissues.

Hemolysis. Red blood cell (RBC) destruction.

Hemolytic anemia. A low red blood cell count due to hemolysis.

Hepatic. Pertaining to the liver.

Hepatic adenoma. A benign liver tumor composed of liver cells (hepatocytes).

Hepatic artery. The artery that carries blood to the liver.

Hepatic bruit. A harsh, musical sound heard when a stethoscope is placed over the liver; suggestive of liver cancer.

Hepatic vein. The vein that carries blood away from the liver.

Hepatitis. Inflammation of the liver.

Hepatocellular carcinoma (HCC). A primary malignant tumor of the liver (liver cancer); also known as hepatoma.

Hepatocellular liver injury. Inflammation and/or injury to liver cells; typically indicated by elevated levels of ALT and/or AST.

Hepatocytes. Cells that make up the liver.

Hepatorenal syndrome (HRS). Progressive deterioration of kidney function, leading to kidney failure, occurring in a person with liver failure.

Hepatoma. *See* Hepatocellular carcinoma.

Hepatomegaly. Enlargement of the liver.

Hepatotoxic. Harmful or damaging to the liver.

Herbs. Plants or plant parts that are used for healing purposes.

Heterozygote. A person who has inherited one gene for a genetic disease.

HFE. The candidate gene for hereditary hemochromatosis.

Hirsutism. Excessive hair growth.

HLA. *See* Human leukocyte antigen.

Homozygote. A person who has inherited two genes for a genetic disorder.

HRS. *See* Hepatorenal syndrome.

Human leukocyte antigen (HLA). Special antigens located on chromosomes that are believed to be a factor in the hereditary predisposition of people to different diseases.

Hyperlipidemia. Elevated levels of lipids (triglycerides and cholesterol) in the blood.

Hyperpigmentation. Increased pigment or melanin in the skin, causing a bronze appearance.

Hypersomnia. Excessive sleeping.

Hypertension. High blood pressure.

Hyperthyroidism. A disorder that occurs when the thyroid produces too much thyroid hormone, speeding up the body systems; an overactive or fast thyroid.

Hypervitaminosis A. A toxic overload of vitamin A that can lead to cirrhosis.

Hypnogonadism. Impaired production of the sex hormones.

Hypokalemia. A low potassium level.

Hypothyroidism. A disorder that occurs when the thyroid produces too little thyroid hormone, slowing down the body systems; an underactive or slow thyroid.

Idiosyncractic drug reaction. An abnormal unexpected hypersensitivity to a normal dose of a drug.

Immunity. The state of being immune or incapable of further infection.

Immunocompromised. Having a poorly functioning immune systems; also known as immunosuppressed.

Immunoglobulins. Proteins associated with the immune system, some of which are made by the liver. Antibodies are examples of immunoglobulins.

Immunomodulatory. Having the ability to regulate and stimulate the immune system.

Immunosuppresive substances. Medications or other substances that stifle the actions of the immune system.

Incubation period. The time between the entrance of the virus into the body and the initial appearance of symptoms and signs of the disease.

Induction therapy. Daily dosing of a medication, such as interferon, during the initial treatment period (one to three months) usually at higher than normal doses.

Infectious. Contagious; the capability to transmit infections to others.

Infectious hepatitis. The old name for hepatitis A.

Insomnia. The inability to sleep.

Interferons. A family of proteins that are made naturally by the body and that have antiviral, antitumor, and immunomodulatory activity; also manufactured synthetically.

Interleukin. A natural protein made in the body that can regulate the intensity and duration of the immune response.

Intractable. Incapable of being relieved.

Intrahepatic. Within the liver.

Intrahepatic cholestasis. Bile duct blockage or injury within the liver.

Intramuscular. Into or within the muscle.

Intravenous (IV). Into or within the vein.

Investigational drug. A drug that is considered experimental and is not yet approved by the FDA. It is only available to people who voluntarily enter a clinical drug trial, which involves the evaluation of the drug's effectiveness and potential side effects.

Iron studies. Blood tests that show levels of iron, ferritin, and transferrin saturation percent; also known as iron profile.

Jaundice. Yellow discoloration of the skin and eyes due to a buildup of bilirubin.

Laparoscope. A thin lighted tube inserted through a small incision in the abdominal wall in order to directly view the liver or other organs.

Leukocytes. White blood cells (WBC).

LFTs. *See* Liver function tests.

Lipid. Fat.

Lipid peroxidation. Iron-induced oxidation of cellular membranes.

Liver. A wedge-shaped gland located on the upper right side of the body, lying beneath the rib cage; the largest organ in the body with numerous functions.

Liver biopsy. The removal of a tiny piece of liver tissue using a special needle; performed for the purpose of examination under a microscope by a pathologist to determine the presence and extent of liver inflammation or damage.

Liver cancer. *See* Hepatocellular carcinoma.

Liver failure. Cessation of normal liver function.

Liver function tests (LFTs). Blood tests that give some indication of, although are not diagnostic of, what is going on inside the liver by measuring the levels of liver enzymes, bilirubin, and liver proteins.

Liver-kidney-microsomal antibody (LKMAb). An autoantibody that occurs in people with type II autoimmune hepatitis.

Liver palms. *See* Palmar erythema.

Liver spots. Brown spots most commonly located on the back of the hand that occur with aging and are not related to liver disease.

Liver-assist device. A form of temporary dialysis for the liver, involving removal of toxins from the blood of people with liver failure.

LKMAb. *See* Liver-kidney-microsomal antibody.

Lymphoma. A malignant tumor of lymph tissue.

Macrocytosis. Large red blood cells.

Macronodular cirrhosis. Cirrhosis in which the cirrhotic nodules in the liver are very large.

Magnetic resonance imaging (MRI). An imaging study that utilizes electromagnetic radiation to create a picture.

Malabsorption/maldigestion. Impaired or inadequate absorption or digestion of foods.

Malignant. Cancerous.

MCV. *See* Mean corpuscular volume.

Mean corpuscular volume (MCV). The volume of the average red blood cell in a sample of blood.

Melanin. Dark brown to black pigment in the skin.

Melatonin. A hormone produced by the pineal gland that is involved in the sleep cycle.

Melena. Black, foul-smelling stool indicative of upper intestinal bleeding.

Metabolism. The sum of the changes of the buildup and breakdown occurring in tissues of living organisms.

Metastasis. The spread of tumor cells from the organ of origin to another organ, most commonly the liver.

Metastasize. The spread of tumor cells to other organs.

Micronodular cirrhosis. Cirrhosis in which the cirrhotic nodules in the liver are numerous and very small.

Mineral. A substance that originates in the soil and water, and eventually becomes incorporated into all animal and plant life through the food chain.

Monotherapy. Treatment with only one drug or agent.

MRI. *See* Magnetic resonance imaging.

Muscle wasting. Loss of muscle mass, most prominent in the arms and upper body; associated with cirrhosis, and general poor nutrition.

Mutation. A permanent alteration of genetic material.

Myalgias. Muscle aches.

Mycophagist. An expert mushroom picker.

Myoglobin. A protein responsible for delivery of oxygen to muscles.

Myopathy. Sore, swollen muscles.

NANB. *See* Non A non B hepatitis.

Non-A non-B hepatitis (NANB). The old name for hepatitis C.

Non-invasive. No surgery required.

Nonresponder. A person with hepatitis C whose transaminase levels do not normalize and who continues to have detectable levels of HCV RNA in the blood while on therapy.

Nonsuppurative. Not pus producing.

Nucleoside/nucleotide. Compounds that form the building blocks of DNA and RNA.

Oral hypoglycemic. Sugar-lowering medication taken orally.

Osteomalacia. A softening of the bones.

Osteoporosis. A decrease in bone quantity.

Overdiuresis. The excessive use of diuretics.

Palmar erythema. Bright red coloring of the palms, particularly at the base of the thumb and pinky; often a sign of chronic liver disease; also called liver palms.

Pancreatitis. Inflammation of the pancreas.

Paper money skin. A condition in which the upper body is covered with numerous thin blood vessels that resemble the silk threads on a United States dollar bill.

Paracentesis. The removal of large amounts of ascitic fluid through a needle inserted into the abdomen.

Paraneoplastic syndrome. The manifestation of tumor symptoms in other parts of the body.

Parenteral. Introduced into the body by any way other than via the intestinal tract.

Parotid gland enlargement. A condition in which the parotid gland enlarges, causing the earlobes to protrude at right angles to the jaw; often a sign of alcoholic cirrhosis.

PCR. *See* Polymerase chain reaction.

Pedal edema. Swollen ankles.

Percutaneous. Through the skin.

Perinatal transmission. Transmission of disease during childbirth.

Peritoneal cavity. The space between the abdominal organs and the skin.

Peritonitis. An infection of abdominal fluids.

Phlebotomy. Removal of blood through a vein; often used as a form of iron-reduction therapy.

Placebo. An inert, harmless substance that has no actual medical effect on a person's illness, but is identical in appearance to a medication under investigation.

Placebo effect. Improvement in the condition of a person in response to treatment that is due to a "dummy drug" or "sugar pill" and not to the active ingredient of the substance being tested.

Platelets. Blood cells that promote blood clotting.

Polymerase chain reaction (PCR). A laboratory test used to detect hepatitis C virus RNA levels in the blood.

Polypeptide. A group of amino acids linked together.

Portal hypertension. High blood pressure in the liver and the portal circulation commonly due to cirrhosis.

Portal vein. The vein that carries blood to the liver.

Portal vein thrombosis. A blood clot in the portal vein.

Prognosis. The anticipated course of a disease without treatment.

Proof. The alcoholic strength of an alcoholic beverage expressed by a number that is double the percentage of alcohol present.

Protein. The basic element of living tissue essential for the growth and repair of tissues; composed of amino acids.

Prothrombin (factor II). A protein produced by the liver that is involved in the process of blood clotting.

Prothrombin time. A blood test that measures the time it takes blood to clot; prolonged in liver failure.

Pruritus. Medical term for itching.

Pseudo tumor. A fake tumor.

Pyruvate dehydrogenase. An enzyme involved in carbohydrate metabolism; a component of the major antigen against antimitochondrial antibody (AMA).

Quasispecies. Genetic variations of the hepatitis C virus due to mutations of the virus.

Raynaud's phenomenon. A rheumatic disorder characterized by the fingertips turning blue and numbness upon excessive exposure to cold weather or emotional stress.

RBCs. *see* Red blood cells.

Recidivism. Relapsing back to old negative behavior, such as drinking alcohol.

Recombinant immunoblot assay (RIBA). A laboratory technique used to detect antibodies to hepatitis C in the blood.

Red blood cells (RBCs). Cells in the blood that carry oxygen to organs and tissues.

Refractory ascites. Ascites that does not respond to treatment with dietary restrictions and medications.

Relapse. The recurrence of disease after a period of improvement.

Relapser. A person with hepatitis C who initially responded to therapy but when taken off therapy, HCV RNA again becomes detectable in the blood and transaminase levels again become elevated.

Resection. Surgical removal of part of an organ or tissue.

Responder. A person with hepatitis C who normalizes transaminase levels and eradicates HCV RNA while on therapy.

RIBA. *See* Recombinant immunoblot assay.

Ribonucleic acid (RNA). A component of chromosomes that carries genetic and hereditary information.

Ribozyme. A type of RNA molecule with the unique ability to cut targeted genetic material.

Right upper quadrant pain or tenderness (RUQT). Pain or tenderness over the liver; occurs most commonly in the acute stages of liver disease, due to acute inflammation, irritation, and distension of the liver's surface.

RNA. *See* Ribonucleic acid.

RUQT. *See* Right upper quadrant pain or tenderness.

Salt. Sodium chloride.

Sampling error. The uncommon occurrence of a liver sample taken during a liver biopsy looking better or worse than the rest of the liver.

Sarcoidosis. A disease characterized by the formation of granulomas in the lungs, skin, lymph nodes, liver, and bones.

SBP. *See* Spontaneous bacterial peritonitis.

Scleral icterus. Yellow discoloration of the sclera (whites of the eyes).

Sclerodactyly. Scleroderma of the fingers and toes.

Scleroderma. An autoimmune disease characterized by a thickening and hardening of the skin and internal organs due to excessive collagen deposits.

Sclerotherapy. The injection of a clotting agent directly into a bleeding varix to stop hemorrhage.

Serology. The measure of either antigens or antibodies in the blood.

Serum hepatitis. The old name for hepatitis B.

Shunt. A surgical procedure performed to decrease portal hypertension in the liver and portal circulation by creating an alternative passageway for blood. Portal systemic and splenorenal shunts are two examples.

Signs. Physical clues or findings of a disease.

Sjögren's syndrome. An autoimmune disorder characterized by xerophthalmia and xerostomia, which often occurs in people with primary biliary cirrhosis.

SLE. *See* Systemic lupus erythematosus.

Smooth muscle antibody (SMA). An autoantibody produced in some people with type 1 autoimmune hepatitis.

Sonogram (ultrasound or sono). An imaging study done by a radiologist by a technique that uses sound waves to produce an image.

Spider angiomatas. Enlarged blood vessels found on the upper chest, back, face, and arms, resembling little red spiders.

Spleen. An organ lying directly opposite the liver under the ribcage on the left side of the body; plays a role in the storage of platelets.

Splenomegaly. An enlarged spleen.

Spontaneous bacterial peritonitis (SBP). An infection of ascitic fluid (ascites).

Steatohepatitis. Fatty liver accompanied by inflammation.

Steatonecrosis. Fatty liver accompanied by scarring.

Steatorrhea. Loose, frothy, light-colored stool due to fat malabsorption.

Steatosis. The medical term for fatty liver.

Subcutaneous. Beneath the skin.

Superinfection. Infection with a virus (such as HDV) in a person who already has a chronic viral illness (such as chronic hepatitis B).

Sustained responder. A person with hepatitis C who has eradicated the virus for more than six months beyond the date when therapy was discontinued.

Symptom. Any abnormal sensation experienced by a person that is indicative of a disease or disorder.

Synergistically. In union with.

Systemic lupus erythematosus (SLE). An autoimmune disease affecting multiple organs characterized by fever, skin rash, and arthritis.

Telangiectasia. Small thin red spots on either the skin or mucous membrane.

Teratogenic. Capable of causing birth defects.

Terry's nails. A condition in which the normal pinkish color of the nail bed turns completely white and the half-moon circles at the base of the nails disappear; usually a sign of cirrhosis.

Testicular atrophy. A condition in which the testicles shrink; usually a sign of cirrhosis.

Testosterone. A sex hormone responsible for masculine traits.

Thrombocytopenia. A low platelet count; lower than 150 x 103/microliter.

Thymosin. A hormone involved in the immune system; produced by the thymus gland.

Thymus gland. A gland in the neck that produces thymosin.

TIPS. *See* Transjugular intrahepatic portosystemic shunt.

Transaminases. *See* Alanine aminotransferase (ALT or SGPT); Aspartate aminotransferase (AST or SGOT)

Transferrin. A protein made in the liver that transports iron through the body.

Transferrin saturation percent. The percentage of transferrin that is saturated with iron at any given time.

Transjugular intrahepatic portosystemic shunt (TIPS). A procedure that creates an alternative passageway in the liver between the portal and hepatic veins in an attempt to reduce portal hypertension.

Treatment naïve. A person who has never been treated, for example, with interferon for chronic hepatitis C.

Treatment refractory. A person who does not respond to therapy; a nonresponder.

Triglycerides. The form of fat stored in the liver.

Truncal obesity. Excessive fat around the midsection.

Tumor. A mass that may be either benign or malignant.

Tumor marker. A blood test that is indicative of, but not diagnostic of, cancer.

Ulcerative colitis. An inflammatory disease of the colon.

Ultrasound. *See* Sonogram.

Umbilical hernia. A protrusion of the umbilicus (belly button), often due to massive ascites.

Upper endoscopy. A procedure in which a tube with a light at the end is inserted through a patient's mouth and passed into the esophagus, stomach, and duodenum.

Varices. Enlarged, distended blood vessels that result from the formation of collateral shunts in people with portal hypertension; usually located in the esophagus and stomach.

Varix. A dilated blood vessel usually located in the esophagus and stomach.

Vascular. Full of blood vessels.

Vasculitis. Inflammation of blood vessels.

Veno-occlusive disease. Blockage of the hepatic vein leading to a lack of supply of blood to the liver.

Vertical transmission. Transmission of disease during pregnancy.

Viral load. The amount of viral particles per milliliter of blood.

Vitamins. Organic substances that come from plants and animals.

Vitiligo. An autoimmune skin condition manifested by smooth nonpigmented patches on various parts of the body.

Wilson's disease. A genetic disorder of copper overload, which leads to an accumulation of copper in the liver, eventually resulting in cirrhosis.

Xanthelasmas. A yellow nodule or patch on the eyelids associated with high cholesterol levels; occurs in people with primary biliary cirrhosis.

Xanthomas. An irregular yellow nodule or patch, usually on the elbows and knees, associated with high cholesterol levels; occurs in people with primary biliary cirrhosis.

Xenotransplantation. The use of organs from animals for transplantation into humans.

Xerophthalmia. Dry eyes.

Xerostomia. Dry mouth.

Bibliography

Chapter 3: Tests, Tests, Tests—Learning What You Need to Know

Guicciardi, M.E., et al. "Diurnal Variation of Serum Alanine Transaminase Activity in Chronic Liver Disease." *Hepatology* Vol. 28, No. 6 (1998): pp. 1794–1795.

Chapter 6: A Look at Cirrhosis

Sorensen, Henrik Toft, et al. "Risk of Liver and Other Types of Cancer in Patients with Cirrhosis: A Nationwide Cohort Study in Denmark." *Hepatology* 28 (1998): pp. 921–925.

Chapter 7: An Overall Look at Hepatitis

Desmet, V.G.M., et al. "Classification of Chronic Hepatitis: Diagnosis, Grading and Staging." *Hepatology* 19 (1994): pp. 1513–1520.

Fagen, E.A., et al. "Fulminant Viral Hepatitis." *British Medical Bulletin* 46 (1990): pp. 462–480.

Ikeda, H., et al. "Infection with an Unenveloped DNA Virus (TTV) in Patients with Acute or Chronic Liver Disease of Unknown Etiology and in Those Positive for Hepatitis C Virus RNA." *Journal of Hepatology* No. 2 (February 1999): pp. 205–212.

Lancet 352 (1998): pp. 164, 191–197.

Nanda, S.K., et al. "Etiological Role of Hepatitis E Virus in Sporadic Fulminant Hepatitis." *Journal of Medical Virology* 42 (1994): pp. 133–137.

New York Times Tuesday, July 20, 1999, pp. F1, F4.

Nishizawa, T., et al. "A Novel DNA Virus (TTV) Associated with Elevated Transaminase Levels in Posttransfusion Hepatitis of Unknown Etiology." *Biochemical and Biophysical Research Communications* 241 (1997): pp. 92–97.

Okamoto, Hiroaki. "Fecal Excretion of a Nonenveloped DNA Virus (TTV) Associated with Posttransfusion Non-A-G Hepatitis." *Journal of Medical Virology* 56 (1998): pp. 128–132.

Chapter 8: Understanding and Treating Hepatitis A

Faust, R.L., et al. "Acute Renal Failure Associated with Nonfulminant Hepatitis A Viral Infection." *American Journal of Gastroenterology* 91 (1996): pp. 369–372.

Inman, R.D., et al. "Arthritis, Vasculitis, and Cryoglobulinemia Associated with Relapsing Hepatitis A Virus Infection." *Annals of Internal Medicine* 105 (1986): pp. 700–703.

Hoofnagle, J.H. "Fulminant Hepatic Failure: Summary of A Workshop." *Hepatology* 21 (1995): pp. 240–252.

Huppertz, H.I., et al. "Autoimmune Hepatitis Following Hepatitis A Virus Infection." *Journal of Hepatology* 23(2) (August 1995): pp. 204–208

Keefe, E.B. "Is Hepatitis A More Severe in Patients with Chronic Hepatitis B and Other Chronic Liver Diseases?" *American Journal of Gastroenterology* 90 (1995): pp. 201–205.

Keefe, E.B., et al. "Safety and Immunogenicity of Hepatitis A Vaccine in Patients with Chronic Liver Disease." *Hepatology* (March 1998): pp. 881–886.

Leino, T., et al. "Hepatitis A Outbreak Amongst Intravenous Amphetamine Abusers in Finland." *Scandinavian Journal of Infectious Diseases* 29 (1997): pp. 213–216.

Melnick, J.L. "History and Epidemiology of Hepatitis A Virus." *Journal of Infectious Diseases* 171 (Suppl. 1) (1995): pp. 52–58.

"Prevention of Hepatitis A Through Active or Passive Immunization. Recommendations of the Advisory Committee on Immunization Practices (ACIP)" *Morbidity and Mortality Weekly Report CDC* Vol. 45., No. RR-15 (December 27, 1996).

Mijch, A.M., et al. "Clinical, Serologic and Epidemiologic Aspects of the Hepatitis A Infection." *Seminars in Liver Disease* 6 (1986): pp. 42–45.

Shapiro, C.N., et al. "Epidemiology of Hepatitis A. Seroepidemiology and Risk Groups in the USA." *Vaccine* 10 (1992):59.

Vento, S., et al. "Identification of Hepatitis A Virus as a Trigger for Autoimmune Chronic Hepatitis Type 1 in Susceptible Individuals." *Lancet* 337 (1991): pp. 1183–1186.

Vento, S., et al. "Fulminant Hepatitis Associated with Hepatitis A Superinfection in Patients with Chronic Hepatitis C." *New England Journal of Medicine* 338 (1998): pp. 286–290.

Villano, S.A., et al. "Hepatitis A Among Homosexual Men and Injection Drug Users:

More Evidence for Vaccination." *Clinical Infectious Diseases* 25 (1997): pp. 726–728.

Williams, I., et al. "Association Between Chronic Liver Disease and Death from Hepatitis A, United States, 1989–92." Presented at the Triennial International Symposium on Viral Hepatitis and Liver Disease, Rome, April 21–25, 1996. Abstract.

Willner, I.R. "Serious Hepatitis A: An Analysis of Patients Hospitalized During an Urban Epidemic in the United States." *Annals of Internal Medicine* 128 (1998): pp. 111–114.

Yao, G. "Clinical Spectrum and Natural History of Viral Hepatitis A in A 1988 Shanghai Epidemic." In: Hollinger FB., et al. *Viral Hepatitis and Liver Disease* Baltimore: William and Wilkins, (1991): pp. 76–78.

Chapter 9: Understanding Hepatitis B and D

Bianco, Celso. New York Blood Center Analysis 1998.

Fattovich, B., Giovanna, et al. "Natural Course and Prognosis of Chronic Hepatitis Type." *Viral Hepatitis Reviews* Vol. 2, No. 4 (1996): pp. 263–276.

Denniston, K.J., et al. "Cloned Fragment of the Hepatitis Delta Virus RNA Genome: Sequence and Diagnostic Application." *Science* 232 (1986): pp. 873–875.

DiBisceglie, Adrian M. *Viral Hepatitis Diagnosis, Treatment, Prevention* "Hepatitis C Virus" edited by Richard A. Willson. Marcel Dekker, Inc. (1997): pp. 217–238.

Dienstag, J.L. "Hepatitis B as an Immune Complex Disease." *Seminars in Liver Disease* 1 (1981): pp. 45–57.

Gimson, A.W.Y., et al. "Clinical and Prognostic Differences in Fulminant Hepatitis Type A, B, and Non-A Non-B." *Gut* 24 (1983): p. 1194.

Hoofnagle, J.D.A. "Serologic Diagnosis of Acute and Chronic Viral Hepatitis." *Seminars in Liver Disease* 11 (1991): pp. 73–78.

Inman, R.D. "Rheumatic Manifestations of Hepatitis B Virus Infection." *Seminars in*

Arthritis and Rheumatism 11 (1982): pp. 406–420.

Kowdley, Kris V. "The Role of Iron in Chronic Viral Hepatitis: Implications for Therapy." in *Viral Hepatitis Diagnosis Treatment Prevention* edited by Richard A. Willson. Marcel Dekker, Inc. (1997): pp. 505–520.

Lai, K.N., et al. "The Clinico-Pathologic Features of Hepatitis B Virus-Associated Glomerulonephritis." *Quarterly Journal of Medicine* 63 (1987): pp. 323–333.

Lai, K.N., et al. "Membranous Nephropathy Related to Hepatitis B Virus in Adults." *New England Journal of Medicine* 324 (1991): pp. 1457–1463.

Lee, William M., M.D., "Hepatitis B Virus Infection, " *New England Journal of Medicine* Vol. 337, No. 24 (December 11, 1997): pp. 1733–1745.

Liang, T.J., et al. "A Hepatitis B Virus Mutant Associated with An Epidemic of Fulminant Hepatitis." *New England Journal of Medicine* 324 (1991): pp. 1705–1709.

Lin, H-H, et al. "Natural Course of Patients with Chronic Type B Hepatitis Following Acute Delta Hepatitis Superinfection." *Liver* 9 (1989): pp. 129–134.

Lisker-Melman, M., et al. "Glomerulonephritis Caused by Chronic Hepatitis B Virus Infection: Treatment with Recombinant Human Alpha-Interferon." *Annals of Internal Medicine* 111 (1989): pp. 479–483.

Mcmahon, B.J., et al. "Hepatitis B-Related Sequelae: Prospective Study in 1400 Hepatitis B Surface Antigen-Positive Alaska Native Carriers." *Archives of Internal Medicine* 150 (1990): pp. 1051–1054.

Marcellin, P., et al. "Redevelopment of Hepatitis B Surface Antigen After Renal Transplantation." *Gastroenterology* 100 (1991): pp. 1432–1434.

Margolis, H.S., et al. "Hepatitis B: Evolving Epidemiology and Implications for Control." *Seminars in Liver Disease* 11 (1991): pp. 84–92.

Martin, B.A., et al. "Hepatitis B Reactivation Following Allogenic Bone Marrow Transplantation: Case Report and Review of the Literature." *Bone Marrow Transplantation* 15 (1995): pp. 145–148.

Pease, C., et al. "Arthritis as the Main Or Only Symptom of Hepatitis B Infection." *Postgrad Medicine* 61 (1985): pp. 545–547.

Rehermann, Barbara. "Hepatitis B Virus: Molecular Biology and Immunopathology—Experimental and Clinical Features," edited by Richard A. Willson. Marcel Dekker, Inc. (1997): pp. 85–118.

Rizzetto, M., et al. "Chronic Hepatitis in Carriers of Hepatitis B Surface Antigen with Intrahepatic Expression of Delta Antigen: An Active and Progressive Disease Unresponsive to Immunosuppressive Treatment." *Annals of Internal Medicine* 98 (1983): pp. 437–441.

Rogers, Steven. "Hepatitis B Virus: Clinical Disease—Prevention and Therapy." edited by Richard A. Willson. Marcel Dekker, Inc. (1997): pp. 119–146.

Saracco, G., et al. "Rapidly Progressive Hbsag-Positive Hepatitis in Italy: the Role of Hepatitis Delta Virus Infection." *Journal of Hepatology* 5 (1987): pp. 274–821.

Scott, D.G.I., et al. "Systemic Vasculitis in A District General Hospital 1972–1980: Clinical and Laboratory Features, Clarification and Prognosis in 80 Cases." *Quarterly Journal of Medicine* 203 (1982): pp. 292–311.

Vento, S., et al. "Clinical Reactivation of Hepatitis B in Anti-Hbs-Positive Patients with AIDS." *Lancet* 1 (1989): pp. 332–333.

Wands, J.R., Blum, H. "Primary Hepatocellular Carcinoma." [Editorial]. *New England Journal of Medicine* 325 (1991): pp. 729–731.

Weissberg, J.A.L., et al. "Survivial in Chronic Hepatitis B: An Analysis of 379 Patients." *Annals of Internal Medicine* 101 (1984): pp. 613–616.

Chapter 10: Understanding Hepatitis C

Alter, M.J. "The Epidemiology of Acute and Chronic Hepatitis C." *Clinics in Liver Disease* Vol. 1, No. 3 (November 1997): pp. 559–568.

Associated Press "Blood Recipients Urged to Test for Hepatitis C." *Newsday* August 13, 1997, p. A36.

Bjoro, Kristian, et al. "Hepatitis C Infection in Patients with Primary Hypogammaglobulinemia After Treatment with Contaminated Immune Globulin." *New England Journal of Medicine* Vol. 331., No. 24 (December 15, 1994): pp. 1607–1650.

Bonkovsky, H.L. "Iron and Chronic Viral Hepatitis." *Hepatology* (March 1997): pp. 759–768.

Choo, Q.L., et al. "Isolation of a C DNA Clone Derived from A Blood-Borne Viral Hepatitis Genome." *Science* 244 (1989): pp. 359–362.

Collier, Jane, et al. "Hepatitis C Viral Infection in the Immunosuppressed Patient." *Hepatology* (January 1998): pp. 2–6.

Conry-Cantilena, Cathy, et al. "Routes of Infection, Viremia, and Liver Disease in Blood Donors Found to Have Hepatitis C Virus Infection." *New England Journal of Medicine* Vol. 334, No. 26 (June 27, 1996): pp. 1691–1696.

Davis, Gary L. "Hepatitis C." *Clinics in Liver Disease* Vol. 1 No. 3 (November 1997).

Dickson, Roland C. "Clinical Manifestations of Hepatitis C." *Clinics in Liver Disease* Vol. 1 No.3 (November 1997): pp. 569–585.

Esteban, Juan, et al. "Hepatitis C. in Viral Hepatitis Diagnosis, Treatment, Prevention," edited by Richard A. Willson. Marcel Dekker, Inc. (1997): pp. 147–216.

Farci, Patricia, et al. "Hepatitis C Virus-Associated Fulminant Hepatic Failure." *New England Journal of Medicine* Vol. 335, No. 9, pp. 631–634.

Forns, Xavier, et al. "Methods for Determining the Hepatitis C Virus Genotype." *Viral Hepatitis Reviews* Vol. 4, No. 1 (1998): pp. 1–19.

Fried, Michael, et al. "Absence of Hepatitis C Viral RNA from Saliva and Semen of Patients with Chronic Hepatitis C." *Gastroenterology* 102 (1992): pp.1306–1308.

Gish, Robert. "Hepatitis C Virus: Eight Years Old." *Viral Hepatitis Reviews* Vol. 3, No. 1 (1997): pp. 17–37.

Gitlin, Norman. "Hepatitis C: Risk of a Haircut." Letter to the Editor, *Annals of Internal Medicine* Vol. 126, No.5, March 1 1997.

Gordon, Stuart C. "Clinical Outcome of Hepatitis C as a Function of Mode of Transmission," *Hepatology* Vol. 28, No 2 (1998): pp. 562–567.

Gordon, S., et al. "The Pathology of Hepatitis C as a Function of Mode of Transmission: Blood Transfusion Vs. Intravenous Drug Use." *Hepatology* 18 (1993): pp. 1338–1343.

Gross, John B. "Clinician's Guide to Hepatitis C." *Mayo Clinic Proceedings* 73 (1998): pp. 355–362.

Hadziyannis, S.J. "The Spectrum of Extrahepatic Manifestations in Hepatitis C Virus Infection." *Journal of Viral Hepatitis* 4 (1997): pp. 342–348.

Isaacson, A.H., et al. "Should we Test Hepatitis C Virus Genotype and Viremia Level in Patients with Chronic Hepatitis C?" *Journal of Viral Hepatitis* 4 (1997): pp. 285–292.

Kaito, M., et al. "Hepatitis C Virus Particle Detected by Immunoelectron Microscopic Study." *Journal of General Virology* 75 (1994): pp. 1755–1760.

Kasahara, Akinori, et al. "Risk Factors for Hepatocellular Carcinoma and Its Incidence After Interferon Treatment in Patients with Chronic Hepatitis C." *Hepatology* (May 1998): pp. 1394–1402.

Kuzushita, N., et al. "Influence of HLA Haplotypes on the Clinical Course of Individuals Infected with HCV." *Hepatology* (January 1998): pp. 240–244.

Leevey, Carroll B. "High incidence of Hepatitis C in New Jersey Suburb Prompts Study of Role of Mosquitoes." *Gastroenterology and Endoscopy News* (August 1998): p. 32.

Martinot, Michele, et al. "Influence of Hepatitis G Virus Infection on the Severity of Liver Disease and Response to Interferon-alpha in Patients with Chronic Hepatitis C." *Annals of Internal Medicine* 126 (1997): pp. 874–881.

Mathurin, Phillipe. "Slow Progression of Fibrosis in Hepatitis C Virus patients with Persistently Normal Alanine Transaminase Activity." *Hepatology* (March 1998): pp. 868–872.

NIH Consensus Statement. "Management of Hepatitis C." Vol. 15, No. 3 (March 24–26 1997): pp. 1–41.

Peano, Gianmichele, et al. "HLA-DR5 Antigen A Genetic Factor Influencing the Outcome of Hepatitis C Infection?" *Archives of Internal Medicine* Vol. 154 (December 26, 1994): pp. 2733–2736.

Puoti, Claudio, et al. "Clinical, Histological and Virological Features of Hepatitis C Virus Carriers with Persistently Normal or Abnormal Alanine Transaminase Levels." *Hepatology* (December 1997): pp. 1393–1398.

"Recommendations for Follow-up of Health-Care Workers after Occupational Exposure to Hepatitis C Virus." *Journal of the American Medical Association* Vol. 278, No. 13 (October 1, 1997): pp. 1056–1057.

Shetty, Kirti, et al. "Diagnostic Tests for Viral Hepatitis B and C." *Practical Gastroenterology* (May 1998): pp. 39–47.

Terada, Soichiro, et al. "Minimal Hepatitis C Infectivity in Semen." *Annals of Internal Medicine* Vol. 117, No. 2 (July 15, 1992): p. 171.

Tibbs, C.J. "Methods of Transmission of Hepatitis C." *Journal of Viral Hepatitis* 2 (1995): pp. 113–119.

Tong, Myron J., et al. "Clinical Outcomes After Transfusion-Associated Hepatitis C." *New England Journal of Medicine* Vol. 332, No. 22 (June 1, 1995): pp. 1463–1466.

Vento, Sandro, et al. "Fulminant Hepatitis Associated with Hepatitis A Virus Superinfection in Patients with Chronic hepatitis C." *New England Journal of Medicine* (January 29, 1998): pp. 286–290.

Willson, Richard A. "Extrahepatic Manifestations of Chronic Viral Hepatitis." in *Viral Hepatitis Diagnosis, Treatment, Prevention* Marcel Dekker, Inc., pp. 331–369.

Zein, N.N., et al. "Hepatitis C Genotypes in the United Sates; Epidemiology, Pathogenicity, and Response to Interferon Therapy." *Annals of Internal Medicine* 125 (1996): pp. 634–639.

Chapter 11: Treating Chronic Viral Hepatitis

Bennett, William G., et al. "Estimates of the Cost-Effectiveness of a Single Course of Interferon Alpha 2b in Patients with Histologically Mild Chronic Hepatitis C." *Annals of Internal Medicine* 127 (1997): pp. 855–865.

Dusheiko, G.M., et al. "Treatment of Chronic Type B and C Hepatitis with Interferon Alfa: An Economic Appraisal." *Hepatology* 22 (1995): pp. 1863–1873.

Gross, G., et al. "Genital Warts do not Respond to Systemic Recombinant Interferon Alfa-2a Treatment During Cannabis Consumption." *Dermatologica* 183(3) (1991): pp. 203–207.

Kim, R.W. "Cost-Effectiveness of 6 and 12 Months of Interferon-alpha Therapy for Chronic Hepatitis C." *Annals of Internal Medicine* 127 (1997): pp. 866–874.

Physicians' Desk Reference Edition 53, Montvale, NJ: Medical Economic Company, Inc.

Chapter 12: Treating Hepatitis B and D

Allen, Marchelle, et al. "Identification and

Characterization of Mutations in Hepatitis B Virus Resistant to Lamivudine." *Hepatology* Vol. 27, No. 6 (1998): pp. 1670–1677.

Brook, M.P.L., McDonald J., et al. "Histological Improvement After Anti-Viral Treatment for Chronic Hepatitis B Virus Infection." *Journal of Hepatology* 8 (1989): pp. 218–225.

Chien, Rong-Nan, et al. "Efficacy of Thymosin Alpha 1 in Patients with Chronic Hepatitis B: A Randomized, Controlled Trial." *Hepatology* 27 (1998): pp. 1383–1387.

Dienstag, J.L., et al. "A Preliminary Trial of Lamivudine for Chronic Hepatitis B Infection." *New England Journal of Medicine* Vol. 333 (December 21, 1995): pp. 1657–1661.

Dusheiko, G.M., et al. "Treatment of Chronic Type B and C Hepatitis with Interferon Alfa: An Economical Appraisal." *Hepatology* 22 (1995): pp. 1863–1873.

Farci, P., et al. "Treatment of Chronic Hepatitis D with Interferon Alfa-2a." *New England Journal of Medicine* 330 (1994): pp. 88–94.

Gately, M.K. "Interleukin-12: Potential Clinical Application in the Treatment of Chronic Viral Hepatitis." *Journal of Viral Hepatitis* 4 (Suppl 1) (1997): pp. 33–39.

Greenberg, H.B., et al. "Effect of Human Leukocyte Interferon on Hepatitis B Virus Infection in Patients with Chronic Active Hepatitis." *New England Journal of Medicine* 295 (1976): pp. 517–522.

Honkoop, P., et al. "Lamivudine Resistance in Immunocompetent Chronic Hepatitis B: Incidence and Patterns." *Journal of Hepatology* 26 (1997): pp. 1393–1395.

Honkoop, P., et al. "Histological Improvement in Patients with Chronic Hepatitis B Virus Infection Treated with Lamivudine." *Liver* 76 (1997): pp. 103–106.

Hoofnagle, J.H., and D. Lau. "New Therapies for Chronic Hepatitis B." *Journal of Viral Hepatitis* 4 (Suppl. 1) (1997): pp. 41–50.

Huo, Teh-ia, et al. "Sero-Clearance of Hepatitis B Surface Antigen in Chronic Carriers Does Not Necessarily Imply A Good Prognosis." *Hepatology* 36 (July 1998): pp. 231–236.

Keefe, Emmet B., et al. "Is Hepatitis A More Severe in Patients with Chronic Hepatitis B and Other Liver Diseases?" *American Journal of Gastroenterology* 90 (1995): pp. 201–205.

Lai, C., et al. "A One-Year Trial of Lamivudine for Chronic Hepatitis B." *New England Journal of Medicine* Vol. 339, No. 2 (1999): pp. 286-297.

Lee, William. "Hepatitis B Virus Infection." *New England Journal of Medicine* Vol. 337, No. 24 (1997): pp. 1734–1745.

Mutchnick, Milton G., et al. "Thymosin Treatment of Chronic Hepatitis B: A Placebo-Controlled Pilot Trial." *Hepatology* 14 (January 1993): pp. 409–415.

Niederau, Claus, et al. "Long-Term Follow-up of HBeAg-Positive Patients Treated with Interferon Alfa for Chronic Hepatitis B." *New England Journal of Medicine* Vol. 334, No. 22 (May 30, 1996): pp. 1422–1427.

Neiderau, Claus, et al. "Long-term Follow-up of HBeAg-Positive Patients Treated with Interferon Alfa for Chronic Hepatitis B." *New England Journal of Medicine* Vol. 334, No. 22 (May 30, 1996): pp. 173–179.

Perrillo, Robert P. "Treatment of Chronic Hepatitis B with Interferon: Experience in Western Countries." *Seminars in Liver Disease* Vol. 9, No. 4 (1989): pp. 144–151.

Perrilo, Robert, et al. "A Randomized Controlled Trial of Interferon Alfa 2b Alone and After Prednisone Withdrawal for the Treatment of Chronic Hepatitis B." *New England Journal of Medicine* Vol. 323, No. 5 (1993): pp. 295–301.

Pol, S., et al. "Efficacy of ImmunoTherapy with Vaccination Against Hepatitis B Virus on Virus B Multiplication." *CR Acad Sci III* 316: (1993): pp. 688–691.

Puoti, M., et al. "Treatment of Chronic Hepatitis D with Interferon Alfa-2b in Patients with Human Immunodeficiency

Virus Infection." *Journal of Hepatology* July 29(1): pp. 45–52.

Rosenberg, Peter, et al. "Therapy with Nucleoside Analogues for Hepatitis B Virus Infection." *Clinics in Liver Disease Hepatitis B* Vol. 3, No. 2 (May 1999): pp.349–361.

Van Leeuwen, R., et al. "Evaluation of Safety and Efficacy of 3 TC (Lamivudine) in Patients with Asymptomatic or Mildly Symptomatic Human Immunodeficiency Virus Infection: A Phase I/II Study." *Journal of Infectious Diseases* 171 (1995): pp. 1166–1171.

Chapter 13: Treating Hepatitis C

Abdelmalek, Manal, et al. "Treatment of Chronic Hepatitis C with Interferon with or Without Ursodeoxycholic Acid. A Randomized Prospective Trial." *Journal of Clinical Gastroenterology* 26(2) (1998): pp. 130–134.

Alter, M.J. "The Epidemiology of Acute and Chronic Hepatitis C." *Clinics in Liver Disease* 1(3) (1997): pp. 559–568.

Andreone, P., et al. "A Double-Blind, Placebo-Controlled, Pilot Trial of Thymosin Alfa 1 for the Treatment of Chronic Hepatitis C." *Liver* 16 (1996): pp. 207–210.

Bacon, R.P., et al. "Beneficial Effect of Iron Reduction Therapy in Patients with Chronic Hepatitis C Who Have Failed to Respond to Interferon Therapy" *Hepatology* 18 (1993): p. 373.

Bodenheimer, H.C., et al. "Tolerance and Efficacy of Oral Ribavirin Treatment of Chronic Hepatitis C: A Multicenter Trial." *Hepatology* 26 (1997): pp. 473–477.

Bonkovsky, Herbert, et al. "Reduction of Health-Related Quality of Life in Chronic Hepatitis C and Improvement with Interferon Therapy." *Hepatology* 29 (1999): pp. 264–270.

Camma, C., et al. "Long-term Course of Interferon-Treated Chronic Hepatitis C." *Journal of Hepatology* 28 (1998): pp. 531–537.

Chemello, L., et al. "The Effect of Interferon on Alfa and Ribavirin Combination Therapy in Naive Patients with Chronic Hepatitis C." *Journal of Hepatology* 23 (suppl 2) (1995): pp. 8–12.

Davis, Gary, et al. "Interferon alfa-2b Alone or in Combination with Ribavirin for the Treatment of Relapse of Chronic Hepatitis C." *New England Journal of Medicine* 339 (1998): pp. 1493–1499.

Di Bisceglie, Adrien, et al. "Ribavirin as Therapy for Chronic Hepatitis C." *Annals of Internal Medicine* Vol. 124 (December 15, 1995): pp. 126–132

Dusheiko, G., et al. "Ribavirin Treatment for Patients with Chronic Hepatitis C; Results of A Placebo-Controlled Study." *Journal of Hepatology* 25 (1996): pp. 591–598.

Gately, M.K. "Interleukin-12: Potential Clinical Application in the Treatment of Chronic Viral Hepatitis." *Journal of Viral Hepatitis* 4 (Suppl. 1) (1997): pp. 33–39.

Gavier, B., et al. "Viremia After One Month of Interferon Therapy Predicts Treatment Outcome in Patients with Chronic Hepatitis C." *Gastroenterology* 113 (1997): pp. 1647–1653.

Hassanein, T., et al. "Induction Therapy with Interferon Alfa-2b Induces Rapid Clearance of Hepatitis C Viremia in Naive Patients." *Hepatology* 26 (Suppl.) 521A Abstract (1997): p. 1,572.

Hwang, S.J., et al. "A Randomized Controlled Trial of Recombinant Interferon Alfa 2b in the Treatment of Chinese Patients with Acute Post-Transfusion Hepatitis C." *Journal of Hepatology* 21 (1994): p. 861

Ikeda, Kenji, et al. "Effect of Interferon Therapy on Hepatocellular Carcinogenesis in Patients with Chronic Hepatitis Type C: A Long-Term Observation Study of 1,643 Patients Using Statistical Bias Correction with Proportional Hazard Analysis." *Hepatology* 29 (1999): pp. 1124–1130.

Imai, Yasuharu, et al. "Relation of Interferon Therapy and Hepatocellular Carcinoma in Patients with Chronic Hepatitis C." *Annals of Intern Medicine* 129 (1998): pp. 94–99.

Jubin, R., et al. "Amantadine and Rimantadine Have No Specific Inhibitory Activity Against Hepatitis C." *Hepatology* Vol. 28, No. 4 (1998): Abstract 829, p. 370A.

Khalili, M., et al. "A Comparison of Combination Therapy with Interferon and Ribavirin versus Interferon and Amantadine in Interferon Non-responders with chronic hepatitis C." *Hepatology* Vol. 28, No. 4 (1998): Abstract 26, p. 169A.

Kim, Joseph, et al. "Hepatitis C Virus NS3 RNAS Helicase Domain with a Bound Oligonucleotide: the Crystal Structure Provides Insights Into the Mode of Unwinding." *Structure* Vol. 6, No. 1 (1998): pp. 89–100.

Kim, J.L., et al. "Crystal Structure of the Hepatitis C Virus NS3 Protease Domain Complexed with a Synthetic NS4A Cofactor Peptide." *Cell* Vol. 87 (October 18, 1996): pp. 343–355.

Kwong, Ann. "Hepatitis C Virus NS3/4A Protease." *Current Opinion in Infectious Diseases* 10 (1997): pp. 485–490.

Lam, N.P., et al. "Dose-Dependent Acute Clearance of Hepatitis C Genotype 1 Virus with Interferon Alfa." *Hepatology* 26 (1997): pp. 226–231.

Lampertico, R., et al. "A Multicenter Randomized Controlled Trial of Recombinant Interferon Alfa-2b in Patients with Acute Transfusion-Associated Hepatitis C." *Hepatology* 19 (1994): p. 19.

Lau, Daryl T.Y., et al. "10–Year Follow-up After Interferon-alfa Therapy for Chronic Hepatitis C." *Hepatology* 28 (1998): pp. 1121–1127.

Lau, M.Y., et al. "Long-Term Efficacy of Ribavirin Plus Interferon Alfa in the Treatment of Chronic Hepatitis C." *Gastroenterology* 111 (1996): pp. 1307–1312.

Lee, William, et al. "Early Hepatitis C Virus-RNA Response Predict Interferon Treatment Outcomes in Chronic Hepatitis C." *Hepatology* 28 (1998): pp. 1411–1415.

McHutchison, John G., et al. "Interferon Alfa-2b Alone or in Combination with Ribavirin as Initial Treatment for Chronic Hepatitis C." *New England Journal of Medicine* 339 (1998): pp. 1485–1492.

Marcellin, P., et al. "Long-Term Histologic Improvement and Loss of Detectable Intrahepatic HCV RNA in Patients with Chronic Hepatitis C and Sustained Response to Interferon-Alfa Therapy." *Annals of Internal Medicine* 127 (1997): pp. 875–881.

Marcellin, P., et al. "Long-Term Histologic Improvement and Loss of Detectable Intrahepatic HCV RNA in Patients with Chronic Hepatitis C and Sustained Response to Interferon-Alfa Therapy." *Annals of Internal Medicine* 127 (1997): pp. 875–881.

Mathurin, Philippe, et al. "Slow Progression Rate of Fibrosis in Hepatitis C Virus Patients with Persistently Normal Alanine Transaminase Activity." *Hepatology* 32 (March 1998): pp. 868–872.

Nishigucho, S., et al. "Randomized Trial of Effects of Interferon-Alfa on Incidence of Hepatocellular Carcinoma in Chronic Active Hepatitis C with Cirrhosis." *Lancet* 346 (1995): pp. 1051–1055.

Omata, M., et al. "Resolution of Acute Hepatitis C After Therapy with Natural Beta Interferon." *Lancet* 338 (1991): p. 914.

Poynard, Thierry, et al. "Randomized Trial of Interferon Alfa 2b Plus Ribavirin for 48 Weeks or for 24 Weeks Versus Interferon Alfa 2b Plus Placebo for 48 Weeks for Treatment of Chronic Infection with Hepatitis C Virus." *Lancet* 352 (1998): pp. 1426–1432.

Puoti, Claudio, et al. "Clinical, Histological, and Virological Features of Hepatitis C Virus Carriers with Persistently Normal Or Abnormal Alanine Transaminase Levels." *Hepatology* 26 (1997): pp. 1393–1398.

Puoti, C., et al. "Serum HCVRNA Titer Does Not Predict the Severity of Liver Damage in HCV Carriers with Normal Aminotransferase Levels." *Liver* 2 (April 1999): pp. 104–109.

Roche Laboratories. "New Treatment May offer Advance in Treatment of Chronic Hepatitis C." Press Release, November 8th 1998, Chicago.

Sangiovanni, Angelo, et al. "Interferon Alfa Treatment of HCV RNA Carriers with Persistently Normal Transaminase Levels A Pilot Randomized Controlled Study." *Hepatology* (March 1998): pp. 853–856.

Reichard, O., et al. "Randomized, Double-Blind, Placebo-Controlled Trial of Interferon Alfa-2b with and Without Ribavirin for Chronic Hepatitis C." *Lancet* 351 (1998): pp. 83–87.

Rossini, Angelo, et al. "Virological Response to Interferon Treatment in Hepatitis C Virus Carriers with Normal Aminotransferase Levels and Chronic Hepatitis." *Hepatology* 28 (October 1997): pp. 1012–1016.

Rowell, Diana, et al. "Should Chronic Viral Hepatitis with Persistently Normal Aminotransferase Levels be Treated?" *Viral Hepatitis Reviews* Vol. 3, No. 3 (1997): pp. 189–199.

Schalm, S.W., et al. "Ribavirin Enhances the Efficacy but not the Side Effects of Interferon in Chronic Hepatitis C. Meta-Analysis of Individual Patient Data from European Centers." *Journal of Hepatology* 26 (1997): pp. 961–966

Schiffman, Mitchell, et al. "A Controlled, Randomized, Multicenter Descending Dose Phase II Trial of Pegylated Interferon Alfa-2A (PEG) Vs Standard Interferon Alfa-2A(IFN) for Treatment of Chronic Hepatitis C." *Hepatology* (April 1999): Abstract LO418.

Senturk, H., et al. "Amantadine MonoTherapy of Chronic Hepatitis C Patients Infected with Genotype 1b." *Hepatology* Vol. 28, No. 4 (1998): Abstract 842, p. 373A.

Sherman, Kenneth, et al. "Combination Therapy with Thymosin Alfa 1 and Interferon for the Treatment of Chronic Hepatitis C Infection: A Randomized, Placebo-Controlled Double-Blind Trial." *Hepatology* 27 (1998): pp. 1128–1135.

Smith, Jill. "Treatment of Chronic Hepatitis C with Amantadine." *Digestive Diseases and Sciences* 42 (1997): pp. 1681–1687.

Takano, Susumu, et al. "A Multicenter Randomized Controlled Dose Study of Ursodeoxycholic Acid for Chronic Hepatitis C." *Hepatology* 20 (1994): pp. 558–564.

Thevenot, T., et al. "Effects of Cirrhosis, Interferon, and Azathioprine on Adverse Events in Patients with Chronic Hepatitis C Treated with Ribavirin." *Journal of Viral Hepatitis* 4 (1997): pp. 243–253.

Van Thiel, D.H., et al. "Response to Interferon Alfa Therapy is Influenced by the Iron Content of the Liver." *Journal of Hepatology* 20 (1994): pp. 410–415.

Viladomiu, L., et al. "Interferon-Alfa in Acute Posttransfusion Hepatitis C: A Randomized Controlled Trial." *Hepatology* 15 (1992): p. 767.

Weisz, K. "Erythropoietin Use for Ribavirin/Interferon Induced Anemia in Patients with Hepatitis C." *Hepatology* Vol. 28, No 4 (October 1998): Abstract 228A.

Chapter 14: Autoimmune Hepatitis

Al-Fadda, Mohammad, et al. "Idiopathic Chronic Active Hepatitis: A Diagnostic and Therapeutic Dilemma." *Journal of Clinical Gastroenterology* 19(4), (1994): pp. 313–317.

Czaja, Albert J. "The Variant Forms of Autoimmume Hepatitis." *Annals of Internal Medicine* 125 (1996): pp. 588–598.

Danielsson, A., et al. "Oral Budesonide for Treatment of Autoimmune Chronic Active Hepatitis." *Ailment Pharmacology therapies* 8 (1994): pp. 585–590.

Dufour, Jean-Francois, et al. "Reversibility of Hepatic Fibrosis in Autoimmune Hepatitis." *Annals of Internal Medicine* Vol. 127, No.11, pp. 981–985.

Gregorio, Germana, et al. "Autoimmune Hepatitis in Children: A 20–Year Experience." *Hepatology* Vol. 25, No.3 (1997). pp. 99–107.

Huppertz, H.I., et al. "Autoimmune Hepatitis Following Hepatitis A Virus Infection." *Journal of Hepatology* 23 (2) (August 1995): pp. 204–208.

Johnson, P.J., and I.G. McFarlane. "Meeting Report: International Autoimmune Hepatitis Group." *Hepatology* 18 (1993): pp. 998–1005.

Johnson, Philip, et al. "Azathioprine for Long-Term Maintenance of Remission in Autoimmune Hepatitis." *The New England Journal of Medicine* 228 (October 12, 1995): pp. 958–963.

Kamiyama, T. "Autoimmune Hepatitis Triggered by Administration of An Herbal Medicine, " *American Journal of Gastroenterology* 220 (1995) p. 923.

Krawitt, E.L. "Autoimmune Hepatitis," *New England Journal of Medicine* Vol. 334 No.14 pp. 897–903.

Lebovics, Edward. "Autoimmune Chronic Active Hepatitis in Postmenopausal Women." *Digestive Diseases and Sciences* Vol. 30, No. 9 (September 1985).

Lebovics, Edward, and Melissa Palmer. "Outcome of Primary Sclerosing Cholangitis, Analysis of Long-term Observation of 38 Patients." *Archives of Internal Medicine* Vol. 147 (April 1987).

Papo, T., et al. "Autoimmune Chronic Hepatitis Exacerbated by Alpha-interferon." *Annals of Internal Medicine* 116(1) (1992): pp. 51–53.

Van Thiel, D.H., et al. "Tacrolimus: A Potential New Treatment for Autoimmune Chronic Active Hepatitis: Results of an Open-Label Preliminary Trial." *American Journal of Gastroenterology* 90 (1995): pp. 771–776.

Vento, S., et al. "Identification of Hepatitis A Virus as a Trigger for Autoimmune Chronic Hepatitis Type 1 in Susceptible Individuals." *Lancet* 337 (1991): pp. 1183–1186.

Wang, K.K., and A.J. Czaja. "Prognosis of Corticosteroid-Treated Hepatitis B Surface Antigen Negative Chronic Active Hepatitis in Postmenopausal Women: A Retrospective Analysis." *Gastroenterology* 97 (1989): pp. 1288–1293.

Chapter 15: Primary Biliary Cirrhosis

Ahrens, E.J., et al. "Primary Biliary Cirrhosis." *Medicine* 29 (1950): pp. 299–364.

Bach, N., Schaffner, F. "Familial Primary Biliary Cirrhosis." *Journal of Hepatology* 20 (1994): pp. 698–701.

Balasubramaniam, K., et al. "Diminished Survival in Asymptomatic Primary Biliary Cirrhosis: A Prospective Study." *Gastroenterology* 98 (1990): pp. 1567–1571.

Brind, A.M., et al. "Prevalence and Pattern of Familial Disease in Primary Biliary Cirrhosis." *Gut* 36 (1995): pp. 615–617.

Combes, B., et al. "A Randomized, Double-Blind, Placebo-Controlled Trial of Ursodeoxycholic Acid in Primary Biliary Cirrhosis." *Hepatology* 23 (1995): pp. 759–766.

Culp, K.S., et al. "Autoimmune Associations in Primary Biliary Cirrhosis." *Mayo Clinic Proceedings* 57 (1982): pp. 365–370.

D'Amico, E., et al. "Primary Biliary Cirrhosis Induced by Interferon-Alpha Therapy for Hepatitis C Virus Infection." *Digestive Diseases and Sciences* 40 (1995): pp. 2113–2116.

Dickey, W., et al. "High Prevalence of Celiac Sprue Among Patients with Primary Biliary Cirrhosis." *Journal of Clinical Gastroenterology* 25(1) (1997): pp. 328–329.

Heathcote, E.J., et al. "The Canadian Multicenter Controlled Trial of Ursodeoxycholic Acid in Primary Biliary Cirrhosis." *Hepatology* 19 (1994): pp. 1149–1156.

Jones, D.E.J., et al. "Hepatocellular Carcinoma in Primary Biliary Cirrhosis and Its Impact on Outcomes." *Hepatology* 26 (1997): pp. 1138–1142.

Jones, David, et al. "Primary Biliary Cirrhosis, Clinical and Associated Autoimmune Features and Natural History." *Clinics in Liver Disease* Vol. 2, No.2 (May 1998): pp. 265–282.

Kaplan, Marshall. "Primary Biliary Cirrhosis." *The New England Journal of Medicine* (November 21, 1996): pp. 1570–1580.

Kaplan, M.M., et al. "A Prospective Trial of Colchicine for Primary Biliary Cirrhosis." *New England Journal of Medicine* 315 (1986): pp. 1448–1454.

Keefe, E.B. "Sarcoidosis and Primary Biliary Cirrhosis. Literature Review and Illustrative Case." *American Journal of Medicine* 83 (1987): pp. 977–980.

Kim, W.R., and E.R. Dickson. "Predictive Models of Natural History in Primary Biliary Cirrhosis." *Clinics in Liver Disease* Vol. 2, No.2 (May 1998): pp. 313–331.

Klion, F., T. Fabry, M. Palmer, F. Schaffner. Prediction of Survival of Patients with Primary Biliary Cirrhosis. Examination of the Mayo Clinic Model on a Group of Patients with Known Endpoint." *Gastroenterology* 102 (1992): pp. 310–313.

Krawitt, E.L., "Autoimmune Hepatitis," *New England Journal of Medicine* Vol. 334, No.14 (1996) pp. 897–903.

Lindor, K.D., et al. "Effects of Ursodeoxycholic Acid on Survival in Patients with Primary Biliary Cirrhosis." *Gastroenterology* 110 (1996): pp. 1515–1518.

Lindor, K.D., et al. "Ursodeoxycholic Acid in the Treatment of Primary Biliary Cirrhosis." *Gastroenterology* 106 (1994): pp. 1284–1290.

Mahl, T.C., et al. "Primary Biliary Cirrhosis: Survival of a Large Cohort of Symptomatic and Symptomatic Patients Followed for 24 Years." *Journal of Hepatology* 20 (1994): p. 707.

Metcalf, J., J. Oliver, "The Geoepidemiology of Primary Biliary Cirrhosis." *Seminars of Liver Disease* Vol. 17, No. 1 (1997).

Moradjpour, D., et al., "Chlorpromazine Induced Vanishing Bile Duct Syndrome Leading to Primary Biliary Cirrhosis." *Hepatology* 20 (1994): pp. 1437–1441.

Nijhawan, Pardeep, et al. "Incidence of Cancer in Primary Biliary Cirrhosis: The Mayo Experience." *Hepatology* 29 (1999): pp. 1396–1398.

O'Donohue, J., et al. "Antibodies to Atypical Mycobacteria in Primary Biliary Cirrhosis." *Journal of Hepatology* 21 (1994): pp. 887–889.

Poupon, R.E., et al. "Ten-Year Survival in Ursodeoxycholic Acid-Treated Patients with Primary Biliary Cirrhosis." *Hepatology* 29 (1999): pp. 1668–1671.

Poupon, R.E., et al. "Ursodiol for the Long-Term Treatment of Primary Biliary Cirrhosis." *New England Journal of Medicine* 330 (1994): pp. 1342–1347.

Poupon, R.E., et al. "Combined Analysis of Randomized Trials of Ursodeoxycholic Acid in Primary Biliary Cirrhosis." *Gastroenterology* 113 (1997): pp. 884–890.

Shibata, J., et al. "Combination Therapy with Ursodeoxycholic Acid and Colchicine for Primary Biliary Cirrhosis." *Journal of Gastrotroenterology and Hepatology* 7 (1992): pp. 277–282.

Trigor, D.R. "Primary Biliary Cirrhosis: An Epidemiological Study." *British Medical Journal* 281 (1980): pp. 772–775.

Witt-Sullivan, H., et al. "The Demography of Primary Biliary Cirrhosis in Ontario, Canada." *Hepatology* 12 (1990): p. 98.

Chapter 16: Fatty Liver and Nonalcoholic Steatohepatitis

Bacon, B.R. "Nonalcoholic Steatohepatitis: An Expanded Clinical Entity." *Gastroenterology* 107 (1994): pp. 1103–1109.

Buchman, A.L., et al. "Lecithin Increases Plasma Free Choline and Decreases Hepatic Steatosis in Long-Term Total Parenteral Nutrition Patients." *Gastroenterology* 102 (1992): p. 1363,

Gitlin, Norman. *The Liver and Systemic Disease* 1997, Churchill Livingstone, New York, pp. 73–114.

Hourigan, Luke. "Fibrosis in Chronic Hepatitis C Correlates Significantly with Body Mass Index and Steatosis." *Hepatology* 29 (1999): pp. 1215–1219.

Iwamura, K. "Clinical and Pathophysiological Aspects of Fatty Liver of Unknown Etiology in Modern Japan." *Tokai Journal of Experimental and Clinical Medicine* 14 (1989): pp. 61–85.

Keith, George, et al. "Increased Hepatic Iron Concentration in Nonalcoholic Steatohepatitis is associated with increased fibrosis." *Gastroenterology* 114 (1998): pp. 311–318.

Laurin, J., et al. "Ursodeoxycholic Acid or Clofibrate in the Treatment of Non-Alcoholic-Induced Steatohepatitis: A Pilot Study." *Hepatology* 23 (1996): pp. 1464–1467.

Ludwig, J., et al. "Nonalcoholic Steatohepatitis." *Mayo Clinic Proceedings* 55 (1980): p. 434.

McGill, D. "Nonalcoholic Steatohepatitis." *Gastrointestinal Diseases Today* Vol. 6, No. 2 (March-April, 1997): pp. 1–7.

Matteoni, Christi. "Nonalcoholic Fatty Liver Disease: A Spectrum of Clinical and Pathological Severity." *Gastroenterology* 116 (1999): pp. 1413–1419.

Neuschwander-Tetri, B. "Nonalcoholic Steatohepatitis." *Clinics in Liver Disease* Vol. 2, No. 1 (February 1998): pp. 149–173.

Sheth, S., et al. "Nonalcoholic Steatohepatitis." *Annals of Internal Medicine* 126 (1997): pp. 137–145.

Palmer, M., et al. "Excessive Weight Gain After Transplantation." *Transplantation* 57 (1991): pp. 797–800.

Palmer, M., et al. "Effect of Weight Reduction on Hepatic Abnormalities in Overweight Patients." *Gastroenterology* 99 (1990): pp. 1408–1413.

Powell, E.E., et al. "The Natural History of Nonalcoholic Steatohepatitis: A Follow-Up of Forty-Two Patients for Up to 21 Years." *Hepatology* 11 (1990): p. 74.

Propst, A., et al. "Prognosis in Nonalcoholic Steatohepatitis." *Gastroenterology* 108 (1995): p. 1607.

Rosenbaum, M., et al. "Obesity." *New England Journal of Medicine* 6, 337 (1997): pp. 396–407.

VanItallie, T.B. "The Perils of Obesity in Middle-Aged Women." *New England Journal of Medicine* 322 (1990): pp. 928–929

Chapter 17: Alcohol and the Liver

Adachi, Y., et al. "Antibiotics Prevent Liver Injury in Rats Following Long-Term Exposure to Ethanol." *Gastroenterology* 108 (1995): pp. 218–224.

Annoni, G., et al. "Serum Type III Procollagen Peptide and Laminin [Lam-P1. Detect Alcoholic Hepatitis in Chronic Alcohol Abusers." *Hepatology* 9 (1989): p. 693.

Boyer, C.S., and D.R. Petersen, "Potentiation of Cocaine-Mediated Hepatotoxicity by Acute and Chronic Alcohol." *Alcoholism: Clinical and Experimental Research* 14 (1990): pp. 28–31.

Carithers, R.L., et al. "Methylprednisolone Therapy in Patients with Severe Alcoholic Hepatitis: A Randomized Multicenter Trial." *Annals of Internal Medicine* 110 (1989): pp. 685–688.

Frezza, M., et al. "High Blood Alcohol Levels in Women: the Role of Decreased Gastric Alcohol Dehydrogenase Activity and First-Pass Metabolism." *New England Journal of Medicine* 322 (1990): pp. 95–99.

Fong, T.L., et al. "Clinical Significance of Concomitant Hepatitis C Virus Infection in Patients with Alcoholic Liver Disease." *Hepatology* 19 (1994): pp. 554–557.

Jenkins, P., S. Cromie, et al. "Chronic Hepatitis C, Alcohol and Hepatic Fibrosis" (Abstract). *Hepatology* 24 (1996): p. 153 A.

Kershenobich, D., et al. "Colchicine in the Treatment of Cirrhosis of the Liver." *New England Journal of Medicine* 318 (1988): pp. 1709–1711.

Kwoh-Gain, I., et al. "Desialylated Transferrin and Mitochondrial Aspartate Aminotransferase Compared as Laboratory Markers of Excessive Alcohol Consumption."

Clinical Chemistry 36, 6 (1990): pp. 841–845.

Lieber, C. "Biochemical Factors in Alcoholic Liver Disease." *Seminars in Liver Disease* Vol. 13, No. 2 (1993) pp. 182–189.

Mayfield,, D., et al. "The CAGE Questionnaire: Validation of A New Alcoholism Screening instrument." *American Journal of Psychiatry* 131 (1974): pp. 1121–1123.

Morse, R.M., D.K. Flavin, for the Joint Committee of the National Council on Alcoholism and Drug Dependence and the American Society of Addiction Medicine to Study the Definition and Criteria for the Diagnosis of Alcoholism. "The Definition of Alcoholism." *Journal of the American Medical Association* 268 (1992): pp. 1012–1014.

Niemela, O., et al. "Markers of Fibrogenesis and Basement Membrane Formation in Alcoholic Liver Disease. Relation to Severity, Presence of Hepatitis, and Alcohol Intake." *Gastroenterology* 98 (1990): p. 1612.

Orrego, H., et al. "Effect of Short-Term Therapy with Propylthiouracil in Patients with Alcoholic Liver Disease." *Gastroenterology* 75 (1978): pp. 105–111.

Ostapowicz, George, et al. "Role of Alcohol in the Progression of Liver Disease Caused by Hepatitis C Virus Infection." *Hepatology* Vol. 27 No. 6, (1998): pp. 1730–1735.

Pessione, Fabienne, et al. "Effect of Alcohol Consumption on Serum Hepatitis C Virus RNA and Histological Lesions in Chronic Hepatitis C." *Hepatology* Vol. 27, No. 6, (1998): pp. 1717–1722.

Poynard, T., et al. "Natural History of Liver Fibrosis Progression in Patients with Chronic Hepatitis C." *Lancet* 349 (1997): pp. 825–832.

Raymond, M.J., et al. "A Randomized Trial of Prednisolone in Patients with Severe Alcoholic Hepatitis." *New England Journal of Medicine* 326 (1992): pp. 507–510.

Robbins, C. "Sex Differences in Psychosocial Consequences of Alcohol and Drug Abuse." *Journal of Health and Social Behavior* 30 (1989): pp. 117–130.

Smith-Warner, S.A., et al. "Alcohol and Breast Cancer in Women." *Journal of the American Medical Association* 279 (1998): pp. 535–540.

Stedmans Medical Dictionary 26th Edition Weights and Measures Appendix, p. 1986.

Viitala, K., et al. "Serum IgA, IgG and IgM Antibodies Directed Against Acetaldehyde-Derived Epitopes: Relationship to Liver Disease Severity and Alcohol Consumption." *Hepatology* Vol. 35 (June 1997): pp. 1418–1424.

Chapter 18: Hemochromatosis

Adams, Paul, and Chakrabarti Subrata. "Genotypic/Phenotypic Correlation's in Genetic Hemochromatosis: Evolution of Diagnostic Criteria." *Gastroenterology* 114 (1998): pp. 319–323.

Adams, Paul C., M.D., and Leslie S. Valberg, M.D. "Evolving Expression of Hereditary Hemochromatosis." *Seminars in Liver Disease* Vol. 16, No. 1. (1996): pp. 47–54.

American Liver Foundation pamphlet "Hemochromatosis: Not So Rare," 1997.

Bacon, Bruce R. "Diagnosis and Management of Hemochromatosis." *Gastroenterology* 113 (1997): pp. 995–999.

Beutler, E., T. Gelbart, C. West, et al. "Mutational Analysis in Hereditary Hemochromatosis." *Blood Cells, Molecules, and Diseases* 22, 16. (1996): pp. 187–194.

Bonkovsky, Herbert L.M.D., et al. "Iron in Liver Diseases Other than Hemochromatosis." *Seminars in Liver Disease* Vol. 16, No.1, pp. 65–82.

Brissot, P., et al. "A Genotypic Study of 217 Unrelated Probands Diagnosed as Genetic Hemochromatosis on Classical Phenotypic Criteria." *Hepatology* 28 (1998): 1105–1107

Fargion S., et al. "Survival and Prognostic Factors in 212 Italian Patients with Genetic Hemochromatosis." *Hepatology* 15 (1992): p. 655.

Feder, J.N., A. Gnirke, W. Thomas, et al. "A Novel MHC Class I-Like Gene Is Mutated in Patients with Hereditary Hemochromatosis." *Nature Genetics* 13 (1996): pp. 399–408.

Iron Overload Disease Association—statistics 1998, Internet website, www.ironoverload.org.

Kowdley, K.V., et al. "Primary Liver Cancer and Survival in Patients Undergoing Liver Transplantation for Hemochromatosis." *Liver Transplantation and Surgery* 1 (1995): p. 237.

Niederau, C., et al. "Survivial and Causes of Death in Cirrhotic and in Noncirrhotic Patients with Primary Hemochromatosis." *New England Journal of Medicine* 313 (1985): p. 1256.

Niederau, Claus, et al. "Hemochromatosis and the Liver." *Journal of Hepatology* 30 (1999): pp. 6–11.

Olynyk, J.K., et al. "Hereditary Hemochromatosis Diagnosis and Management in the Gene Era." *Liver* 2 (April 1999): pp. 73–80.

Powell, L.W., J.F.R. Kerr, "Reversal of Cirrhosis in Idiopathic Hemochromatosis Following Long-Term Intensive Venesection Therapy." *Australian Annals of Medicine* 19 (1970): p. 54.

Powell, Lawrie W., M.D., et al. "Hemochromatosis: Genetics and Pathogenesis." *Seminars in Liver Disease* Vol. 16, No.1 (1996): pp. 55–63.

Wallace, Daniel, et al. "A Novel Mutation of HFE Explains the Classical Phenotype of Genetic Hemochromatosis in a C282Y Heterozygote." *Gastroenterology* 116 (1999): pp. 1409–1412.

Chapter 19: Benign and Malignant Liver Tumors

Arnold, William. "Hepatic Resection for Metastatic Lesions," *Practical Gastroenterology* (December 1996): pp. 6–12

Bruix, Jordi. "Treatment of Hepatocellular Carcinoma." *Hepatology* Vol. 25, No. 2 (1997)

Castells, A., et al. "Treatment of Small Hepatocellular Carcinoma in Cirrhotic Patients: A Cohort Study Comparing Surgical Resection and Percutaneous Ethanol Injection." *Hepatology* 28 (1993): pp. 1121–1126.

Castells, A., et al. "Treatment of Hepatocellular Carcinoma with Tamoxifen: A Double Blind Placebo-Controlled Trial in 120 Patients." *Gastroenterology* 109 (1995): pp. 917–922.

Collier, Jane, et al. "Screening for Hepatocellular Carcinoma." *Hepatology* Vol. 27, No.1. (1998).

Colombo, M. "Treatment of Hepatocellular Carcinoma." *Journal of Viral Hepatitis* 4 (Suppl.10) (1997): pp. 125–130.

Di Bisceglie, Adrien. "Hepatitis C and Hepatocellular Carcinoma." *Seminars in Liver Disease* Vol. 15, No.1, (1995): pp. 64–69.

Fattovich, Giovanna. "Natural Course and Prognosis of Chronic Hepatitis Type B." *Viral Hepatitis Reviews* Vol. 2, No. 4, (1996): pp. 263–276

El-Serag, Hashem, et al. "Rising Incidence of Hepatocellular Carcinoma in the United States." *New England Journal of Medicine* Vol. 340, No. 10 (March 11, 1999): p. 745–750.

Goritsas, Constantin, P., et al. "The Leading Role of Hepatitis B and C Viruses as Risk Factors for the Development of Hepatocellular Carcinoma." *Journal of Clinical Gastroenterology* 20 3 (1995): pp. 220–224.

Groupe d'Etude et de Traitement du Carcinome Hepatocellylaire. "A Comparison of Lipiodol Chemoembolization and Conservative Treatment for Unresectable Hepatocellulare Carcinoma." *New England Journal of Medicine* 332 (1995): pp. 1256–1261.

Iwatsuki, S., T.E. Starzl, D.G. Sheahan, et al. "Hepatic Resection Versus Transplantation for Hepatocellular Carcinoma." *Annals of Surgery* 214 (1991): pp. 221–229.

Jenkins, Roger L., et al. "Surgical Approach to Benign Liver Tumors." *Seminars in Liver Disease* Vol. 14, No.2 (1994): 347–353.

Lai, C.L., et al. "Recombinant Interferon Alpha in Inoperable Hepatocellular Carcinoma: A Randomized Controlled Trial." *Hepatology* 17 (1993): pp. 389–394.

Livraghi, T., et al. "Percutaneous Injection in the Treatment of Hepatocellular Carcinoma in Cirrhosis: A Study on 207 Patients." *Cancer* 69 (1992): pp. 925–929.

Manesis, E.K. "Treatment of Hepatocellular Carcinoma with Combined Suppression and Inhibition of Sex Hormones: A Randomized, Controlled Trial." *Hepatology* 21 (1995): pp. 1535–1542.

Matsuzaki, Y., et al. "A New, Effective and Safe Therapeutic Option Using Proton Irradiation for Hepatocellular Carcinoma." *Gastroenterology* 106 (1994): pp. 1032–1041.

Palmer, M., et al. "Fatty Liver Effect of Weight Reduction on Hepatic Abnormalities in Overweight Patients." *Gastroenterology* 99 (1990): p. 1,408.

Raoul, J.L., et al. "Randomized Controlled Trial for Hepatocellular Carcinoma with Portal Vein Thrombosis: Intr-Arterial Iodine-131–Iodinized Oil Versus Medical Support." *Journal of Nuclear Medicine* 35 (1994): pp. 1782–1787.

Reddy, K. Rajender M.D., and Eugene R. Schiff, M.D. "Approach to a Liver Mass." *Seminars in Liver Disease* Vol. 13, No. 4 (1993): 127–138.

Reynolds, Telfer, B. "Hepatomegaly in a Menopausal Woman: Differential Diagnosis of Liver Tumors." *Gastrointestinal Diseases Today* Vol. 1, No. 3 (November-December, 1992): 42–50.

Ros, Pablo, Gary Davis. "The Incidental Focal Liver Lesion: Photon, Proton, or Needle?" *Hepatology* (May 1998): pp. 1183–1190.

Seki, T., et al. "Ultrasonically Guided Pertcutaneous Microwave Coagulation Therapy for Small Hepatocellular Carcinoma." *Cancer* 74 (1994): pp. 817–825.

Vilana, R., et al. "Tumor Size Determines the Efficacy of Percutaneous Ethanol Injection for the Treatment of Small Hepatocellular Carcinoma." *Hepatology* 16 (1992): pp. 353–357.

Wands, J.R, and H.E. Blum. "Primary Hepatocellular Carcinoma." [Editorial] *New England Journal of Medicine* 325 (1991): pp. 729–731.

Chapter 20: Treatment of Common Symptoms and Complications

Bergasa, Nora, et al. "The Pruritus of Cholestasis. Evolving Pathogenic Concepts Suggest New Therapeutic Options." *Clinics in Liver Disease* Vol. 2, No. 2 (May 1998): pp. 391–405.

Betts, A., et al. "Beta-blockers and Sleep: A Controlled Trial." *European Journal of Clinical Pharmacology* 28 (Suppl.) (1985): pp. 65–68.

Bonkovsky, Herbert, et al. "Prevalence and Prediction of Osteopenia in Chronic Liver Disease." *Hepatology* 12 (1990): pp. 273–280.

Cordoba, Juan, et al. "High Prevalence of Sleep Disturbance in Cirrhosis." *Hepatology* 27 (1998): pp. 339–345.

Cummings, Steven, et al. "Effect of Alendronate on Risk of Fracture in Women with Low Bone Density but Without Vertebral Fractures." *Journal of the American Medical Association* 280 (1998): pp. 2077–2082.

Dasani, B.M., et al. "The Role of *Helicobacter Pylori* in the Pathogenesis and Treatment of Chronic Hepatic Encephalopathy" (Abstract). *Hepatology* 22 (1995): p. 161.

Garfinkel, D., et al. "Improvement of Sleep Quality in Elderly People by Controlled-Release Melatonin." *Lancet* 346 (1995): pp. 541–544.

Hay, J. Eileen. "Osteoporosis." *Clinics in Liver Disease* Vol. 2, No.2 (May 1998): pp. 407–419.

McDonald, Jennifer, et al. "Bone Loss After Transplantation." *Hepatology* 14 (1991): pp. 613–619.

Merkel, C., et al. "Randomized Trial of Nadolol Alone or with Isosorbide Mononitrate for Primary Prophylaxis of Variceal Bleeding in Cirrhosis." *Lancet* 348 (1996): pp. 1677–1681.

Pawlikowska, T., et al. "Population Based Study of Fatigue and Psychological Distress." *British Medical Journal* 308 (1994): pp. 763–766.

Quero, J.C., et al. "Does Subclinical Hepatic Encephalopathy Affect Quality of Life?" (Abstract). *Gastroenterology* 108 (1995): p. 1151A.

Ring, Ernest, et al. "Using Transjugular Intrahepatic Portosystemic Shunts to Control Variceal Bleeding before Liver Transplantation." *Annals of Internal Medicine* 116 (1992): pp. 304–309.

Roosle, M., et al. "The Transjugular Intrahepatic Portosystemic Stent-Shunt Procedure for Variceal Bleeding." *New England Journal of Medicine* 330 (1994): pp. 165–171.

Rosen, H.M., et al. "Plasma Amino Acid Patterns in Hepatic Encephalopathy of Differing Etiology." *Gastroenterology* 72 (1977): p. 483.

Schreiber, A.J., et al. "Estrogen-Induced Cholestasis: Clues to Pathogenesis and Treatment." *Hepatology* 3 (1983): pp. 607–613.

Steindl, P.E., et al. "Disruption of the Diurnal Rhythm of Plasma Melatonin in Cirrhosis." *Annals of Internal Medicine* 123 (1995): pp. 274–277.

Van Der Rijt, C.C.D., et al. "Overt Hepatic Encephalopathy Precipitated by Zinc Deficiency: A Double-Blind Crossover Study." *Gastroenterologie Clinique Et Biologique* 19 (1995): pp. 572–580.

Chapter 21: Herbs and Other Alternative therapies

Abbot, Neil, et al. *International Journal Risk Safety Medicine* 11 (1998): pp. 99–106.

Abe, Y., et al. "Effectiveness of Interferon, Glycyrrhizin Combination Therapy in Patients with Chronic Hepatitis C." *Nippon Rinsho* 52(7) (July 1994): pp. 1817–1822.

Albrecht, M., et al. "Therapy of Toxic Liver Pathologies with Legalon." *Zeitschrift fur Klinische Medizin* 47 (1992): pp. 87–92.

Alderman, Sheri, et al. "Cholestatic Hepatitis After Ingestion of Chaparral Leaf: Confirmation by Endoscopic Retrograde Cholangiopancreatography and Liver Biopsy." *Journal of Clinical Gastroenterology* 19(3) (1994): pp. 242–247.

Anderson, I.B., et al. "Pennyroyal Toxicity: Measurement of Toxic Metabolite Levels in Two Cases and Review of the Literature." *Annals of Internal Medicine* 124 (1996): p. 726.

Awang, D.V.C. "Atropine as Possible Contaminant of Comfrey Tea." *Lancet* (July 1, 1989): p. 44.

Bach, Nancy, et al. "Comfrey Herb Tea-Induced Hepatic Veno-occlusive Disease." *The American Journal of Medicine* (July 1989): pp. 97–99.

Bar-Meir, S., et al. "Effect of (+) –Cyanidanol-3 (Catechin) on Chronic Active Hepatitis: A Double Blind Controlled Trial." *Gut* Vol. 26 (9) (1985): Pp. 975–979.

Berkson, B. "Thioctic Acid in the Treatment of Hepatotoxic Mushroom Poisoning" (letter). *New England Journal of Medicine* (1979): pp. 300–371.

Betz, Joseph, et al. "Determination of Pyrrolizidine Alkaloids in Commercial Comfrey Products (Symphytum sp.)." *Journal of Pharmaceutical Sciences* Vol. 83, No. 5 (May 1994): pp. 649–653.

Beuers, Ulrich, et al. "Hepatitis After Chronic Abuse of Senna." *Lancet* Vol. 337 (Feb. 9, 1991): pp. 191–199.

Blumenthal, M., ed. "The Complete German Commission E Monographs: Therapeutic Guide to Herbal Medicines." Austin, Tex.: American Botanicals Council, 1998.

Boari, C., et al. "Silymarin in the Protection Against Exogenous Noxae." *Drugs Under Experimental and Clinical Research* 7 (1981): pp. 115–120.

Bosisio, E., et al. "Effect of the Flavanolignans of Silybum Marianum L. on Lipid Peroxidation in Rat Liver Microsomes and Freshly Isolated Hepatocytes." *Pharmacological Research* 25 (1992): pp. 147–154.

Brevoort, P. "The U.S. Botanical Market— An Overview." *Herbalgram* 1996 36: pp. 49–57.

Burgstiner, C.B. "Complete Thymic Formula (Label) Duluth, GA: "Preventive Therapeutic, Inc.

Carini, R., et al. "Lipid Peroxidation and Irreversible Damage in the Rat Hepatocyte Model: Protection by the Silybin-Phospholipid Complex IdB 1016." *Biochemical Pharmacology* 43 (1992): pp. 2111–2115.

Colin-Jones, D.G., et al. "Mistletoe Hepatitis." *British Medical Journal* Vol. 284 (1982): p. 744.

Colman, J.C., et al. "Treatment of Alcohol-Related Liver Disease With(+) –Cyanidanol-3 (Catechin): A Randomized Double-Blind Trial." *Gut* Vol. 21(11) (1980): pp. 965–969.

Daschner, F.D., et al. "Hepatitis C and Human Immunodeficiency Virus Infection Following Ozone AutohaemoTherapy." *European Journal of Clinical Microbiology and Infectious Disease* 16(8) (August 1997): p. 620.

Despalces, A., et al. "The Effects of Silymarin on Experimental Phalloidine Poisoning." *Araneimittel-Forschung* 25 (1975): pp. 89–96.

Dietary Supplement Health and Education Act of 1994.

Farnsworth, N.R., et al. "Mistletoe Hepatitis." *British Medical Journal* Vol. 282 (1981): p. 1058.

Fau, Daniel, et al. "Diterpenoids from Germander, An Herbal Medicine, Induce Apoptosis in Isolated Rat Hepatocytes." *Gastroenterology* 113 (1997): pp. 1334–1346.

Feher, J., et al. "Hepatoprotective Activity of Silymarin (Legalon) Therapy in Patients with Chronic Liver Disease." *Orvosi Hetilap* 130 (1989): pp. 2723–2727.

Ferenzi, P., et al. "Randomized Controlled Trial of Silymarin Treatment in Patients with Cirrhosis of the Liver." *Journal of Hepatology* 9 (1989): pp. 105–113.

Fletcher, Hyde F., et al. "Mistletoe Hepatitis." *British Medical Journal* Vol. 282 (1981): p. 1058.

Floersheim, G.L., et al. "Poisoning by the Deathcap Fungus (Amanita Phalloides): Prognostic Factors and Therapeutic Measures." *Schweiz Med Wochenschrift* 112 (1982): pp. 1164–1177.

Flora, Kenneth, et al. "Milk Thistle (*Silybum marianum*) for the Therapy of Liver Disease." *The American Journal of Gastroenterology* Vol. 93, No. 2 (1998): pp. 139–143.

Foster, S. *Milk Thistle: Silybum Marianum* Austin, TX: American Botanical Council, No. 305, 1991.

Gabriel, C., et al. "Transmission of Hepatitis C by Ozone Enrichment of Autologous Blood." *Lancet* 347 (9000) (February 24, 1996): p. 541.

Goldman, J.A., et al. "Chinese Herbal Medicine Camouflaged Prescription Antiinflammatory Drugs, Corticosteroids, and Lead." *Arthritis and Rheumatism* 34 (1991): p. 1207.

Gordon, Dafna, et al. "Chaparral Ingestion: the Broadening Spectrum of Liver Injury Caused by Herbal Medications." *Journal of the American Medical Association* Vol. 273 (1995): pp. 489–490.

Greive, M. *A Modern Herbal.* Vol. 2, New York: Dover Publications, 1981.

Gross, G., et al. "Genital Warts do Not Respond to Systemic Recombinant Interferon Alfa-2a Treatment During Cannabis Consumption." *Dermatologica* 183(3) (1991): pp. 203–207.

Graham-Brown, Robin. "Toxicity of Chinese Herbal Remedies." *Lancet* Vol. 340 (September 12, 1992): p. 673.

Green, Saul. "A Critique of the Rationale for Cancer Treatment with Coffee Enemas and Diet." *Journal of the American Medical Association* Vol. 268, No. 22 (December 1992)

Gross, G., et al. "Genital Warts do Not Respond to Systemic Recombinant Interferon Alfa-2a Treatment During Cannabis Consumption." *Dermatologica* 183(3) (1991): pp. 203–207.

Hamid, S. "Protracted Cholestatic Hepatitis After the Use of Prostata." *Annals of Internal Medicine* 127 (1997): p. 169.

Harvey, J., et al. "Mistletoe Hepatitis." *British Medical Journal* Vol. 282 (6259) (January 17, 1981): pp.186–187.

"Herbal Roulette," *Consumer Reports* (November 1995) pp. 698–705.

Hobbs, C. *Milk Thistle: The Liver Herb.* Capitola, CA: Botanical Press, 1992.

Horowitz, Rivka, et al. "The Clinical Spectrum of Jin Bu Huan Toxicity." *Archives of Internal Medicine* Vol. 156 (April 22 1996): pp. 899–903.

Hruby, C. "Silibinin in the Treatment of Deathcap Fungus Poisoning." *Forum* 6 (1984): pp. 23–26.

Huxtable, R.J., et al. "The Myth of Beneficent Nature: the Risks of Herbal Preparation." *Annals of Internal Medicine* 117 (1992): pp. 165–166.

Katz, M., et al. "Herbal Hepatitis: Subacute Hepatic Necrosis Secondary to Chaparral Leaf." *Journal of Clinical Gastroenterology* 12 (1990): pp. 203–206.

Keeling, P.W., et al. "Trial of (+) –Cyanidanol-3 (Catechin)" *JR Soc Med* Vol. 79 (8) (August 1986): pp. 460–461.

Khakoo, S.I., et al. "Hepatotoxicity and Accelerated Fibrosis Following 3, 4–Methylenedioxymetamphetamine ('Ecstasy')

Usage." *Journal of Clinical Gastroenterology* 20(3) (1995): pp. 244–247.

Koul, Indu Bala, et al. "Evaluation of the Liver Protective Potential of Piperine an Active Principle of Black and Long Peppers." *Planta Medica* Vol. 59 (1993): pp. 413–417.

Kumana, C.R., et al. "Hepatic Veno-Occlusive Disease Due to Toxic Alkaloid Herbal Tea." *Lancet* (1983): pp. 1360–1361.

Lagnado, L. "Oxford to Create Alternative-Medicine Network." *Wall Street Journal* (October 7 1996): p. B9.

Laliberte, Lyne, et al. "Hepatitis After the Use of Germander, A Herbal Remedy." *Canadian Medical Association Journal* 154(11) (June 1, 1996).

Larrey, Dominique, et al. "Hepatitis After Germander (Teucrium Chamaedrys) Administration: Another Instance of Herbal Medicine Hepatotoxicity." *Annals of Internal Medicine* Vol. 117 (1992): pp. 129–132.

Larrey, D., et al. "Hepatotoxicity of Herbal Remedies and Mushrooms." *Seminars in Liver Disease* 15 (1995): p. 183.

Larrey, D. "Hepatotoxicity of Herbal Remedies." *Journal of Hepatology* 26 (1997): p. 47.

McGarey, William. "The Oil That Heals." A.R.E. Clinic, Phoenix, Arizona, 85018.

MacGregor, F.B., et al. "Hepatotoxicity of Herbal Remedies." *British Medical Journal* Vol. 299, No. 4 (1989): pp. 1156–1157.

Matsunami, Hidetoshi, et al. "Use of Glycyrrhizin for Recurrence of Hepatitis B after Liver Transplantation," Letters to the Editor. *American Journal of Gastroenterology* Vol. 88, No. 1 (1993).

Miquez, M.P., et al. "Hepatoprotective Mechanism of Silymarin: No Evidence for Involvement of Cytochrome P 450 2E1." *Chemico-Biological Interactions* 91(1) (April 1994): pp. 51–63.

Mira, L., et al. "Scavenging of Reactive Oxygen Species by Silibinin Dihemisuccinate."

Biochemical Pharmacology 48 (1994): pp. 753–759.

Mostefa-Kara Nacim, et al. "Fatal Hepatitis After Herbal Tea." *Lancet* Vol. 340 (September 12, 1992): p. 674.

Mourelle, M., et al. "Prevention of CCL4–Induced Liver Cirrhosis by Silymarin." *Fundamental Clinical Pharmacology* Vol. 3 (3) (1989): pp. 183–191.

Nadir, A., et al. "Acute Hepatitis Associated with the Use of A Chinese Herbal Product, Ma-huang." *American Journal of Gastroenterology* 91 (1996): p. 1436.

Nippon Rinsho, et al. "Efficacy of Interferon Combined Glycyrrhizin Therapy in Patients with Chronic Hepatitis C Resistant to Interferon Therapy." *Gut* 52 (7) (July 1994): pp. 1823–1827.

Oetari, S., et al. "Effects of Curcumin on Cytochrome P450 and Glutathione S-Transferase Activities in Rat Liver." *Biochemical Pharmacology* Vol. 51(1) (January 12, 1996): pp. 39–45.

Perharic-Walton, L., et al. "Toxicity of Chinese Herbal Remedies." *Lancet* 340 (1992): p. 674.

Pietrangelo, A., et al. "Antioxidant Activity of Silybin in Vivo During Long-Term Iron Overload in Rats." *Gastroenterology* 109 (1995): pp. 1941–1949.

Plomteux, G. "Hepatoprotector Action of Silymarin in Human Acute Viral Hepatitis." *Int Res Common Syst* 5 (1977): p. 259.

Rasi, G., et al., "Combination Thymosin Alfa 1 and Lymphoblastoid Interferon Treatment in Chronic Hepatitis C." *Gut* 39 (1996): pp. 679–683.

Raymond, Robert, et al. "Oral Thymic Extract for Chronic Hepatitis C in Patients Previously treated with Interferon." *Annals of Internal Medicine* (November 15, 1998): pp. 797–800.

Reddy, A.C., et al. "Effect of Curcumin and Eugenol on Iron-Induced Hepatic Toxicity in Rats." *Toxicology* Vol. 107 (1) (January 22 1996): pp. 39–45.

Rezkovic, I., et al. "A Pilot Study of Thymosin Alpha Therapy in Chronic Active Hepatitis C." (Abstract) *Hepatology* 18 (1993): p. 252A.

Ridker, Paul, et al. "Comfrey Herb Tea and Hepatic Veno-Occlusive Disease." *Lancet* (March 25, 1989): p. 657.

Rui, Yao-Cheng. "Advances in Pharmacological Studies of Silymarin." *Memorias Do Instituto Oswaldo Cruz* Vol. 86, Suppl II, (1991): pp. 79–85.

Russel S. "HMO's Try Dose of Alternative Medicine." *San Francisco Chronicle* January 22, 1996, p. A1.

Segivelman, Alvin, et al. "Sassafras and Herb Tea." *Journal of the American Medical Association* Vol. 236, No. 5 (August 2, 1976): pp. 477.

Sherman, K.E.G., et al. "Thymosin Alpha-1 Plus Interferon Combination Therapy for Chronic Hepatitis C: Results of a Randomized Controlled Trial." (Abstract) *Hepatology* 24 (1996): p. 402A.

Slifman, Nancy R., et al. "Contamination of Botanical Dietary Supplements by Digitalis Lanata." *New England Journal of Medicine* (September 17, 1998), pp. 29–37.

Soni, K.B., et al. "Reversal of Aflatoxin Induced Liver Damage by Tumeric and Curcumin." *Cancer Letters* Vol. 66 (2) (Sept. 30, 1992): pp. 115–21.

Stirpe, F. "Mistletoe Toxicity." *Lancet* 97 (1983): p. 295.

Szilard, S., et al. "Protective Effect of Legalon in Workers Exposed to Organic Solvents." *Acta Medica Hungarica* 45 (1988): pp. 249–256.

Takahara, E., et al. "Stimulatory Effects of Silibinin on the DNA Synthesis in Partially Hepatectomized Rat Livers: Non-Response in Hepatoma and Other Malignant Cell Lines." *Biochemical Pharmacology* 35 (1986): pp. 538–541.

Valenzuela, A., et al. "Biochemical Bases of the Pharmacological Action of the Flavonoid Silymarin and of Its Structural Isomer Silibinin." *Biological Research* 27 (2) (1994): pp. 105–112.

Vogel, G., et al. "Protection by Silybinin Against Amanita Phalloides Intoxication in Beagles." *Toxicology Applications Pharmacology* 73 (1984): pp. 355–362.

Weston, C.F., et al. "Veno-Occlusive Disease of the Liver Secondary to Ingestion of Comfrey." *British Journal of Medicine* Vol. 295 (1987): p. 183.

Winship, K.A., et al. "Toxicity of Comfrey." *Adverse Drug Reactions and Toxicological Review* (1991): pp. 47–59.

Wolf, Graham, et al. "Acute Hepatitis Associated with the Chinese Herbal Product Jin Bu Huan." *Lancet* Vol. 121, No.10 (November 15, 1994): pp. 729–735.

Yamamura, Y., et al. "The Relationship Between Pharmokinetic Behavior of Glycyrrhizin and Hepatic Function in Patients with Acute Hepatitis and Liver Cirrhosis." *Biopharmalogical Drug Disp* 16 (1) (January 1995): pp. 13–21.

Yeong, Mee Ling, et al. "Hepatic Veno-Occlusive Disease Associated with Comfrey Ingestion." *Journal of Gastroenterology and Hepatology* Vol. 5 (1990): pp. 211–214.

Yoshida, E.M., et al. "Chinese Herbal Medicine, Fulminant Hepatitis and Liver Transplantation." *American Journal of Gastroenterology* 91 (1996): p. 2647.

Chapter 22: Liver Transplantation

Ash, S.R., et al. "Clinical Effects of A Sorbent Suspension Dialysis System in the Treatment of Hepatic Coma (the Biologic-DT)." *International Journal of Artificial Organs* 15 (1992): pp. 151–161.

Belle, Steven, et al. "Changes in Quality of Life After Liver Transplantation Among Adults." *Liver Transplantation and Surgery* Vol. 3, No. 2 (1997): pp. 93–104.

Belle, S.H., et al. "Liver Transplantation in the United States: Results from the National Pitt-UNOS Liver Transplantation Registry." In: Terasaki PI, Cecka JM (eds) *Clin-ical Transplants* 1994. Los Angeles: UCLA Tissue Typing laboratory (1995): pp. 19–35.

Belli, L., et al. "Early Cyclosporine Mono-Therapy in Liver Transplantation: A 5 Year Follow-Up of A Prospective Randomized Trial." *Hepatology* 27 (1998): pp. 1524–1529.

Bizollon, T., et al. "Pilot Study of Combination of Interferon Alfa and Ribavirin as Therapy of Recurrent Hepatitis C After Liver Transplantation." *Hepatology* 26 (1997): pp. 500–504.

Broznick, B.A. "Organ Procurement: Fulfilling A Need." *Transplantation Proceedings* 20 (Suppl 1) (1988): p. 1010.

Burke, Anne, et al. "Liver Transplantation for Alcoholic Liver Disease." *Clinics in Liver Disease* Vol. 2, No. 4 (November 1998): pp. 839–850.

Charlton, Michael, et al. "Predictors of Patient and Graft Survival Following Liver Transplantation for Hepatitis C." *Hepatology* 28 (1998): pp. 823–830.

Colledan, Michelle, et al. "A New Splitting Technique for Liver Grafts." *Lancet* Vol. 353 (May 22, 1999): pp. 39–43.

Czaja, A.J., et al. "Natural History, Clinical Features and Treatment of Autoimmune Hepatitis." *Seminars in Liver Disease* 4 (1984): pp. 1–12.

Dickson, E.R., et al. "Prognosis in Primary Biliary Cirrhosis: Model for Decision Making." *Hepatology* 10 (1989): pp. 1–7.

Eastell, R., et al. "Rates of Vertebral Bone Loss Before and After Liver Transplantation in Women with PBC." *Hepatology* 14 (1991): p. 296.

Emond, JC., et al. "Improved Results of Living-Related Liver Transplantation with Routine Application in A Pediatric Program." *Transplantation* 55 (1993): pp. 835–840.

European Mycophenolate Mofetil Cooperative Study Group. "Placebo-Controlled Study of Mycophenolate Mofetil Combined with Cyclosporine and Corticosteroids for

Prevention of Acute Rejection." *Lancet* 345 (8961) (May 27, 1995): pp. 1321–1325.

Farmer, D.G., et al. "Current Treatment Modalities for Hepatocellular Carcinoma." *Annals of Surgery* 219 (1994): p. 236.

Feray, C. "An Open Trial of IFN Alpha Recombinant for Hepatitis C After Liver Transplantation." *Hepatology* 22 (1995): pp. 1084–1089

Fox, I.J., et al. "Treatment of the Crigler-Najjar Syndrome Type I with Hepatocyte Transplantation." *New England Journal of Medicine* 338 (1998): pp. 1422–1426.

Gane, Edward, et al. "Long-Term Outcome of Hepatitis C Infection After Liver Transplantation." *New England Journal of Medicine* 334 (1996): pp. 815–820.

Gerlach, J.C., et al. "Hepatocyte Culture Between Three Dimensionally Arranged Biomatrix-Coated Independent Artificial Capillary Systems and Sinusoidal Endothelial Cell C0–Culture Compartments." *International Journal of Artificial Organs* 17 (1994): pp. 301–306.

Gish, R.G., et al. "Ganciclovir Treatment of Hepatitis B Virus Infection in Liver Transplant Recipients." *Hepatology* 23 (1996): pp. 1–7.

Greenson, J.K., et al. "Histologic Progression of Recurrent Hepatitis C in Liver Transplant Allografts." *American Journal of Surgical Pathology* 20 (1996): pp. 731–738.

Heathcote, E.J., et al. "The Canadian Multicenter Double-Blind Randomized Controlled Trial of Ursodeoxycholic Acid in Primary Biliary Cirrhosis." *Hepatology* 19 (1994): pp. 1149–1156.

Heneine, W., et al. "No Evidence of Infection with Porcine Endogenous Retrovirus in Recipients of Porcine Islet-Cell Xenografts." *Lancet* 352 (1998): pp. 695–698.

Hoofnagle, J.H., et al. "Liver Transplantation for Alcoholic Liver Disease: Executive Statement and Recommendations." Summary of a National Institutes of Health Workshop Held December 6–7 1996, Bethesda, Maryland. Liver Transplantation and Surgery Vol. 3, No. 3 (May 1997): pp. 347–350.

Houssin, D., et al. "Controlled Liver Splitting for Transplantation in Two Recipients: Technique, Results and Prospectives." *British Journal of Surgery* 80 (1993): p. 75.

Hughes, R.D., et al. "Evaluation of the Biologic-DT Sorbent-Suspension Dialyser in Patients with Fulminant Hepatic Failure." *International Journal of Artificial Organs* 17 (1994): pp. 657–662.

Jurim, O., et al. "Liver Transplantation for Chronic Hepatitis B in Asians." *Transplantation* 57 (1994): pp. 1393–1395.

Klion, F.M., et al. "Prediction of Survival of Patients with PBC." *Gastroenterology* 102 (1992): pp. 310–313.

Kowdley, K.V., et al. "Primary Live Cancer and Survival in Patients Undergoing Liver Transplantation for Hemochromatosis." *Liver Transplantation and Surgery* 1 (1995): p. 237.

Kruger, M., et al. "Famciclovir Treatment of Hepatitis B Virus Recurrence After Orthotopic Liver Transplantation-A Pilot Study." *Hepatology* 22 (1995): p. 449A.

Lindor, K.D., et al. "Effects of Ursodeoxycholic Acid on Survival in Patents with Primary Biliary Cirrhosis." *Gastroenterology* 110 (1996): pp. 1515–1519.

Makowka, L., et al. "Pig Liver Xenografts as a Temporary Bridge for Human Allografting." *Xenobiotics* 1 (1993): p. 27.

Marcellin, P., et al. "Pretransplantation Interferon Treatment and Recurrence of Hepatitis B Virus Infection Liver Transplantation for Hepatitis B-Related End-Stage Liver Disease." *Hepatology* (1994): pp. 6–12.

Margarit, C., et al. "Maintenance Immunosuppression Without Steroids in Pediatric Liver Transplantation." *Transplant Proceedings* 21 (1989): pp. 2230–2231.

Markowitz, et al. "Prophylaxis Against Hepatitis B Recurrence Following Liver Transplantation Using Combination lamivudine and Hepatitis B Immune Globulin." *Hepatology* 28 (1998): pp. 585–589.

Mazariegos, G.V., et al. "Weaning of Immunosuppression in Liver Transplant Recipients." *Transplantation* 63 (1997): pp. 243–249.

Metselaar, H.J., et al. "Recovery of Failing Liver After Auxiliary Heterotopic Transplantation." *Lancet* 335 (1990): p. 115.

Molloy, R. Michael, et al. "Recurrent NASH and Cirrhosis after Liver Transplantation." *Liver Transplantation and Surgery* Vol. 3, No. 29 (March 1997): pp. 177–178.

Moritz, M.J., et al. "Heterotopic Liver Transplantation for Fulminant Hepatic Failure: Bridge to Liver Regeneration." *Transplantation* 50 (1991): p. 524.

Niederau, C., et al. "Survival and Causes of Death in Cirrhotic and in Noncirrhotic Patients with Primary Hemochromatosis." *New England Journal of Medicine* 313 (1985): p. 1256.

Osorio, R.W., et al. "Predicting Recidivism After Orthotopic Liver Transplantation." *Clinical Research* 41 (1993): p. 86A.

Padbury, R.T.A., et al. "Steroid Withdrawal from Long-Term Immunosuppression in Liver Allograft Recipients." *Transplantation* 55 (1993): pp. 789–794.

Padbury, R., et al. "Withdrawal of Immunosuppression in Liver Allograft Recipients." *Liver Transplantation and Surgery* 4 (1998): pp. 242–248.

Porayko, M.K., et al. "Bone Disease in Liver Transplant Recipients: Incidence, Timing and Risk Factors." *Transplantation Proceedings* 23 (1991): pp. 1462–1465.

Poulos, P. "Liver Transplantation for Hereditary Hemochromatosis." *Digestive Diseases and Sciences* 14 (1996): p. 316.

Powell, L.W., et al. "Does Transplantation of the Liver Cure Genetic Hemochromatosis?" *Journal of Hepatology* 16 (1992): p. 259.

Prottas, J.M., et al. "The Willingness to Give:

the Public and the Supply of Transplantable Organs." *Journal of Health, Political Policy & Law* 16 (1991): pp. 121–134.

Samuel, D., et al. "Liver Transplantation in European Patients with the Hepatitis B Surface Antigen." *New England Journal of Medicine* 329 (1993): p. 1842.

Sanches-Urdazpal, L., et al. "Prognostic Features and Role of Liver Transplantation in Severe Corticosteroid-Treated Autoimmune Chronic Active Hepatitis." *Hepatology* 15 (1992): pp. 215–220.

Shapiro, J.M., et al. "Serum Bilirubin: A Prognostic Factor in PBC." *Gut* 20 (1979): p. 137.

Sheiner, Patricia, et al. "The Efficacy of Prophylactic Interferon Alfa-2b in Preventing Recurrent Hepatitis C After Liver Transplantation." *Hepatology* 28 (1998): pp. 831–838.

Siminoff, L.A., et al. "Public Policy Governing Organ and Tissue Procurement in the United States. Results from the National Organ and Tissue Procurement Study." *Annals of Internal Medicine* 123 (1995): pp. 10–17.

Sollinger, H.W., et al. "Mycophenolate Mofetil for the Prevention of Acute Rejection in Primary Renal Allograft Recipients." U.S. Renal Transplant Mycophenolate Mofetil Study Group. *Transplantation* 60 (3) (August 15, 1995): pp. 225–232.

Starzl, T.E., et al. "Liver Transplantation." *New England Journal of Medicine* 329 (1989): pp. 1014–1022, 1092–1099.

Starzl, T.E., et al. "Baboon to Human Liver Transplantation." *Lancet* 341 (1993): p. 65.

Stolberg, Sheryl Gay. "Pennsylvania Set to Break Taboo on Reward for Organ Donations." *The New York Times National* Thursday, May 6, 1999, pp. A1, A30.

Strom, S.C., et al. "Hepatocyte Transplantation as A Bridge to Orthotopic Liver Transplantation in Terminal Liver Failure." *Transplantation* 63 (1997): pp. 559–569.

Sussman, N.L., et al. "Hepatix Extracorporeal Liver Assist Device: Initial Clinical Experience." *International Journal of Artificial Organs* 18 (1994): pp. 390–396.

Teperman, L., et al. "The Successful Use of Older Donors for Liver Transplantation." *Journal of the American Medical Association* 262 (1989): p. 2837.

Terpstra, O.T., et al. "Auxiliary Partial Liver Transplantation for End-Stage Chronic Liver Disease." *New England Journal of Medicine* 319 (1988): pp. 1507–1511.

Todo, S., et al. "Orthotopic Liver Transplantation for Patients with Hepatitis B Virus-Related Liver Disease." *Hepatology* 13 (1991): pp. 619–626.

Trevisani, F., et al. "The Use of Donor Fatty Liver for Liver Transplantation: A Challenge or a Quagmire?" *Journal of Hepatology* 24 (1996): p. 114.

US and European Multicenter FK 506 Liver Study Groups; 3 Year Experience. Abstract presented at the American Society of Transplant Physicians Annual Meeting, Chicago, IL 1997.

The U.S. Multicenter FK 506 Liver Study Group. "A Comparison of Tacrolimus (FK506) and Cyclosporine for Immunosuppression in Liver Transplantation." *New England Journal of Medicine* 331 (1994): pp. 1110–1115.

Watanabe, F.D., et al. "Clinical Experience with A Bioartificial Liver in the Treatment of Severe Liver Failure." *Annals of Surgery* 225 (1997): pp. 484–494.

Whitington, P.F., et al. "Orthotopic Liver Transplantation for Crigler-Najjar Syndrome Type 1." *Lancet* 342 (1993): pp. 779–780.

Chapter 23: Diet, Nutrition, and Exercise

Anderson, K.E.G., et al. "Nutritional Influences on Chemical Biotransformation in Humans." *Nutritional Reviews* 40 (1982): pp. 161–171.

Andreone, Pietro. "Vitamin E for Chronic Hepatitis B." *Annals of Internal Medicine* Vol. 128, No. 2, pp. 156–157.

Ashar, Bimal, et al. "Shark Cartilage-Induced Hepatitis." *Annals of Internal Medicine* Vol. 125 (November 1996): pp. 53–56

Balch, James, F., P.A. Balch. *Prescription for Nutritional Healing* Second Edition, Garden City Park, New York: Avery Publishing Group, 1997.

Bonkovsky, Herbert, et al. "Prevalence and Prediction of Osteopenia in Chronic Liver Disease." *Hepatology* 12 (1990): pp. 273–280.

Crippin, Jeffrey, et al. "Hypercholesterolemia and Atherosclerosis in Primary Biliary Cirrhosis: What Is the Risk?" *Hepatology* 15 (1992): pp. 858–862.

Feinman, L., et al. "Nutrition and Liver Disease." *Hospital Medicine* (April 1990): pp. 150–166.

Hendriks, H.F.J., et al. "Fat-Storing Cells: Hyper and Hypovitaminosis A and the Relationships with Liver Fibrosis." *Seminars in Liver Disease* Vol. 13, No.1 (1993): pp. 72–80.

Herbert, Victor. *The Mount Sinai School of Medicine Complete Book of Nutrition*. St. Martin's Press/New York, 1990.

Hourigan, Luke., et al. "Fibrosis in Chronic Hepatitis C Correlates Significantly with Body Mass Index and Steatosis." *Hepatology* 29 (1999): pp. 1215–1219.

Krishnamachari, K.A.V.R., et al. "Hepatitis Due to Aflatoxicosis: An Outbreak in Western India." *Lancet* 1 (1975): pp. 1061–1064.

Meyers, David, et al. "Safety of Antioxidant Vitamins." *Archives of Internal Medicine* 156 (1996): pp. 925–935.

Mezey, Esteban. "Dietary Fat and Alcoholic Liver Disease." *Hepatology* Vol. 28, No. 4 (October 1998): pp. 901–905.

Naveau, S., et al. "Obesity, A Risk Factor for Alcoholic Cirrhosis." *Hepatology* 22 (1995): p. 246A.

Negro, Francesco, et al. "Hepatotoxicity of Saccharin." *New England Journal of Medicine* (July 14, 1994): pp. 133–135.

Newberne, P.M., et al. "Chemical Carcinogenesis: Mycotoxins and Other Chemicals to which Humans are Exposed." *Seminars in Liver Disease* 4 (1989): pp. 122–135.

Rothman, Kenneth. "Teratogenicity of High Vitamin A Intake." *New England Journal of Medicine* 333 (1995): pp. 1369–1373.

Chapter 24: Pregnancy, Sex, Medications, and Prevention

Bach, Nancy, et al. "Sexual Behavior in Women with Nonalcoholic Liver Disease." *Hepatology* 9 (1989): pp. 698–703.

Benhamou, J.P. "Drug-Induced Hepatitis: Clinical Aspects." in Fillastre JP (ed): *Hepatotoxicity of Drugs* Rouen, University of Rouen, 1986, pp. 23–30.

Black, Martin. "Drug-Induced Liver Disease." *Clinics in Liver Disease* Vol. 2, No. 3 (August 1998): pp. 457–643.

Celso, Bianco, New York Blood Center Analysis, (1998).

Cheng, Y.S. "Pregnancy in Liver Cirrhosis and/or Portal Hypertension." *American Journal of Obstetrics and Gynecology* 128 (1977): pp. 812–822.

Choo, Q.L., et al. "Vaccination Against Hepatitis C Virus Infection: Miles to Go Before We Sleep." *National Academy of Scineces USA* 91 (1994): pp. 1294–1298.

Coole, I., et al. "Remission of Autoimmune Hepatitis During Pregnancy: A Report of Two Cases." *Liver* 1 (February 1999): pp. 55–57.

Crespo, Javier, et al. "Severe Clinical Course of De Novo Hepatitis B Infection After Liver Transplantation." *Liver Transplantation and Surgery* Vol. 5, No. 3 (May 1999): pp. 175–183.

Das, Ananya. "An Economic Analysis of Different Strategies of Immunization Against Hepatitis A Virus in Developed Countries." *Hepatology* 29 (1999): pp. 548–552.

Fidler, H., et al. "Chronic ecstasy (3.4.methylenededioxyamphetamine) Abuse: A Recurrent and Severe Cause of Acute Hepatitis." *Journal of Hepatology* 25 (1996): pp. 563–567.

Gavaler, Judith, et al. "Sexuality of Older Women After Liver Transplantation: Interrelationships of Prednisone use, Sex Steroid Hormone Levels, Body Image and Intimacy." *Liver Transplantation and Surgery* Vol. 1, No. 5, Supple 1 (September 1995): pp. 74–83.

Gluud, C., et al. "No Effect of Oral Testosterone Treatment on Sexual Dysfunction in Alcoholic Cirrhotic Men." *Gastroenterology* 95 (1988): pp. 1582–1587.

Haimov-Kochman, R., et al. "The Contraceptive Choice for a Wilson's Disease Patient with Chronic Liver Disease." *Contraception* 56 (1997): pp. 241–244.

Hutin, Yvan J.F., et al. "A Multistate Foodborne Outbreak of Hepatitis A." *New England Journal of Medicine* 340 (1999): pp. 595–602.

Inchauspe, Genevieve. "DNA Vaccine Strategies for Hepatitis C." *Journal of Hepatology* 30 (1999): pp. 339–346.

Kane, M. "Implementing Universal Vaccination Programs: USA." *Vaccine* 13 (1995): pp. S75–76.

Keefe, E.B., et al. "Safety and Immunogenicity of Hepatitis A Vaccine in Patients with Chronic Liver Disease." *Hepatology* 27 (1998): pp. 881–886.

Lee, M., et al. "Pregnancy in Chronic Active Hepatitis with Cirrhosis." *Journal Tropical Medicine and Hygiene* 90 (1987): pp. 245–248.

Lee, S., et al. "Role of Cesarean Section in Prevention of Mother-Infant Transmission of Hepatitis B Virus." *Lancet* (October 8, 1988): pp. 833–834.

Lee, William. "Drug-Induced Hepatotoxicity." *New England Journal of Medicine* (October 26, 1995): pp.1118–1127.

Lee, W.L. "Pregnancy in Patients with Chronic Liver Disease." *Gastroenterology Clinics of North America* 21 (1992): pp. 889–903.

Leiken, E.L., et al. "Intrauterine Transmission of Hepatitis A Virus." *Obstet Gynecol* 88 (1996): p. 690.

Lemon, Stanley, et al. "Vaccines to Prevent Viral Hepatitis." *New England Journal of Medicine* (January 16, 1997): pp. 196–204.

Levy, M., et al. "Hepatitis B Vaccine in Pregnancy: Maternal and Fetal Safety." *American Journal of Perinatol* 8 (1991): pp. 227–232.

Lewis, James H. "Drug-Induced Liver Disease." *Gastroenterology Clinics of North America* Vol. 24, No. 4 (December 1995).

Lin, H.H., et al. "Absence of Infection in Breast-Fed Infants Born to Hepatitis C Virus-Infected Mothers." *Journal of Pediatrics* 126 (1995): pp. 589–591.

Maged, D., et al. "Noncystic Liver Mass in the Pregnant Patient." *Southern Medical Journal* 83 (1990): pp. 51–53.

Molmenti, Ernesto P. "Liver Transplantation and Pregnancy." *Clinics in Liver Disease* Vol. 3, No.1 (February 1999): pp. 163–173.

Morrell, D.G., et al. "Laparoscopic Cholecystectomy During Pregnancy in Symptomatic Patients." *Surgery* 112 (1992): p. 856.

National Digestive Diseases Information Clearinghouse (NIDDKS): "Smoking and Your Digestive System." *Practical Gastroenterology* (July 1998): p. 42.

Nir, A., et al. "Pregnancy and Primary Biliary Cirrhosis." *International Journal of Gynecology and Obstetrics* 28 (1989): pp. 279–282.

Ohto, H., et al. "Intrauterine Transmission of Hepatitis B Virus is Closely Related to Placental Leakage." *Journal of Medical Virology* 21 (1987): pp. 1–6.

Palmer, M., et al. "Pregnancy in Autoimmune Chronic Active Hepatitis." *Hepatology* Vol. 10, No. 4 (October1989): p. 684.

"Prevention of Hepatitis A Through Active or Passive Immunization." *Morbidity and Mortality Weekly Report CDC* Vol. 45, No. RR-15 (December 27, 1996).

Rabinowitz, Mordechai, et al. "Primary Biliary Cirrhosis Diagnosed During Pregnancy: Does it Have a Different Outcome?" *Digestive Diseases and Sciences* Vol. 40, No. 3 (March 1995): pp. 571–574.

Radomski, John, et al. "National Transplantation Pregnancy Registry: Analysis of Pregnancy Outcomes in Female Liver Transplant recipients." *Liver Transplantation and Surgery* Vol. 1, No. 5 (September 1995): pp. 281–284.

Rawal, B.K., et al. "Symptomatic Reactivation of Hepatitis B in Pregnancy." *Lancet* 337 (1991): p. 364.

Reinus, John, et al. "Viral Hepatitis in Pregnancy." *Clinics in Liver Disease* Vol. 3, No. 1 (February 1999).

Reutter, J., et al. "Production of Antibody to Hepatitis A Virus and Hepatitis B Surface Antigen Measured After Combined Hepatitis A/Hepatitis B Vaccination in 242 Adult Volunteers." *Journal of Viral Hepatitis* 5 (1998): pp. 205–211.

Roudot-Thoraval, Francoise, et al. "Lack of Mother-to-Infant Transmission of Hepatitis C Virus in Human Immunodeficiency Virus-Seronegative Women: A Prospective Study with Hepatitis C Virus RNA Testing." *Hepatology* 17 (1993): pp. 772–777.

Shimizu, Y.K., et al. "Neutralizing Antibodies Against Hepatitis C Virus and the Emergence of Neutralization Escape Viruses." *Journal of Virology* 68 (1994): pp. 1494–1500.

Steven, M.M., et al. "Pregnancy in Chronic Active Hepatitis." *Quarterly Journal of Medicine* 48 (1979): pp. 519–531.

Thaler, M.M., et al. "Vertical Transmission of Hepatitis C Virus." *Lancet* 338 (1991): pp. 17–18.

"Updated Recommendations from the Advisory Committee on Immunization Practices: Prevention of Hepatitis A through Active Immunization" (Draft 1/25/99).

Van Thiel, D.H. "Vaccination of Patients with Liver Disease: Who, When and How

Liver Transplantation and Surgery," Vol. 4, No. 2 (March 1998): pp. 185–187.

Wanless, I.R., et al. "Histopathology of Cocaine Hepatotoxicity." *Gastroenterology* 98 (1990): pp. 497–501.

Watson, J.C., et al. "Vertical Transmission of Hepatitis A Resulting in an Outbreak in a Neonatal Intensive Care Unit." *Journal of Infectious Diseases* 167 (1993): p. 567.

Willner, I., et al. "Serious Hepatitis A: An Analysis of Patients Hospitalized During an Urban Epidemic in the United States." *Annals of Internal Medicine* 128 (1998): pp. 111–114.

Zanetti, A.R., et al. "Perinatal Transmission of the Hepatitis B Virus Associated Delta Agent from Mothers to Offspring in Northern Italy." *Journal of Medical Virology* 9 (1982): p. 139.

Zhang, R.L., et al. "Survey of 34 Pregnant Women with Hepatitis A and their Neonates." *Chin Med J* 103 (1990): p. 522.

Zifroni, Abraham, et al. "Sexual Function and Testosterone Levels in Men with Non-alcoholic Liver Disease." *Hepatology* 14 (1991): p. 479–482.

About the Author

Melissa Palmer, M.D., is a nationally renowned hepatologist who maintains a private practice devoted to liver disease. Dr. Palmer graduated from Columbia University with a B.A. and obtained her medical degree from Mount Sinai Medical School. After training in internal medicine at Beth Israel Hospital, Dr. Palmer completed a hepatology fellowship at Mount Sinai Hospital. She then went on to complete a gastroenterology fellowship and is currently board-certified in both internal medicine and gastroenterology.

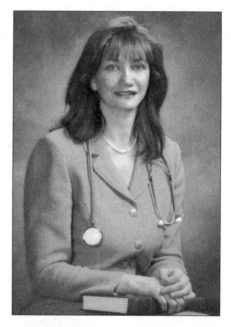

Dr. Palmer has authored numerous scientific publications in the field of hepatology. She is frequently called upon by the media for her opinion on various topics related to liver disease. Dr. Palmer has appeared many times on television as a liver disease expert, and has been quoted in such publications as *TIME Magazine, Prevention Magazine, The Los Angeles Times,* and *Newsday.* She also has appeared in videos aimed at educating the public about hepatitis C.

Dr. Palmer lectures to the medical and general public on liver disease-related topics on a regular basis. She also serves as a liver consultant to four major pharmaceutical companies. In addition, Dr. Palmer sits on the medical advisory board of the New York chapter of the American Liver Foundation (ALF), and on the nutrition education subcommittee of the national chapter of ALF.

Dr. Palmer has performed trials on various experimental medications for the treatment of hepatitis. She is currently conducting research on new therapies for liver disease, specifically in the area of hepatitis C. She maintains a popular Internet website, liverdisease.com. Dr. Palmer currently treats patients with both liver and digestive problems in her three offices located on Long Island, New York.

Index